Handbook of Outcomes Measurement in Audiology

Handbook of Outcomes Measurement in Audiology

By
Carole E. Johnson, Ph.D., CCC-A, FAAA
Professor
Department of Communication Disorders
Auburn University
Auburn University, Alabama

and

Jeffrey L. Danhauer, Ph.D., CCC-A, FAAA
Professor
Department of Speech and Hearing Sciences
University of California, Santa Barbara
Santa Barbara, California

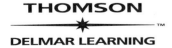

Australia Canada Mexico Singapore Spain United Kingdom United States

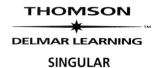

THOMSON

™

DELMAR LEARNING

SINGULAR

Handbook of Outcomes Measurement in Audiology
by
Carole E. Johnson and Jeffrey L. Danhauer

Executive Director,
Health Care Business Unit:
William Brottmiller

Executive Editor:
Cathy L. Esperti

Acquisitions Editor:
Candice Janco

Editorial Assistant:
Maria D'Angelico

Executive Marketing Manager:
Dawn F. Gerrain

Channel Manager:
Jennifer McAvey

Technology Project Manager:
Laurie Davis

Project Assistant:
Sherry McGaughan

Production Editor:
Mary Colleen Liburdi

Library of Congress
Cataloging-in-Publication Data
on file.

ISBN: 0-7693-0102-9

CONTENTS

Chapter 3   Levels of Evidence   **33**

Section III: Outcomes Measurement Across Service-Delivery Sites

AUTHORS' BIOGRAPHICAL SKETCHES

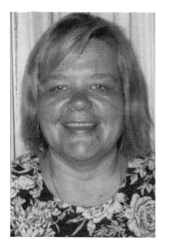

Carole E. Johnson, Ph.D., CCC-A, FAAA, is a Professor of Communication Disorders and Coordinator of the Au.D. Program at Auburn University where she has been a faculty member since 1992. She also taught at the University of Oklahoma Health Sciences Center from 1989 to 1992. Dr. Johnson earned B.A. degrees in Psychology and Speech and Hearing Sciences from the University of California at Santa Barbara, and her M.A. (Audiology) and Ph.D. (Speech and Hearing Sciences) from the University of Tennessee at Knoxville. Dr. Johnson has been principal investigator on research grants from the American Speech-Language-Hearing Foundation (ASHF), the National Organization for Hearing Research (NOHR), and the National Institute of Deafness and other Communicative Disorders of the National Institutes of Health (NIDCD-NIH). She has published 2 books, over 25 articles, and made over 60 research presentations to professional societies on various topics related to aural rehabilitation and practice management. She is a biographee in *Who's Who in Science and Engineering* and *Who's Who Among America's Teachers.* Dr. Johnson is a licensed audiologist in the State of Alabama.

Jeffrey L. Danhauer, Ph.D., CCC-A, FAAA, ASHA-F, is Professor of Audiology and Chair of the Department of Speech and Hearing Sciences at the University of California at Santa Barbara where he has been a faculty member since 1978. He also taught at Bowling Green State University from 1974 to 1978. Dr. Danhauer earned his B.A. from the Ohio State University, and his M.A. and Ph.D. from Ohio University. Dr. Danhauer has directed numerous dissertations and theses for his students. He has published over 100 articles and 5 books, made over 100 presentations at professional societies, edited over 60 books as Editor of Audiology for Singular Publishing Group, served as reviewer for several journals, is a member of several audiologic associations, and was one of the founders and past Chair of Education for the California Academy of Audiology. He has served on the Membership Committee of the American Academy of Audiology, and was a

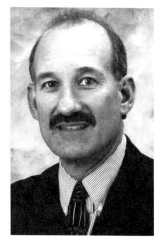

member and Chair of the Student Research Forum for the Academy. He has served as research consultant to the House Ear Institute. He is a licensed audiologist and hearing aid dispenser in California. He has been the owner of Hearing Consultants of California, a private practice, since 1978 through which he has served thousands of patients with hearing impairments and their families. His special interests include aural rehabilitation, hearing aids, otoacoustic emissions, diagnostic speech perception tests, and editing.

PREFACE

All audiologists, whether teaching students; conducting research; screening newborns; diagnosing hearing loss, balance problems, or tinnitus; selecting, evaluating, and fitting hearing aids, FM systems, cochlear implants, or assistive listening devices; providing aural habilitative or rehabilitative treatment; or establishing hearing conservation programs across varied service-delivery sites and models (e.g., hearing networks, private practice, hospital clinic, otolaryngology office, public school, health- and long-term residential care facilities for the elderly, and university training programs) know it or not are involved in outcomes measurement. Outcomes are usually thought of as the end result of treatment, but they actually occur throughout the continuum of hearing health-care from screening, to diagnosis, to intervention. This textbook has been written for audiologists at all levels to increase their awareness of the importance of outcomes measurement to the profession.

During the past several years, outcomes measurement has received increasing attention in the field of audiology. When encountering the words "outcomes measurement," audiologists think of the use of self-assessment scales and consumer satisfaction measures. However, outcomes measurement is much more than that, and it plays a major role in both the day-to-day and future viability of the profession. Recently, the hearing health-care industry has faced challenges, such as the Food and Drug Administration's edict to hearing aid manufacturers to substantiate their advertising claims through research, erosion of the scientific base of the profession, and the need to document positive patient outcomes in an era of managed care.

At the same time, audiology is transitioning to a doctoral-level profession declaring that the Doctor of Audiology, the Au.D., is a clinical degree, not to be confused with the Ph.D., which is to prepare students for a career in higher education involving teaching and research, for example. Faculty designing Au.D program curricula are in disagreement regarding the level of research competence to require from students. Some academicians believe that inclusion of words even remotely associated with research might discourage students from applying to their Au.D. programs. Although possible, this attitude may be the death knell for the profession when considering the dwindling enrollments in audiology Ph.D. programs. Will the profession rely on scientists from other professions to do its research? We are not advocating that the Au.D. necessarily must involve extensive research training, but believe that clinicians must understand the dynamics of outcomes measurement to compete in a health-care arena that demands evidence-based practice. Therefore, we believed that the field was in need of a comprehensive textbook on outcomes measurement.

What should a handbook on outcomes measurement contain? Should it contain a few chapters on the use of self-assessment scales and a computer disk of the most widely used outcome measures? The answer to this question is yes. This textbook contains a companion CD-ROM that is packed with useful forms that include handy tools and the most widely used outcome measures. Moreover, we believe that the use of outcome measures must be based on strong theoretical underpinnings that are linked to specific areas of practice across challenging service-delivery sites. This vision serves as the rationale for the three major sections of the book.

The first section, "Foundations for Outcomes Measurement," provides readers with practical and theoretical underpinnings. For example, Chapter 1 speaks directly to audiologists by showing the relevance of outcomes measurement to everyday clinical situations through a series of short scenarios. Chapter 2, "An Introduction to Outcomes Measurement," introduces key terms; explains the importance of outcomes measurement to the profession; and discusses shared responsibilities by the profession, training programs, and practitioners. Chapter 3, "Levels of Evidence," establishes a hierarchy of scientific rigor for clinicians to use when evaluating procedures, products, and treatments, for example. Chapter 4, "Methods of Measurement," provides a perspective on the levels, reliability, and validity of measurement; the ins and outs of critiquing measurement tools; and the advantages, disadvantages, and steps in designing an original instrument. Chapter 5, "Use of Computers in Outcomes Measurement," concludes this section of the book by discussing use of computer-based data management systems in outcomes measurement.

The second section of the book, "Outcomes Measurement in Specific Areas of Practice," focuses on the aspects of outcomes measurement in specific areas of practice. For example, Chapter 6, "Outcomes Measurement in Early Hearing Detection and Intervention (EHDI) Programs," discusses the importance of outcomes measurement in identifying, diagnosing, and following of young children having hearing impairment utilizing the benchmarks and quality indicators established by the, "*Joint Committee on Infant Hearing (JCIH) Year 2000 Position Statement.*" Chapter 7,"Outcomes Measurement in Diagnostic Audiology," discusses the evaluation of diagnostic procedures and the importance of positive patient outcomes in an area not traditionally associated with outcomes measurement. Chapter 8, "Outcomes Measurement in Hearing Conservation," discusses two approaches to outcomes measurement (i.e., prescriptive versus outcome-based), the role of comprehensive record keeping, the effect of service-delivery model, and strategic planning for outcomes measurement in hearing conservation. Chapter 9, "Outcomes Measurement in Aural Habilitation," explores reasons for the lack of reliable and valid outcome measures for children, considers complications in outcomes measurement in aural habilitation, reviews objective and subjective pediatric outcome measures, acknowledges alternative approaches, and discusses the complexity of outcomes measurement for early intervention programs. Chapter 10, "Outcomes Measurement in Aural Rehabilitation," concludes this section by assisting readers to acknowledge conceptual frameworks, select self-report instruments, apply outcomes measurement in clinical practice/research, consider outcomes measurement within the context of recommended hearing aid fitting guidelines, and use outcome measures in tinnitus and vestibular/ balance therapy.

The last section of the book, "Outcomes Measurement Across Service-Delivery Sites," discusses the unique situations encountered in challenging service-delivery sites. Some of the most compelling service-delivery sites have been considered in this textbook. For example, Chapter 11, "Outcomes Measurement in Hearing Health-Care Networks," discusses aural rehabilitation support programs in a hearing network and the use of outcomes measurement for meeting rigorous accreditation standards of groups, such as the National Committee on Quality Assurance (NCQA). Chapter 12 discusses outcomes measurement in health- and long-term residential care facilities for the elderly to help audiologists provide quality hearing health-care services to the steadily increasing elderly segment of the population. Chapter 13, "Outcomes Measurement in the Public Schools," assists clinicians in understanding and meeting the challenges of outcomes measurement for improving audiologic services to school-aged children despite inadequacies of current service-delivery models. Chapter 14 discusses the importance of outcomes measurement in university training programs in reference to the development and accreditation of Au.D. programs.

The last chapter of the book discusses the future of outcomes measurement in the field of audiology. This chapter ties some loose ends together, and encourages readers to stay the course and to take information presented in this textbook to higher and higher levels of excellence in clinical practice. This textbook should be ideal for use in Au.D. courses and has learning activities, recommended readings, and review exercises at the end of each chapter. Practicing audiologists should keep the *Handbook of Outcomes Measurement in Audiology* close at hand as an easy reference for assistance in achieving positive patient outcomes and to enhance their professionalism, profitability, and self-esteem.

Carole E. Johnson
Auburn, Alabama

Jeffrey L. Danhauer
Santa Barbara, California

LIST OF APPENDICES
FOR THE COMPANION CD-ROM

Readers are advised to print out all of the appendices on the companion CD-ROM for placement into a notebook to refer to when reading the textbook.

Appendix I-A:	Evaluation of Treatment Procedures, Products, and Programs
Appendix II-A:	Ph.D. Program Evaluation Checklist
Appendix II-B:	Au.D. Program Evaluation Checklist
Appendix III-B:	Checklist for Evaluating Scientific Articles
Appendix III-C:	Checklist for Evaluating or Designing Single-Subject Studies
Appendix IV-B:	Checklist for Evaluation of Self-Assessment Tools
Appendix IV-C:	Worksheet for Writing Questionnaires and Interviews
Appendix V-C:	Checklist for Evaluating Webpages
Appendix VI-C:	Outcome Checklist for Implementing Early Hearing Detection and Intervention (EHDI) Programs
Appendix VI-D:	Worksheet for Evaluating Quality Early Hearing Detection and Intervention (EHDI) Programs
Appendix VII-A:	Checklist for Evaluating Investigations of Diagnostic Tests
Appendix VIII-A:	Important Prescriptive Outcomes for Comprehensive Hearing Conservation Programs (HCPs)
Appendix VIII-B:	Strategic Planning for Outcomes Measurement in Hearing Conservation Programs (HCPs)
Appendix X-A:	Abbreviated Profile of Hearing Aid Benefit (APHAB)
Appendix X-B:	Hearing Performance Inventory (HPI)
Appendix X-C:	Hearing Aid Performance Inventory (HAPI)
Appendix X-D:	Shortened Hearing Aid Performance Inventory (SHAPI)
Appendix X-E:	Client Oriented Scale of Improvement (COSI)
Appendix X-F:	The Hearing Handicap Inventory for the Elderly (HHIE)
Appendix X-G:	The Hearing Handicap Inventory for Adults (HHIA)
Appendix X-H:	The Hearing Handicap Inventory for the Elderly— Screening Form (HHIE—S)

CHAPTER 1

Outcomes Measurement and the Audiologist

LEARNING OBJECTIVES

This chapter will enablere aders to:

- Understand the complexity of outcomes measurement
- Analyze problems regarding outcomes measurement in clinical scenarios
- Acknowledge critical questions regarding outcomes measurement for audiologists

INTRODUCTION

At first thought, the writing of a handbook of outcomes measurement in audiology seemed like it would be no big deal. How difficult could it be? Simply collect data about what outcome measures are being used, in what areas of practice, by whom, when, where, and why. Better yet, inventory outcome measures on an accompanying CD-ROM for user application, which should be relatively easy to compile. The phrase, "outcome measures," is one of the most popular "buzz words" in health care today. Therefore, we should be able to assume that everyone knows what outcome measures are. Or, if

not, a reasonable definition of outcome measures could be provided by quoting some nice, concise statement in the literature. So, at first consideration, we envisioned this textbook to be short and sweet, maybe a bit dry, but, hey—a piece of cake!

Well, guess what? When trying to plan this undertaking, we soon discovered that the process was not going to be easy. For example, discussing the multiple roles of the Self-Help for the Hard of Hearing People, Inc. (SHHH) consumer organization, Vignette 1-1 was presented to one of our undergraduate aural rehabilitation courses and we were

1

surprised at our students' reactions to the passage.

We had discussed the role of the Food and Drug Administration (FDA) regarding consumer protection and the dispensing of hearing aids, and the students had a keen interest in the idea of a surgically implantable hearing aid. However, students had numerous questions about the process of FDA approval of new medical technology:

- Why do manufacturers have to be approved by the FDA to try new technology?
- What is "efficacy?"
- What are Level 1 clinical trials?
- What are "realistic performance outcomes?"
- What is "cost-benefit ratio?"

We answered these questions using an analogy of the process involved in the approval of new drugs in the fight against cancer. Surprisingly, our answers to students' questions generated even more areas for discussion.

Intrigued by our undergraduate students' questions, we presented the same passage to a group of second-year audiology graduate students enrolled in an advanced amplification course and asked them to define efficacy, Level 1 clinical trials, outcome measures, and cost-benefit ratio. The graduate students recalled hearing about some of the terms in their research methods course that had been thorough, but had little practical connection to the real world. After a brief explanation of these concepts, a discussion ensued which generated insightful questions from the class:

- Are clinical trials ethical? Is it fair to withhold a treatment that could save lives from those patients assigned to a control group?

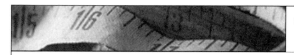

VIGNETTE 1-1

TESTIMONY ON IMPLANTABLE HEARING AIDS

In June 1999, SHHH presented written and oral testimony before the Food and Drug Administration Ear-Nose-Throat Devices Panel on safety and efficacy of implantable middle-ear hearing aids. Three manufacturers have already been approved by the FDA for Level 1 clinical trials. SHHH's comments focused on the consumer perspective. We urged the FDA to ensure that potential candidates be provided with realistic performance outcomes and appropriate and sufficient rehabilitation following surgery for comfortable and successful use of the device. SHHH's testimony also stressed that the device be designed to be used/coupled with assistive listening devices and telephones. It is vital that research is done to ensure that the device has immunity to electromagnetic interference, including the ability to use with digital phones without interference. A cost-benefit ratio for middle-ear implantable devices should be done. Consumers' expectation will be high given that it requires surgery and costs more than conventional amplification devices. There must be a significant benefit to justify the additional expense. Other speakers presenting were representatives of companies developing the devices and representatives from ASHA, AAO-HNS, and the House Ear Institute.

(SHHH: Self-Help for Hard of Hearing People, Inc. (1999). SHHH National Action, Hearing Loss, 20(5), 5).

- Why have we only heard about clinical trials for amplification devices that require surgery (i.e., cochlear implants and implantable hearing aids)?
- Why aren't outcome measures, efficacy data, and clinical trials required of all audiologic procedures?
- Does the lack of efficacy data in our profession have anything to do with third-party payers viewing audiologic services as elective rather than necessary health care?

By the end of class that day, students made the transition from believing that research had really nothing to do with the practice of audiology to realizing its fundamental role in hearing health care for patients and the future of the profession.

Surprisingly, the initial reactions of our students were not unlike those of the clinical faculty in discussions of the role of outcomes measurement in a future Au.D. program. We were reminded that the Au.D. degree is a clinical degree and not a research degree. Indeed, although their point was well taken, it displayed a lack of understanding regarding the many facets of outcomes measurement in clinical practice. So, wait a minute. Had we missed something here? Are we just assuming that our colleagues have a complete understanding of outcomes measurement and its importance to clinical service provision (e.g., accreditation, development of clinical practice guidelines, and reimbursement) *and* research? Moreover, do third-party payers and granting agencies assume that audiologists have a grasp on outcomes measurement? Is there a mismatch between their assumptions and our profession's competence in outcomes measurement? Maybe the task of writing this textbook is not going to be so easy after all.

Have we failed to educate our students about these important concepts? For that matter, did our professors and clinical supervisors forget to tell us about outcomes meas-

urement in our own academic preparations? Is the topic of outcomes measurement so new that it was not even an option for coverage back then in our own course work? Is there room for course work in outcomes measurement in traditional and distance-learning Au.D. programs? Uh oh—here we go thinking and wondering again—we already know this can be dangerous. Can it be that we have uncovered yet another weakness in our professional training and application?

To test our assumptions, we constructed a survey of information about outcomes measurement and administered it to a representative sample of the members of our profession to help us in designing this textbook on outcomes measurement (Johnson & Danhauer, 2001). The data gleaned from the survey were quite interesting to say the least. For example, the vast majority of respondents believed that outcomes measurement was important to the profession and should be taught to those in training. Some of the results of the survey are presented later in this text. The results indeed helped guide us in our mission. The purpose of this chapter is to demonstrate the need for audiologists' involvement in outcomes measurement. Two scenarios are presented and analyzed and several questions are posed for readers to consider.

So, why should audiologists be concerned about outcomes measurement? Perhaps the following two scenarios will help answer this question. These examples may sound familiar. After reading them, see if you can come up with other examples from your own clinical experience (see Vignette 1-2).

ANALYSIS OF SCENARIO ONE

Well, what's wrong with this scenario and what does it have to do with outcomes measurement? Before the equipment representative is dismissed as incompetent and the

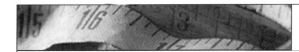

VIGNETTE 1-2

SCENARIO 1

Recently, an audiologic equipment manufacturers' sales-and-service representative confided to us that he was becoming increasingly disappointed with several audiologists' apparent incompetence and lack of preparation in making rational clinical decisions about purchases and day-to-day business operations for their practices.

One of his recent customers was interested in purchasing a newly devised otoacoustic emissions (OAE) screener for the well-baby nurseries and neonatal intensive care units (NICUs) in local hospitals for which he had just landed a new screening contract by impressing hospital administrators with a dazzling presentation of his proposed screening program. Supposedly, the audiologist already had and was familiar with diagnostic OAE equipment, but was now interested in a faster, cheaper screening version. He was actually going to buy 10 such instruments so that he and his support personnel could screen hundreds of infants over the next few months as part of the massive program. The screener was faster (although more limited in capacity), and cheaper than the diagnostic model, which would greatly enhance the audiologist's profit margin. Moreover, the screener was so easy for both well-baby nursery and NICU staff to use that the audiologist could manage the program without leaving the office. By projecting the number of babies to be screened, the length of time required for executing the protocol, and the fee to be charged for testing each ear, he quickly calculated that the screeners would pay for themselves within a few months.

The audiologist planned to use three of these screeners at two of the smaller hospitals to initiate the program, but only attended a quick inservice on use of the new equipment during delivery of the devices. The audiologist stated that he really could not take the time from his already busy schedule to attend an in-depth inservice. Thus, because he was already familiar with the diagnostic OAE model, he instructed the directors of the well-baby nurseries and NICUs on how to use the screeners, and they, in turn, were to instruct the support staff. The audiologist felt that the NICU directors would learn best "on the job." When the audiologist made his first attempt to use the screener on a three-hour-old premature infant having several life-support tubes and cables attached through his incubator, he found that the infant failed the screening. He then tried to use the equipment on two full-term infants in the well-baby nursery, who had also been born that morning. One passed; the other did not. "See, it works!" instructed the audiologist, "Just do what I do and record the results ... " Over the next two weeks, the well-baby nursery and NICU directors and the support staff screened all newborns in each hospital and sent the screening reports to the audiologist.

After reviewing the initial data, surprisingly, the audiologist called the manufacturers' representative and told him to come and get the three screeners and to cancel the order for the remaining seven units. When the representative asked why and what had happened, the audiologist replied that the screener was unreliable and "no damn good." One hospital had no failures while the other had a 50% fail rate. How could two hospitals give such disparate results? The audiologist had also tried to use the screener on a young patient in his office with a known "sensorineural" hearing loss and he passed! Little did

CONTINUES

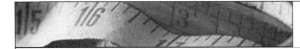

VIGNETTE 1-2

SCENARIO 1   (CONTINUED FROM PAGE 4)

he know, that this young patient actually had an auditory neuropathy (he should have expected to see OAEs in that case). According to the audiologist, the screener failed patients who should have passed and passed patients who should have failed. When the representative attempted to probe further about the screening protocol, the audiologist became arrogant and irritated that a lowly representative would question his audiologic acumen. The audiologist ended the conversation abruptly promising never to do business with him again, and to be sure, he would tell all his colleagues not to use this product.

As promised, the equipment representative did not hear from the audiologist again. However, he did hear from one of his colleagues that eventually the audiologist decided to relinquish the contract to one of his competitors. Apparently, he had similar troubles with the screening equipment made by another manufacturer as well. Furthermore, unnecessary hearing evaluations from false positives, complaints from aggravated parents, and inadequately trained and unsupervised support personnel led to the audiologist's conclusion that newborn screening programs create more problems than they are worth.

OAE screener discarded, some other possibilities should be examined to determine the source of the problem. Does one need to know about research design or outcomes measurement to determine what may be happening here? Maybe not, but these topics are related to the problem and may provide some insight to the answer.

Was the audiologist unfamiliar with outcomes measurement? The answer to this question is yes and no. Audiologists need to know that there are different types of outcomes (as we will discuss in this textbook). Two types of outcomes are *program outcomes* and *process outcomes* (Weinstein, 2000). Program outcomes are relevant to the administration of a practice or a facility, such as patient demographics, number of treatment sessions, and financial aspects of managing a profitable business (Weinstein, 2000). Process outcomes are the *how* and the *why* of clinical practice (Weinstein, 2000). The audiologist in our scenario had such an excellent grasp of program outcomes that he was able to impress hospital administrators with a winning presentation regarding projected cost-benefit ratios of the proposed program versus those of his competitors to secure the contract. In fact, his practice was one of the most successful in the metropolitan area specializing in the dispensing of hearing instruments. According to his projections, the management of these universal newborn hearing screening (UNHS) programs through his practice should be a lucrative venture.

The audiologist did not take the time to master the process outcomes or the *how* and the *why* of managing successful UNHS programs, however. The audiologist may not have felt the need to be familiar with "cutting edge" research in otoacoustic emissions (OAE), but certainly he should have consulted the latest outcomes data on the establishment of UNHS programs prior to initiation of the trial run with the new screeners. The audiologist could have reviewed the procedural data collected by the National Center on Hearing Assessment and Management

(NCHAM) on all viable UNHS programs in 1996, for example. Similarly, he could have logged onto the American Speech-Language-Hearing Association's (ASHA's) Website to download the most current information on UNHS programs from their National Outcomes Measurement System (NOMS). Even more fundamental was the audiologist's lack of basic competence with performing OAEs with this population. For example, OAEs are difficult to obtain on any neonate only a few hours old (either in NICUs or well-baby nurseries), and even more so for premature infants hooked up to various tubes, cables, and other life-support equipment. Furthermore, these neonates frequently have ear canals that are filled with vernix and other debris that can preclude obtaining valid OAE screening results in the first few hours of life. A simple otoscopic examination using a speculum tip or insertion and removal of the probe tip can often create enough of an opening to allow for successful OAE screening. Experienced audiologists know that retesting a few hours or days later before discharge results in "passes" for many of these infants who may not have passed an initial screening only a few minutes or hours after birth.

The audiologist was not prepared to use support personnel (Johnson & Danhauer, 1999) during the initial trial period with the equipment. The audiologist correctly assumed that he could supervise UNHS programs and that support personnel with varied backgrounds could conduct the screenings (Joint Committee on Infant Hearing [JCIH], 2000; Robinette & White, 1998). However, he did not consult guidelines for the use of audiologic support personnel in this capacity, which resulted in several oversights. First, he did not interview well-baby nursery or NICU staff regarding their suitability to participate in the screening program. Johnson, Maxon, White, and Vohr (1993) stated that the three key factors in selecting screening personnel are their:

- comfort level in working with newborns and computers,
- conscientiousness in learning the screening protocol, and
- willingness to make adaptations within the specified protocol to obtain a valid screening result.

Second, the audiologist did not consult the "Position Statement and Guidelines of the Consensus Panel on Support Personnel in Audiology" (AAA, 1997) nor "Use of Support Personnel for Hearing Screening (Proposed Guidelines)" (American Academy of Audiology's Committee on Infant Hearing, 1998) regarding appropriate training and supervision of the program participants. For example, he inadequately instructed both the well-baby nursery and NICU directors on the use of the screening equipment, and then expected them to provide proper inservices to their staff. Only licensed and/or certified audiologists should provide training to support personnel.

The audiologist was perplexed that the two hospitals participating in the equipment trial achieved different screening results. He erroneously assumed that both hospitals should achieve similar results and that the OAE screener at the hospital recording no referrals during the trial period must have been malfunctioning. Had he been familiar with the latest statistical models for assessing UNHS programs, he would not have been surprised to find no screening referrals for one hospital after the two-week trial period (Burrows & Owen, 1999). Similarly, benchmarks for UNHS programs state that the referral rate for audiologic and medical evaluation following the screening process should be 4% or less within one year of program initiation for both birth admission and outpatient follow-up (JCIH, 2000). In fact, a recently hired NICU nurse at the hospital had re-instructed the staff on the procedures she had learned at another hospital with a successful UNHS program. Thus, the audiologist should have been concerned about the hospital with the high referral rate. Moreover, had he been adequately supervising the support personnel, he would have discovered that it was not the screening equipment that was the problem, but his lack of knowledge and instruction of the well-baby nursery and NICU directors that caused the high referral rate.

So, in the end, after relinquishing the contract, the audiologist learned both the value of and the relationship between process and program outcome data. The value of any program is the link between these data (Robertson & Colburn, 1997; Weinstein, 2000). The two types of data are obviously dependent on each other according to the laws of a market economy. Recall that the audiologist was adept at projecting program outcome data (e.g., cost of equipment, amount of audiologist involvement, support personnel needed) for his hypothetical screening program, assuming there were no problems. However, without carefully considering process outcomes (e.g., the how and the why) of screening programs, the audiologist unwisely initiated a trial program with unfamiliar OAE screening equipment. When things did not go well, he was quick to blame the manufacturer's representative and the screening equipment. Some audiologists are inclined toward pushing buttons on screening devices and allowing simple "pass-fail" indicator lights to do their thinking for them, without having a thorough understanding of how and why the equipment works and what the results mean. Thus, many audiologists unknowingly relegate themselves to "technician's status," which cannot be good for the future of the profession. The audiologist had the same difficulty with other equipment, but before he realized the root of his problems, the newborn hearing screening contract had become a drain on his practice. The audiologist was not a bad clinician, as evidenced by his successful practice which had primarily consisted of diagnostic services and dispensing hearing instruments. Indeed, his office walls were covered with testimonies from satisfied patients of all ages whom he had served over the past 20 years. He had simply failed to do his homework on this particular area in his field.

We are increasingly annoyed by audiologists who have no interest in and want nothing to do with research. Often, these clinicians complain that current audiologic equipment and test protocols are outdated and inefficient. Do they really think that our current technology "just fell out of the sky?" Without Carhart, Fletcher, Harris, Jerger, Kemp, von Bekesy, and scores of other clinicians and researchers, where would our field be? Our field needs to educate new researchers to take their place and clinicians to implement their findings. Doing research does not just mean conducting formal research investigations. It means doing one's homework; it means being prepared. It means critically reviewing available data prior to using any new treatment procedure, product, or clinical programs. Are audiologists prepared to do this? Do they know how to access databases on the Internet? Did they pay attention in their introductory research courses? Can they critically evaluate all the data available to them? Appendix I-A on the companion CD-ROM contains a tool adapted from ASHA (1999) that readers can use when evaluating any treatment procedure, product, or program. Use of this Appendix is discussed again in Chapter 9. It includes such words as reliability, validity, population, sample, outcomes, peer-reviewed, control groups, FDA, clinical trials ... But don't worry, the Foundations section of this textbook first introduces readers to outcomes measures, the various levels of evidence, methods of measurement, and computer-based data management systems.

Scenario one dealt with the importance of clinician preparation (e.g., familiarity of equipment, access of available outcome measures, review of clinical practice guidelines) prior to the initiation of clinical programs. Scenario two has to do with a clinician's role in collecting outcomes measures (see Vignette 1-3).

ANALYSIS OF SCENARIO TWO

What is wrong with scenario two? In what ways does this example relate to outcomes measurement? The audiologist was surprised to find that only a few months after completion of the clinical trial, the manufacturer would be marketing the new circuit design as enhancing patients' performance. The audiologist wondered if other study sites

had achieved results similar to those found in his own laboratory, in which only 6 out of 10 patients had preferred the new circuit design. Hmmm, well, 6 out of 10 is a majority, isn't it? However, at least 2 of the patients who said they preferred the new circuit design really were not sure. The audiologist scratched his head and wondered how the manufacturer could make such claims in its advertising campaign for the new circuit design. Was this false advertising? Was it ethical? Did he have enough information to be suspicious? Was the manufacturer to blame or the audiologist?

We should remember that both manufacturer and all clinical trial personnel at all study sites need to understand that clinical trials research has definitive connotations

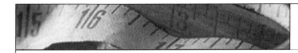

VIGNETTE 1-3

SCENARIO 2

A research audiologist conducted studies that had applications to cochlear implants for patients with severe-to-profound hearing loss as part of a multisite clinical trial sponsored by a manufacturer investigating the efficacy of various circuit settings on cochlear implant designs. He related his frustrations with his clinical trials research. After countless hours in the laboratory with several patients who served as subjects, the researcher was unable to discern any clear differences among three or more processing schemes available with the new circuit design. He felt that he had wasted a lot of time carefully administering the manufacturer's protocol for each patient. Being perplexed by his lack of definitive results and pressured by his employer, who in turn was being harassed by the manufacturer to deliver a product to market, the researcher slighted steps in the protocol and actually left many empty cells in his data entries. Because the objective (e.g., test results in the laboratory) outcome measures failed to show significant differences, he turned to a more subjective means of assessment (i.e., patient preferences) by simply asking the patients which of the three device settings they preferred. Six of the 10 subjects preferred the processing schemes made possible through the new circuit design. However, two of the six favoring the new product feature really were not sure about their preference. Nevertheless, the researcher turned the results over to the employer who passed them on to the manufacturer. Ultimately, a new processor with the new circuit design was to be made available for current cochlear implant users and marketed to them with the implication that the new circuit design should enhance their performance with their implants.

and ground rules for implementation and interpretation. Evidence-based health-care practice relies on research results that are organized according to a hierarchy of evidence by the Agency of Health Policy Research (Beck, 1999). Clinical trial research is at the highest level of experimental stringency and provides a basis for treatment options and referrals for care, and is fast becoming the "gold standard" for our profession (Beck, 1999). The development of clinical practice guidelines that recommend the performance or exclusion of specific procedures and services requires the rigorous methodologic requirements of clinical trial research (Beck, 1999). Unfortunately, neither the manufacturer nor the audiologist in our example appeared to be cognizant of these rigid "ground rules."

First of all, clinical trial research requires "double-blinding," such that participating investigators and subjects are masked with regard to the administration of the different treatment conditions. The audiologist was not masked as to the administration of the independent variable and was discouraged that the new circuit design did not result in improved performance for patients. Second, the manufacturer should have ensured that personnel at all participating sites were "on board" regarding the strict adherence to the experimental protocol. The audiologist felt so pressured by his employer (who felt pushed by the manufacturer) to obtain "positive outcomes" for the new circuit design that important data were omitted from the final report.

Did the audiologist commit scientific misconduct? Well, yes and no. Although no data were falsified, the audiologist should have reported the actual data that were collected rather than just leaving empty cells. The omission of these data may have severely compromised the validity of the clinical trial. Moreover, the manufacturer may have been negligent by advertising enhanced patient performance with the new circuitry. Did some study sites find different outcomes from those of the audiologist in our scenario? On what evidence did the manufacturer feel justified in making these claims in its advertising? Was this clinical trial doomed for failure?

Clinicians may be thinking—well, they are not picking on us this time, but, in fact, these issues carry over to clinical practice. Often, clinicians must convince their patients and third-party payers that both hearing aids and/or cochlear implants provide benefits that justify their cost. Clinicians must be critical consumers of the research substantiating the alleged efficacy of these devices prior to offering new products to their patients. Clinicians' skills need to go far beyond just reading manufacturers' specification sheets before fitting hearing instruments to patients. Indeed, manufacturers offer attractive incentives (e.g., cruises) for audiologists who sell high volumes of their products. We hope this textbook will encourage readers to understand the importance of and to master the skills for objectively evaluating outcome measures, regardless of attractive marketing campaigns or handsome bonuses from manufacturers. As middlemen, clinicians must be involved in outcomes measurement on both ends of the rehabilitation process, namely, evaluating manufacturers' data from the research and development of a product, and then collecting data on benefits provided to their own patients.

FOOD FOR THOUGHT

At this point, we will dispense with further scenarios, assuming that readers are sufficiently convinced of the need for outcomes measurement. So far, this chapter has discussed some issues regarding outcomes measurement in a few areas of clinical practice. It is important to understand, though, that outcomes measurement is important throughout all areas of practice and across all service-delivery sites. Indeed, practicing audiologists' days are filled with various incidents of either evaluating or collecting these data. Unfortunately, outcomes measurement involves tasks or experiences that are considered to be unpleasant by both students-in-training and practicing professionals. Unless clinicians are forced to use outcome measures by third-party payers, audiologists may only choose to use them if the benefit is commensurate with the required administration time (Dillon & So, 2000). These day-to-day endeavors may become more palatable to readers when they understand the importance of outcomes measurement not only to the autonomy of the profession, but also to the fiscal viability of their practices. Unfortunately, some of the outcome measures that audiologists collect are meaningless and wasteful of our most precious commodity—time. Indeed, the goal of this text is both to stress the importance of outcomes measurement and to provide readers with the mindset and skills to use these practices for their benefit. However, before progressing to the how and why of outcomes measurement, we would like to present some "food for thought" or questions for readers to consider. Our aim is for readers to play "devil's advocate" and question the very foundations of outcomes measurement prior to embracing these practices as a necessary part of audiologic practice. We will now present some questions regarding the use of, tools for, and implications of outcomes measurement. Some of the questions may be answered at face value, and others will become clearer in future chapters of this textbook.

Ponder these questions. The first set of questions has to do with the use of outcomes measurement:

- What happens if the profession does not use outcomes measurement?

- What happens if a particular audiologist decides not to use outcomes measurement?
- In what areas of practice and in what service-delivery sites are outcomes measurement required?
- Who or what is requiring outcomes measurement (e.g., patients, their families, third-party payers, facilities, accrediting agencies)? Are these requirements reasonable? If not, is there any way for audiologists to effect their change?
- Are there any mechanisms at the local, state, or national level that audiologists can use to record, share, and/or compare results for benchmarking?
- Should the profession develop guidelines for referral and care that designate appropriate outcomes measures?
- In what ways have the American Speech-Language-Hearing Association, the American Academy of Audiology, and other professional organizations promoted outcomes measurement for the profession?
- Are there any information management systems (e.g., software) available for audiologists' use in outcomes measurement?
- How can audiologists use the resulting outcomes data to improve service-delivery to patients and to enhance their practices?

The next set of questions has to do with outcomes measurement tools:

- What types of tools are available for audiologists' use?
- Are some tools better than others? What makes a tool reliable and valid? What other criteria can we use to evaluate these tools?
- What is the difference between subjective (e.g., patient ratings) versus objective (i.e., test results) measures? Is one better than the other? What happens if one shows improvement as a result of treatment while the other does not?
- How much change is needed for a significant difference? How much change is

needed for clinical significance? Is there a difference between statistical and clinical significance?

■ How, when, and why should outcome measures be reported and to whom or what?

■ How can audiologists construct their own valid and reliable outcomes measurement tools?

The above-stated questions are but a handful that the profession and audiologists must consider in incorporating a seamless outcomes measurement program into their daily practices. Read on.

SUMMARY

Outcomes measurement is presently a very popular concept for the profession. Everyone says it is important to do it, but there are no established ground rules or frameworks to guide clinicians in using these practices to their best advantage. This chapter has introduced readers to the complexity of key issues, provided two scenarios for demonstrating the important role of outcomes measurement in the profession, and provided some questions to keep in mind while reading this textbook.

LEARNING ACTIVITIES

■ Review the latest issues of two trade journals and select two advertisements. Carefully review their content and underline any claims the manufacturer has made regarding either the performance or benefits of the product to patients. Contact the manufacturer either on-line or by phone to inquire about access to experimental evidence supporting advertising claims.

■ Use the "Evaluation of Treatment Procedures, Products, and Programs" (ASHA, 1999) tool in Appendix I-A found on the companion CD-ROM to evaluate a relatively new product, such as the following (Advertisement appears in Appendix I-B which can be used for this activity).

Keith, R.L. (1999). SCAN-C: Test for auditory processing disorders in children—revised. San Antonio, TX: The Psychological Corporation: A Harcourt Assessment Company.

RECOMMENDED READINGS

Weinstein, B.E. (2000). Outcome measures in rehabilitative audiology. In J.G. Alpiner and P.A. McCarthy (Eds.), *Rehabilitative audiology: Children and adults* (3rd ed., pp. 575–594). Baltimore, MD: Lippincott, Williams, & Wilkins.

Wilson, B., & Cleary, P. (1995). Linking clinical variables with quality of life: Conceptual model of patient outcomes. *Journal of the American Medical Association, 273,* 59–65.

REVIEW EXERCISES

Fill-in-the-Blank

Instructions: Please fill-in-the-blank with the correct term from the word bank below.

1. _____ outcomes are relevant to the administration of a practice or a facility, such as patient demographics, number of treatment sessions, and financial aspects of managing a profitable business.

2. _____ outcomes deal with the how and the why of clinical practice.

Word Bank:

Process   Program

Matching

Instructions: Please match the following items with the correct statements and terms below.

I. Process outcomes
II. Program outcomes

1. ___ NICU protocol
2. ___ Patient demographics
3. ___ Calibration procedures
4. ___ Number of treatment sessions
5. ___ Overhead

ANSWERS

Fill-in-the-Blank:	Matching:	
1. Program	1. II	4. I
2. Process	2. I	5. I
	3. II	

REFERENCES

American Academy of Audiology. (1997). Position statement and guidelines of the consensus panel on support personnel in audiology. *Audiology Today, 9*(3), 27–28.

American Academy of Audiology Committee on Infant Hearing. (1998). Use of support personnel for newborn hearing screening (proposed guidelines). *Audiology Today, 10*(6), 21–23.

American Speech-Language-Hearing Association. (1999). *Questions to ask when evaluating a procedure, product, or program.* Available Internet: www.asha.org/audiology/evaluation.html.

Beck, L. (1999). *The NIDCD/VA hearing aid clinical trial and evidence based decision-making in the VA.* Paper presented at the Annual Convention of the American Speech-Language-Hearing Association, San Francisco, CA.

Burrows, D.L., & Owen, W. (1999). *A statistical model for assessing universal newborn hearing screening programs.* Paper presented at the Annual Convention of the American Speech-Language Hearing Association, San Francisco, CA.

Dillon, H., & So, M. (2000). Incentives and obstacles to the routine use of outcomes measures by clinicians. *Ear and Hearing, 21*(Suppl. 4), 2S–14S.

Johnson, C.E., & Danhauer, J.L. (1999). *Guidebook for support programs in aural rehabilitation.* Clifton Park, NY: Delmar Thomson Learning.

Johnson, C.E., & Danhauer, J.L. (2001). *A survey of audiologists on outcomes measurement.* Poster presented at the 13th Annual Convention and Exposition of the American Academy of Audiology, San Diego, CA.

Johnson, M.J., Maxon, A.B., White, K.R., & Vohr, B.R. (1993). Operating a hospital-based universal newborn hearing screening program using transient evoked otoacoustic emissions. *Seminars in Hearing, 14*(1), 46–55.

Joint Committee on Infant Hearing (2000). Year 2000 position statement: Principles and guidelines for early hearing detection and intervention programs. *American Journal of Audiology: A Journal of Clinical Practice 9*(1), 9–29.

Robertson, S., & Colburn, A. (1997). Outcomes research for rehabilitation: Issues and solutions. *Journal of Rehabilitation Outcomes Measurement, Application, Methodology, & Technology. 1,* 15–24.

Robinette, M.S., & White, K.R. (1998). The state of newborn hearing screening. In F. Bess (Ed.), *Children with hearing impairment: Contemporary trends* (pp. 45–67). Nashville, TN: Vanderbilt Bill Wilkerson Center Press.

Weinstein, B.E. (2000). Outcome measures in rehabilitative audiology. In J.G. Alpiner and P.A. McCarthy (Eds.), *Rehabilitative audiology: Children and adults* (3rd ed., pp. 575–594). Baltimore, MD: Lippincott, Williams, & Wilkins.

APPENDIX I-A

Evaluation of Treatment Procedures, Products, and Programs

(Adapted with permission © American Speech-Language-Hearing Association, 1999: Available Internet: www.asha.org/audiology/evaluation.html)

The above-referenced Appendix can be found on the companion CD-ROM.

APPENDIX I-B

Ad for Scan—C:
Test for Auditory Processing Disorders in Children—Revised

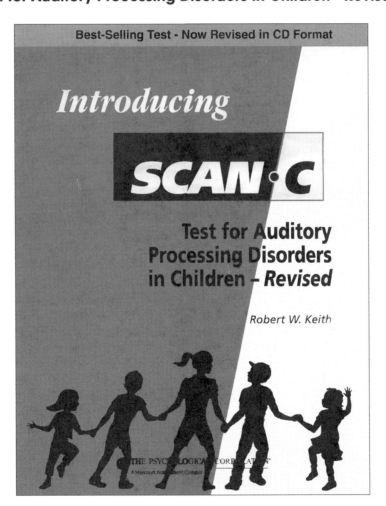

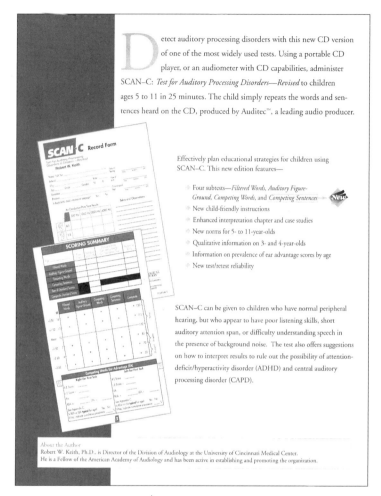

Detect auditory processing disorders with this new CD version of one of the most widely used tests. Using a portable CD player, or an audiometer with CD capabilities, administer SCAN–C: *Test for Auditory Processing Disorders—Revised* to children ages 5 to 11 in 25 minutes. The child simply repeats the words and sentences heard on the CD, produced by Auditec™, a leading audio producer.

Effectively plan educational strategies for children using SCAN–C. This new edition features—

- Four subtests—*Filtered Words, Auditory Figure-Ground, Competing Words,* and *Competing Sentences*
- New child-friendly instructions
- Enhanced interpretation chapter and case studies
- New norms for 5- to 11-year-olds
- Qualitative information on 3- and 4-year-olds
- Information on prevalence of ear advantage scores by age
- New test/retest reliability

SCAN–C can be given to children who have normal peripheral hearing, but who appear to have poor listening skills, short auditory attention span, or difficulty understanding speech in the presence of background noise. The test also offers suggestions on how to interpret results to rule out the possibility of attention-deficit/hyperactivity disorder (ADHD) and central auditory processing disorder (CAPD).

About the Author
Robert W. Keith, Ph.D., is Director of the Division of Audiology at the University of Cincinnati Medical Center. He is a Fellow of the American Academy of Audiology and has been active in establishing and promoting the organization.

CHAPTER 2
An Introduction to Outcomes Measurement

LEARNING OBJECTIVES

This chapter will enable readers to:

- Define and compare key terms in outcomes measurement
- Discuss the importance of outcomes measurement to the profession of audiology
- Understand critical responsibilities of the profession, training programs, and practitioners in outcomes measurement that will ensure the viability of the profession

INTRODUCTION

The United States health-care system is rapidly and dramatically undergoing changes that challenge practitioners (Hicks, 1998). Service delivery in health-care and educational settings is becoming more complex caused, in part, by the development of new paradigms of service delivery (Johnson, 1996). Third-party payers expect coordinated services, facilities, and systems, as well as providers, to be accountable and to demonstrate quality (Hicks, 1998).

The availability of a variety of audiologic services for the diagnosis and treatment of auditory disorders has raised important questions of, "What works? When does it work? How much does it cost?" (Johnson, 1996). Donabedian (1980) believed that quality of care requires a unifying framework involving structure (e.g., audiologists, tools, resources, and organizational settings), process (e.g., activities that go on between and among hearing health-care providers and patients), and outcomes (e.g., changes in patients' current and future health status and quality of life that can be tied to prior audiologic care). In an era of managed care, the status of outcomes measurement in communication sciences and disorders has moved from need to imperative (Robcy & Dalebout, 1998). Third-party payers are demanding efficacy research documenting the effectiveness of diagnostic and therapeutic protocols in highly controlled clinical experiments prior to reimbursement, for example (ASHA, 1996). Clearly, the destiny of the professions is tied to these types of data (Boston, 1994).

Hearing health-care providers must understand basic principles of outcomes measurement and implications of these practices in the real world of service delivery. The purposes of this chapter are to: (1) define and compare key terms in outcomes measurement; (2) emphasize the importance of these practices to the profession of audiology; and (3) propose critical responsibilities for the profession, training programs, and practitioners for ensuring the viability of the profession.

OUTCOMES MEASUREMENT: DEFINITIONS

Outcomes

The first step toward a better understanding of outcomes measurement is to define and compare key terms. Traditionally, an *outcome* has been defined simply as the result of an intervention (Frattali, 1996). Outcomes occur between two points in time (Wertz, 1999), and are measured usually near the beginning and at the end of service delivery (Johnson, 1996). Audiologists and speech-language pathologists have been measuring outcomes for decades by stating goals, applying treatment, and then measuring patients' progress (Johnson, 1996). Moreover, outcomes measurement can differ along several dimensions (Frattali, 1998). For example, "outcomes" in its plural form (i.e., outcomes) can only be defined in terms

of its *agent* (i.e., the consumer) involving patients, their families, clinicians, teachers, employers, and administrators (Frattali, 1998). However, in this text, we have broadened the definition to include the outcomes of clinical service delivery in areas, such as early hearing detection and intervention (EHDI) programs (Chapter 6), diagnostic audiology (Chapter 7), and hearing conservation (Chapter 8). Outcomes measurement can be (Frattali, 1998):

- clinically driven (e.g., ability to speechread),
- functional (e.g., ability to manipulate personal hearing aids, or to understand speech in noisy listening situations),
- administrative (e.g., patient referral rates, number of staff members satisfied with inservice program),
- financial (e.g., cost-effective care, average length of appointments),
- social (e.g., employability, reduction of hearing handicap), and
- patient defined (e.g., satisfaction with service provision, quality of life).

Johnson (1996) presented three aspects of outcomes measurement that have not traditionally been applied in the professions (audiology and speech-language pathology). First, practitioners are now asked to identify patient outcome measures to verify the benefit of treatment. Second, the identified outcome measures must be functional for patients. Third, many third-party payers now require outcome measures for reimbursement.

Measurement Methods

Primary and Secondary (i.e., Synthetic) Methods

Outcomes data are usually submitted to some method of measurement. Methods of measurement can either be primary or secondary (synthetic). *Primary* methods are those in which the clinician/investigator both collects and analyzes data. Outcomes measurement also uses *secondary* or *synthetic* methods for data analysis involving information that is already available (e.g., prior existing data) in order to gain new insight (Frattali, 1998). Synthetic methods can be of three types:

1. meta-analysis,
2. cost-benefit or cost-effectiveness analysis, or
3. technology assessment.

Meta-analysis is a means of objectively synthesizing the outcomes of many investigations, positive and negative, in order to weigh the scientific evidence for a particular treatment (Robey & Dalebout, 1998). Robey and Dalebout (1998) completed a meta-analysis of the results of current studies investigating changes in self-perceived hearing difficulty pre- and post-hearing aid fitting, for example. *Cost-benefit* or *cost-effectiveness* analysis involves assessing the costs of health services in relation to the magnitude of patient benefit. Insurance companies may want to investigate the cost of cochlear implantation to the long-term benefit for a child with a severe-to-profound hearing loss, for example. Frattali (1998) stated that *technology assessment* is multifaceted and concerned with advances in health care regarding safety; efficacy; feasibility; use; cost-effectiveness; and social, economic, and ethical consequences.

Outcomes Research and Efficacy Research

Outcomes measurement involves two types of research: outcomes and efficacy (Frattali, 1998). *Outcomes research* involves studies of specific treatments or other general services under "real world conditions," precluding

rigid control of experimental variables (Frattali, 1996) and lower levels of evidence. *Levels of evidence* is a hierarchy of stringency or quality used in evaluating various measurement methods in research, which are summarized in Table 2-1 and discussed in Chapter 3.

Class I or experimental methods are the most rigorous. Outcomes research often utilizes Class II (quasi-experimental) or Class III (non-experimental) methods, and, therefore, can only make statements about trends, associations, and estimates (Frattali, 1996). Audiologists can state that patients' self-report of hearing handicap decreased when measured before versus after a four-week group hearing aid orientation program, but cannot claim a cause-and-effect relationship between treatment and positive patient outcomes, for example. Researchers primarily conduct Class I and Class II investigations. Although subjective and void of experimental controls, Class III or non-experimental methods offer some important advantages for audiologists serving patients in clinical settings (Frattali, 1998):

- everyone (e.g., practitioners and managers) can participate,
- results can lend support to quasi-experimental and experimental studies of treatment efficacy or outcome, and
- findings can shape causal hypotheses.

Efficacy research answers questions about the process of intervention requiring assessment of treatment under ideal or laboratory conditions at the Class I or experimental level of evidence. Therefore, efficacy research can prove cause-and-effect relationships among variables. Efficacy involves three aspects of accountability or documentation (ASHA, 1996; Frattali, 1998; Olswang, 1998):

- *Treatment effectiveness* addresses whether treatments work.

Table 2-1. Levels of evidence

LEVELS OF EVIDENCE

CLASS I: Experimental with one or more prospective, randomized, and controlled trials (PRCT) including:
- A meta-analysis of two or more randomized control trials
- Other PRCT studies with good internal and external validity
- Time-series research (single-subject design)

CLASS II: Quasi-experimental (non-random assignment) clinical studies with data collection prospectively or retrospectively with reliability and generalization of the findings including:
- Case-controlled studies
- Cohort studies
- Observational studies
- Prevalence studies
- Program evaluations
- Quality improvement studies

CLASS III: Non-experimental retrospectively collected data with historical controls or non-randomized clinical trials including:
- Case reports
- Case reviews/studies
- Clinical series
- Databases or registries

NON-CLASSIFIED STATUS: includes:
- Clinical opinion
- Consensus
- Standards of practice
- Studies that do not meet Class III criteria

(Adapted from the American Academy of Neurology, 1994; American Speech-Language-Hearing Association, 1999c; Fineburg, 1990; Frattali, 1998; Haldorn, Baker, Hodges, & Hicks, 1996).

- *Treatment efficiency* assesses the relative effectiveness of two or more treatments within a given period of time.
- *Treatment effects* seek to establish a cause-and-effect relationship between treatments and changes in patients' behavior.

Variables

Use of experimental and quasi-experimental designs requires knowledge of research methodology and consideration of dependent, independent, and confounding variables. *Dependent* variables are those that are measured. *Independent* variables are those that are manipulated. *Confounding* variables are those that must either be controlled for or eliminated. In clinical trails, for example, researchers investigate the effectiveness of treatments for patients who have some sort of affliction or pathologic condition and are assigned randomly either to an experimental (i.e., receives treatment) or control group (i.e., receives placebo or standard care).

Careful planning requires consideration of possible confounding variables (e.g., subject selection criteria) that could influence results. Researchers may choose to recruit socially active elderly patients (e.g., daily demands of communicating in noisy environments) with similar degrees of hearing loss to assess possible differences between reduction of self-reported hearing handicap using digital signal processing (DSP) hearing aids with and without multi-microphone technology, for example. In this scenario, the use of multi-microphone technology is the independent variable.

Reliability and Validity

Researchers must select a dependent variable that both consistently and accurately documents patients' hearing handicap in "real life," listening conditions involving noise, for example. Recall that *reliability* is the consistency of measurement. A reliable measure is one that will provide a consistent measure of patients' self-reported hearing handicap. *Validity*, on the other hand, is the truth in measurement. Researchers, for example, must use an accurate measure of patients' hearing disability in realistic listening conditions. A dependent variable can be reliable, but not valid. For a measure to be valid, it must also be reliable, however. The *Hearing Handicap Inventory for the Elderly* (HHIE) (Ventry & Weinstein, 1982) may be a reliable measure of social and emotional consequences of hearing handicap, but may not be as true a measure of patients' communication abilities in background noise as the *Abbreviated Profile of Hearing Aid Benefit* (APHAB) (Cox & Alexander, 1995), for example. Thus, although a reliable measure, the HHIE may not be the most valid for use in such an experiment.

Dependent variables are administered to both groups of subjects (i.e., patients) pretreatment and post-treatment. Statistical analyses determine the existence of any significant differences in reduction of self-reported hearing disability in noise by elderly users of digital signal processing (DSP) hearing aids with and without multi-microphone technology, for example. In summary, cause-and-effect relationships between specific interventions and positive outcomes (e.g., reduction of hearing disability in noise) must be established by well-controlled studies of treatment efficacy.

IMPORTANCE OF OUTCOMES MEASUREMENT TO THE PROFESSION OF AUDIOLOGY: SHARED RESPONSIBILITIES

Importance of Outcomes Measurement

In an era of managed care, audiologists must be skilled in outcomes measurement to demonstrate positive patient outcomes to third-party payers for reimbursement of services. Competition is fierce among health-care practitioners whose professions are not usually classified as "medical" (e.g., rehabilitative therapy) (Boston, 1994). Audiologists must be critical reviewers of efficacy research, assessing the effectiveness of the wide variety of treatments and technology available for use. Unfortunately, many hearing health-care providers have little or no time to review the literature or for direct participation in research. However, Boston (1994) stated that health-care professionals who can demonstrate the effectiveness of their services through hard data will have the competitive edge. So, it may be worthwhile, or even necessary, for us to make time for such measures.

Frattali (1996) stated that clinical fields that strive to prove treatment effectiveness must have a scientific base. Audiologists who fail to document patient outcomes create uncertainty and mistrust among key decision-makers in the provision of care (Frattali, 1996). Historically, audiologists have not sufficiently subjected their diagnostic and rehabilitative protocols to both scientific inquiry and scrutiny, thereby flirting with ethical issues (Frattali, 1996). Our patients deserve better! Outcomes measurement of both diagnostic and aural rehabilitation protocols should be readily available for patients, providers, and third-party payers to make informed decisions. The profession, training programs, and practitioners share in the responsibility of outcomes measurement for the future viability of audiology.

Shared Responsibilities

Responsibilities of the Profession

Leadership in outcomes measurement must start with the professions. Boston (1994) provided several reasons for the lack of an information base in audiology and speech-language pathology:

- A history of focusing on process-assurance versus outcomes-assurance
- Confusions between cause and effect for patients with multiple problems
- Incompatible software programs for registering and aggregating data
- Lack of a common language for reporting data
- Lack of training in data collection
- No central data clearinghouse
- No standardized format for outcomes measurement
- No strong networks for data sharing

Professional organizations must assume leadership roles in outcomes measurement at the national level. Toward this aim, the American Speech-Language-Hearing Associ-

ation has developed the National Center for Treatment Effectiveness in Communication Disorders (NCTECD) that operates the National Outcomes Measurement System (NOMS). NOMS is a database that assists practitioners in comparing their outcome data to national averages. Furthermore, NOMS provides audiologists and speech-language pathologists with the ammunition (i.e., data) to address the challenges and questions posed to the profession from internal and external sources (ASHA, 2001). Vignette 2-1 provides a brief history of ASHA's National Outcomes Measurement System.

The current measurement tool used by NOMS is the Functional Communication Measures (FCM) which are seven-point scales used by speech-language pathologists, for example, at patients' admission and discharge (e.g., pre- and post-measures) (ASHA, 2001; Frattali, Thompson, Holland, Wohl, & Ferketic, 1995). In addition, NOMS collects national and program-specific information about: demographics; diagnoses; service-delivery models; amount, frequency, and intensity of service provision; consumer information; and changes in patients' communication from admission to discharge. Clearly, NOMS has numerous uses for audiology and speech-language pathology, including those that are listed in Table 2-2.

First, NOMS can assist practitioners in advocating and negotiating for speech, language, and hearing services. In the future, an audiologist may convince rehabilitation-hospital administrators into funding aural rehabilitation support programs for patients with hearing impairment by presenting NOMS data regarding the differences between length of stay for stroke patients with and without hearing impairment, for example. Second, NOMS assists audiologists and speech-language pathologists in obtaining information required by various accredit-

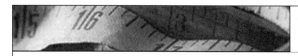

VIGNETTE 2-1

A BRIEF HISTORY OF ASHA'S NATIONAL OUTCOMES MEASURMENT SYSTEM (NOMS)

In 1993, the American Speech-Language-Hearing Association formed a Task Force on Treatment Outcomes and Cost-Effectiveness in response to its members' requests for outcomes data demonstrating the effectiveness of speech-language pathology and audiology services. In doing this, the Task Force reviewed various existing national databases and data collection systems. However, they realized none were comprehensive or sensitive enough to meet the growing needs of the Association. Out of necessity and commitment, the Task Force began working for the next two years on the development of a national database for the professions. To further its efforts, ASHA formed the National Center for Treatment Effectiveness in Communication Disorders (NCTECD). The role of NCTECD became the coordination of all outcomes and efficacy work for the Association.

In 1997, the National Outcomes Measurement System (NOMS) was developed. The purpose of NOMS is to collect aggregated national outcomes data from speech-language pathologists and audiologists working with adults and children in both school and health-care settings. Through the use of NOMS, we are now beginning to demonstrate the value of speech-language pathology and audiology services and provide our members the needed tools to address the challenging questions posed by policy makers, third-party payers, administrators and consumers alike.

(Reproduced with permission © American Speech-Language-Hearing Association, 2001: Available Internet: www.professional.asha.org/nctecd/treatment_outcomes)

Table 2-2. Advantages of NOMS

ASSISTS PRACTITIONERS

- Advocate/negotiate for services
- Gather information required by accrediting agencies
- Benchmark outcomes to aggregated national results
- Identify national trends (e.g., staffing trends)
- Develop preferred practice patterns
- Provide information to third-party payers
- Free of charge
- Undertake tasks of service delivery (e.g., patient satisfaction, demographic information, caseload planning/management, writing functional patient outcomes, optimal allocation of limited financial/personnel resources)

ing agencies. ORYX, a new initiative of the Joint Commission on the Accreditation of Healthcare Organizations (JCAHO), requires that health-care facilities utilize an approved system to collect outcome data and to analyze service provision (ASHA, 2001), for example. Moreover, although discontinued, ASHA's Professional Services Board (PSB) standards required facilities to evaluate the quality of service provision on a systematic and continuing basis. Third, NOMS allows practitioners to compare or benchmark the outcomes of their services to aggregated national results (ASHA, 2001). Benchmarking allows standards for comparisons for continuous quality improvement (Frattali, 1991; Goldberg, 1996). Fourth, NOMS helps practitioners to identify changing trends that might affect staffing patterns (ASHA, 2001). National trends in staffing may be of use to owners of sole-proprietor private practices who must determine how many audiologists to hire for an expanding marketplace. Fifth, NOMS can assist in developing preferred practice patterns to improve the quality of speech, language, and hearing services (ASHA, 2001). Sixth, NOMS provides information to third-party payers regarding the prognosis and functional outcomes of treatment (ASHA, 2001). NOMS can be used by third-party payers (e.g., audiology networks) and audiologists in writing comprehensive hearing plans for various groups, for example. Seventh, NOMS is free and accessible to everyone. Eighth, NOMS can also be used to assist with (ASHA, 2001):

- assessing patient satisfaction with services,
- acquiring demographic information for administrative reports,
- establishing caseload planning and management,
- writing functional patient outcomes, and
- determining optimal allocation of limited financial and personnel resources.

NOMS, to date, has been more focused on the profession of speech-language pathology, than audiology. The expanding scope of practice and service delivery for audiology necessitates the use of this system, however. Numerous mandates for universal newborn hearing screening programs are requiring new innovations in outcomes measurement and other aspects of service delivery, for example. State, institutionally based, and federal agencies are stimulating audiologists

into automating service delivery and collecting outcome measures for follow-up services for individual children, assessing program effectiveness/efficiency, and contributing to state and national data bases (Cherow, 1999). Finitzo, Albright, and O'Neal (1998) found that hospital support and automated data/information management contributed to the achievement of low false-positive rates in these screening programs.

Audiologists can now purchase numerous software packages capable of being customized for specific applications to (Keatley, Miller, & Mann, 1995):

- educate patients, parents, teachers, physicians, third-party payers, legislators, and government officials;
- gather information about patients;
- guide current/future treatment planning; and
- predict outcomes for patients using prognostic variables (e.g., age, sex, communication diagnosis).

Cherow (1999) stated that outcomes measurement will verify appropriate/efficient service delivery and secure the role of audiologists in pediatric service delivery. Therefore, ASHA will begin a treatment outcomes project to define the distinct role of the audiologist in the identification, assessment, and intervention of infants with hearing impairment.

Two other difficult tasks for the professions are to increase participation of practitioners in outcomes/efficacy research and to train the next generation of clinical scientists in the area of outcomes measurement. From 1984 to 1993, ASHA membership increased by 90%, yet the number of ASHA members claiming that research was the primary or secondary employment function increased by only 30% (ASHA, 1994a). In the year 2000, the relative proportion of members declaring research as a major job function decreased even more. Moreover, enrollment in traditional doctoral programs in communication sciences and disorders is at an alarmingly low level, which threatens the future of the professions. Thus, university faculty vacancies created by retirements early in the new millennium may remain unfilled. Clearly, the professions must be proactive in reversing these trends.

The American Speech-Language-Hearing Association has launched several programs to counteract these trends. First, in 1998 and 1999, ASHA held ASHA Leader Live for Speech, Language, and Hearing Scientists and Researchers in a town meeting format to discuss these and other issues at the annual convention. One proposed strategy to recruit for careers in research in communication sciences and disorders is to expose undergraduate and masters degree students to research mentors early in their academic careers. Toward this end, as one of five priority goals in 1999 (ASHA, 1999c), ASHA designated resources to the encouragement of careers in teaching and research in the professions by establishing the Higher Education Mentoring Program (ASHA, 1999a). During the summer of 1999, undergraduate and masters degree students were paired with selected mentors, university-based scientists, for two- to four-week periods to observe these established researchers at work. ASHA's other efforts to stimulate its members' participation in research include; sponsoring research institutes (ASHA, 1999d), travel fellowships to sponsored annual research symposia (i.e., for doctoral and post-doctoral students who are members of under-represented minorities) (ASHA, 1999b), and offer annual grant competitions for students-in-training and new investigators through the American Speech-Language-Hearing Foundation (ASHF). Likewise, The American Academy of Audiology (AAA) offers similar competitions for research grants to stimulate interest in

research in the next generation of professionals. However, as discussed below, some other professional efforts of AAA toward implementation of the Doctor of Audiology degree (Au.D.) may actually decrease future professionals' participation in outcomes measurement, thus further eroding the scientific base of the profession.

For the past 10 years, the AAA has endorsed the doctorate as the minimally acceptable degree for the practice of audiology (AAA, 1990). AAA has worked diligently in clearly designating the difference between the traditional academic doctorate (i.e., Ph.D) and the Doctor of Audiology (i.e., Au.D.) degrees. AAA's position statement on the professional doctorate stated that the Ph.D. is focused on creative scholarship and research in preparation for a career in teaching at a college or university (AAA, 1991), and that the Au.D., on the other hand, is focused on the development of clinical proficiency. The position statement also declares that Au.D. practitioners, however, are supposed to:

- be familiar with the scientific literature,
- have the scientific skills to evaluate and interpret audiologic research studies, and
- synthesize and apply research knowledge to the problems of clinical practice.

Au.D. practitioners, therefore, are not expected to execute outcomes/efficacy research investigations independently. AAA's scope of practice (1993), however, states that audiologists design, implement, analyze, and interpret the results of research. Thus, a discrepancy exists between audiologists' level of research competence stated in their scope of practice (AAA, 1993) and the level of sophistication recommended for training Au.D. practitioners (AAA, 1991). If Au.D. practitioners are not trained to the level of proficiency mentioned in the AAA scope of practice, who will conduct the necessary clinical outcomes/efficacy research investigations needed to ensure the viability of the profession? Certainly not the Ph.D. audiologist if current trends of low enrollment continue for the traditional doctoral programs in communication sciences and disorders. Moreover, if AAA and ASHA do not collaborate in a national student recruitment campaign for both Ph.D. and Au.D. programs, then the profession may even have to rely on researchers from other disciplines for scientific breakthroughs, innovations, and new technology. This could be a potential death knell for the survival of the profession, at least the degree of autonomy that is presently sought by most audiologists. Moreover, who will teach the future generation of audiologists? Clearly, the profession needs to design curricula for these doctoral programs to prepare audiologists to meet the challenges for service delivery in the new millennium.

ASHA and AAA have described optimal components for both Ph.D. and Au.D. training programs, respectively. ASHA (1994a, 1994b) has identified key areas for consideration in the assessment of Ph.D. programs in communication sciences and disorders:

- university-wide curricular resources,
- department level curricular resources,
- financial considerations,
- an available student peer group,
- participation in a variety of research-relevant training experiences,
- mentorship,
- a proven track record in producing successful scientists, and
- physical facilities

The "Ph.D. Program Evaluation Checklist" in Appendix II-A, found on the companion CD-ROM, may be useful for prospective Ph.D. students, faculty, and administrators (ASHA, 1994a, 1994b).

Similarly, the AAA stated that Au.D. programs should be organized within colleges and universities providing an independent school and faculty similar to doctoral degree programs in dentistry, medicine, optometry, veterinary medicine, and so on (AAA, 1990, 1991). Moreover, AAA's Position Statement on the Professional Doctorate states that Au.D. programs should be administered independently from existing graduate schools so that they will develop the highest level of clinical skills in students with emphasis on superior service delivery to patients. Appendix II-B, found on the companion CD-ROM, contains an evaluation checklist of key components for Au.D. programs identified by AAA (AAA, 1990, 1991).

In summary, the training of Ph.D. and Au.D. audiologists should be different. Nevertheless, aspects of both curricula are beneficial to all students regardless of their specific degree aspirations. Ph.D. students in audiology require advanced clinical training in order to conduct clinically relevant, cutting-edge research. Moreover, Au.D. students need advanced training in research methodology to conduct outcomes/efficacy research (e.g., clinical trials). In addition, Ph.D. and Au.D. students would not only learn from cooperative learning experiences, but they could also develop ties for future professional collaboration. Furthermore, the profession must ask who should teach in Au.D. programs. According to the Position Statement on the Professional Doctorate, many Ph.D.-trained audiologists do not have the clinical skills necessary to train Au.D. students. Should Au.D. practitioners primarily teach in Au.D. programs? If so, Au.D. practitioners will not be prepared for careers in university teaching, nor will they solely be able to provide students with the necessary knowledge and skills for outcomes measurement. Similarly, will current master's degree-level clinical supervisors in traditional graduate programs be appropriate instructors for Au.D. students? These and other questions must be addressed as audiology transitions to a doctoral-level profession.

Students in Au.D. programs need to be trained by faculty who are actively involved in clinical pursuits and who have experience in the research bases of our field. Those who insist that Au.D. students should be taught only by individuals having clinical degrees (e.g., an Au.D. degree) must realize that presently, and in the foreseeable future, Au.D. programs are housed within traditional university settings that typically require proof of research productivity (e.g., publication in peer-reviewed journals) for promotion, retention, tenure, and merit raises. Unfortunately, the reality is that most institutions of higher learning do not understand or have mechanisms to evaluate the contributions that clinicians make to our field and to the overall mission of training programs in communication sciences and disorders. Two things must happen in order to help create the dynamic relationships that must exist between clinical and research faculty if Au.D. programs are to prepare future audiologists to practice successfully in tomorrow's health-care arena. Clinical faculty need to be infused into the research process and they must be rewarded for their participation via institutional career ladder programs.

Responsibilities of Training Programs

Ph.D. and Au.D. training programs share the responsibility of ensuring the viability of the profession in part through outcomes measurement. First, program administrators must acknowledge the benefit of both Au.D. and Ph.D. program curricula for all doctoral students, regardless of specific degree candidacy. Both curricula should provide students with adequate training and experience in outcomes measurement. Programs should require courses on the topic, infuse its principles throughout the curricula, and provide students access to the latest software in outcomes measurement, for example. In addition, university speech and hearing clinic and off campus practicum sites should expose students to outcomes measurement within the context of professional practice. Second, training programs must foster scientific inquiry and scrutiny throughout the curricula to develop critical thinking skills in their students. Students must demand efficacy research that demonstrates that proving the benefits of new hearing aid technology actually justifies the increased costs to their patients, for example. Third, academic (Ph.D.) and professional (Au.D.) faculty must be models for enthusiasm and develop an esprit de corps in joint clinical/research endeavors. Future researchers and practitioners need to see that joint collaborations can be successful in achieving significant audiologic breakthroughs. Fourth, administrators need to acknowledge and reward the extracurricular professional efforts (e.g., private practices) of traditional university faculty who may not have had to confront the issue of controlling costs through efficient delivery of services (Vekovius, 1995). Students can benefit from professors' "real world" experiences with outcomes measurement in their private practices. Fifth, training programs must acknowledge the dynamic climate of health care and potential threats to the profession. Students must understand not only managed care, but also the challenge of managing a sole-proprietor private practice in a highly competitive marketplace (Danhauer, 1998). By infusing managed care into the curriculum, training programs can ensure their reputation as being "cutting edge" and their curricular relevance to the health-care climate. Sixth, training programs must tie outcomes measurement and efficacy research to the viability of the profession. For example, students must acknowledge the direct relevance of their courses in outcomes measurement and research methodology to their ability to analyze and select the best diagnostic and aural rehabilitative protocols in service delivery. Appendices II-A and II-B also contain checklists for training Ph.D. and Au.D. students in outcomes measurement, respectively.

Practitioners' Responsibilities

Providers of clinical services also share in the responsibility of outcomes measurement. First, audiologists must educate themselves about outcomes measurement through self-study and continuing education opportunities, and lobby their professional organizations for continuing education opportunities that cover outcomes measurement. Second, audiologists must scrutinize any information or product related to clinical management according to "Levels of Evidence" discussed earlier in this chapter (American Academy of Neurology, 1994; ASHA, 1999e; Fineburg, 1990; Frattali, 1998; Haldorn, Baker, Hodges, & Hicks, 1996). Audiologists should review the levels of evidence for clinical trials to ensure that the high cost of high-performance hearing aid circuitry results in adequate patient bene-

Table 2-3. Activities for audiologists' roles as data gatherers and advocates

AS A DATA GATHERER

- Collect data on consumer satisfaction with treatment services. Share it with legislators, consumer lobbying groups, and other decision-makers.
- Use aggregated data from your own practice as a base. Turn your practice into an "independent study project" and share the results with NOMS.
- Go to professional meetings and attend sessions on outcomes measurement development issues.
- Keep posted on ASHA's progress on NOMS for audiologists and related efforts by AAA and participate in those efforts.

AS AN ADVOCATE

- Write your Congressional representative, senator, and corresponding state officials to advocate for inclusion of audiology services in every piece of health-care legislation.
- Arrange for appointments with your state legislators to explain the value of your professional services. Provide written materials as backup.
- Try to get an opportunity to testify before state legislature committees considering health-care legislation.
- Write letters or public information pieces to the editors of local and regional papers on the importance of audiology services.
- Talk to your patients and encourage them to participate in the above activities.
- Organize a local advocacy group. Include patients, colleagues in the profession, members of the business community, health writers, and members of the media.
- Plan and deliver local programs on professional issues and problems.
- Recruit a high-visibility spokesperson to plead your cause with the public.
- Join a local advocacy group or consumer group addressing health-care reform issues and become a spokesperson for audiology services.
- Join a hearing network and change managed care from the inside out.

(Adapted from Boston, 1994).

fit. Third, audiologists should participate in outcomes measurement in all areas of practice, across service delivery sites, and through national professional organizations. Outcomes measurement should involve both diagnostic and aural rehabilitation protocols, for example. Moreover, audiologists should be aware of the outcomes measurement requirements of the facilities in which they work. For example, audiologists working in nursing homes must be aware of the accountability requirements of the Joint Committee on Accreditation of Healthcare Organizations (JCAHO). Fourth, audiologists should participate in NOMS by gathering data and advocating for its development and use in all areas of practice. Table 2-3 shows important activities for audiologists as data gatherers and advocates not only for NOMS, but also for outcomes management and the profession (Boston, 1994).

Fifth, audiologists should use outcomes measurement to guide their professional practices for success. Outcomes-oriented practices thrive because of their focus on positive patient outcomes and satisfaction. One audiologist can make a difference! We hope readers will find the chapters in this text useful in these pursuits.

SUMMARY

The current climate of health-care demands accountability through outcomes measurement. This chapter has defined and compared key terms that are often confused by audiologists who must understand the importance of outcomes measurement to the viability of the profession in today's competitive health-care arena. The profession, training programs, and practitioners all share responsibilities regarding outcomes measurement.

LEARNING ACTIVITIES

■ List all the ways that your practice or training program engages in outcomes measurement.

■ Classify 10 research studies by the Levels of Evidence.

■ Contact the American Speech-Language-Hearing Association to determine audiologists' current level of participation in NOMS.

■ Determine the American Academy of Audiology's current efforts toward outcomes measurement in the profession.

■ Contact Au.D. programs regarding the training provided for outcomes measurement.

■ Investigate software packages for outcomes measurement in audiology.

RECOMMENDED READINGS

Boston, B.O. (1994). Destiny is in the data: A wake-up call for outcome measures. *ASHA, 36*(11), 35–38.

Frattali, C.M. (1998). Outcomes measurement: Definitions, dimensions, and perspectives. In C. Frattali (Ed.), *Measuring efficacy research in speech-language pathology* (pp. 1–27). New York, NY: Thieme.

Wertz, R.T. (1998). Critical issues in determining efficacious intervention. In F. Bess (Ed.), *Children with hearing impairment: Contemporary trends* (pp. 343–358). Nashville, TN: Vanderbilt, Bill Wilkerson Center Press.

REVIEW EXERCISES

Fill-in-the-Blank

Instructions: Please fill-in-the-blank with the correct term from the word bank below.

1. A(n) _____ is a result of an intervention.
2. _____ methods are those in which the clinician/investigator both collects and analyzes data.
3. _____ methods are those that analyze data that are already available.
4. _____ - _____ is a means of objectively synthesizing the outcomes of many investigations, positive and negative, in order to weigh the scientific evidence for a particular treatment.
5. _____ - _____ analysis involves assessing the costs of health services in relation to the magnitude of patient benefit.
6. _____ _____ is multifaceted and concerned with advances in health care regarding safety; efficacy; feasibility; use; cost-effectiveness; and social, economic, and ethical consequences.
7. _____ research involves studies of specific treatments or general services under "real world" conditions, precluding rigid control of experimental variables.
8. _____ of _____ is a hierarchy of stringency or quality used in evaluating various measurement methods in research.
9. _____ research involves Class I methods (experimental) that can prove cause-and-effect between treatments and patient benefit.
10. _____ variables are those that are measured.
11. _____ variables are those that are manipulated.
12. _____ variables must be controlled for or eliminated.
13. _____ is the truth in measurement.
14. _____ is the consistency of measurement.

Word Bank:

Confounding	Outcome
Cost-benefit	Outcomes
Dependent	Primary
Efficacy	Reliability
Independent	Secondary
Levels of evidence	Technology assessment
Meta-analysis	Validity

Matching

Instructions: Please match the following items with the correct statements below.

I. Class I: Experimental
II. Class II: Quasi-experimental
III. Class III: Non-experimental
IV. Non-classified

1. ___ Cohort studies
2. ___ Time series research (single-subject design)
3. ___ Efficacy research
4. ___ Expert opinion
5. ___ Quality improvement studies
6. ___ Random assignment of subjects to groups
7. ___ Standards of practice
8. ___ Observational studies
9. ___ Databases or registries
10. ___ Case reports

ANSWERS

Fill-in-the-Blank:	Matching:
1. Outcome	1. II
2. Primary	2. I
3. Secondary	3. I
4. Meta-analysis	4. IV
5. Cost-benefit	5. II
6. Technology assessment	6. I
7. Outcomes	7. IV
8. Levels of evidence	8. II
9. Efficacy	9. III
10. Dependent	10. III
11. Independent	
12. Confounding	
13. Validity	
14. Reliability	

REFERENCES

American Academy of Audiology. (1990). Position statement: Graduate education. *Audiology Today, 2*(5), 10.

American Academy of Audiology. (1991). Position statement: The professional doctorate. *Audiology Today, 3*(4), 14–17.

American Academy of Audiology. (1993). Audiology: Scope of practice. *Audiology Today, 5*(1), 16–17.

American Academy of Neurology. (1994). Report of the therapeutics and technology assessment subcommittee on assessment: Melodic intonation therapy. *Neurology, 44,* 566–568.

American Speech-Language-Hearing Association. (1994a). *Handbook of research education in communication sciences and disorders: A guide for program directors, research mentors, and prospective Ph.D. students.* Rockville, MD: Author.

American Speech-Language-Hearing Association. (1994b). *Selecting a doctoral research education program in communication sciences and disorders.* Rockville, MD: Author.

American Speech-Language-Hearing Association. (1996). *Curriculum guide to managed care.* Rockville, MD: Author.

American Speech-Language-Hearing Association. (1999a). Students, mentors selected for new program. *ASHA Leader, 4*(11), 4.

American Speech-Language-Hearing Association. (1999b). Research symposium offers travel fellowships. *ASHA Leader, 4*(11), 4.

American Speech-Language-Hearing Association. (1999c). Association workplans reflect key issues for professions. *ASHA Leader, 4*(12), 3.

American Speech-Language-Hearing Association. (1999d). Researchers will team up at summer institute. *ASHA Leader, 4*(12), 4.

American Speech-Language-Hearing Association. (1999e). *Call for papers.* Rockville, MD: Author.

American Speech-Language-Hearing Association (2001). National Center for Treatment Effectiveness in Communication Disorders. Available Internet: www.professional.asha.org/nctecd/treatment_outcomes.html

Boston, B.O. (1994). Destiny is in the data: A wake-up call for outcome measures. *ASHA, 36*(11), 35–38.

Cherow, E. (1999). Pediatric audiology: Poised for the future. *ASHA, 41*(1), 24–30.

Cox, R.M., & Alexander, G.C. (1995). The abbreviated profile of hearing aid benefit. *Ear and Hearing, 16,* 176–183.

Danhauer, J.L. (1998). Who are those major multi-office groups moving in on us, and—Is this town big enough for the both of us? *Audiology Today, 10*(2), 47–51.

Donabedian, A. (1980). *Explorations in quality assessment and monitoring. Vol. 1: The definition of quality and approaches to its assessment.* Ann Arbor, MI: Health Administration Press.

Fineburg, H.V. (1990). The quest for causality in health services research. In *Research methodology: Strengthening causal interpretations of nonexperimental data.* Rockville, MD: Agency for Health Care Policy and Research, U.S. Department of Health and Human Services.

Finitzo, T., Albright, K., & O'Neal, J. (1998). The newborn with hearing loss: Detection in the nursery. *Pediatrics, 102,* 1452–1460.

Frattali, C.M. (1991). From quality assurance to total quality management. *American Journal of Audiology: A Journal of Clinical Practice. 1*(1), 41–47.

Frattali, C.M. (1996). Outcomes data: Laying the groundwork for efficacy research and outcomes research. In *A practical guide to applying treatment outcomes and efficacy resources* (pp. 9–16). Rockville, MD: American Speech-Language-Hearing Association.

Frattali, C.M. (1998). Outcomes measurement: Definitions, dimensions, and perspectives. In C. Frattali (Ed.), *Measuring outcomes in speech-language pathology* (pp. 1–27). New York, NY: Thieme.

Frattali, C.M., Thompson, C.M., Holland, A.L., Wohl, C.B., & Ferketic, M.M. (1995). The FACS of life: ASHA FACS—A functional outcome measure for adults. *ASHA, 37*(4), 40–46.

Goldberg, B. (1996). Imagining tomorrow: What's ahead for our professions? *ASHA, 38*(3), 22–23, 25–28.

Haldorn, D.C., Baker, D., Hodges, J.S., & Hicks, N. (1996). Rating the quality of evidence for clinical practice guidelines. *Journal of Clinical Epidemiology, 49*, 749–754.

Hicks, P.L. (1998). Outcomes measurement requirements. In C. Frattali (Ed.), *Measuring outcomes in speech-language pathology* (pp. 28–49). New York, NY: Thieme.

Johnson, A. (1996). Outcomes and efficacy: Some considerations for practitioners in audiology and speech-language pathology. In *A practical guide to applying treatment outcomes and efficacy resources* (pp. 1–7). Rockville, MD: American Speech-Language-Hearing Association.

Keatley, M.A., Miller, T.I., & Mann, A. (1995). Treatment planning using outcome data: Fitting the pieces together. *ASHA, 32*(2), 48–52.

Olswang, L.B. (1998). Treatment efficacy research. In C. Frattali (Ed.), *Measuring outcomes in speech-language pathology* (pp. 134–150). New York, NY: Thieme.

Robey, R.R., & Dalebout, S.D. (1998). A tutorial on conducting meta-analysis of clinical outcome research. *Journal of Speech-Language-Hearing Research, 41*(6), 1227–1241.

Vekovius, G.T. (1995). Managed care 101: Introducing managed care into the curriculum. *ASHA,37*(9), 44–47.

Ventry, I.M., & Weinstein, B.E. (1982). The hearing inventory for the elderly: A new tool. *Ear and Hearing, 3*, 128–134.

Wertz, R.T. (1998). Critical issues in determining efficacious intervention. In F. Bess (Ed.), *Children with hearing impairment: Contemporary trends* (pp. 343–358). Nashville, TN: Vanderbilt, Bill Wilkerson Center Press.

APPENDIX II-A

Ph.D. Program Evaluation Checklist

(Adapted with permission © American Speech-Language-Hearing Association, 1994a, 1994b)

The above-referenced Appendix can be found on the companion CD-ROM.

APPENDIX II-B

Au.D. Program Evaluation Checklist

(Adapted from AAA, 1990; 1991)

The above-referenced Appendix can be found on the companion CD-ROM.

CHAPTER 3
Levels of Evidence

LEARNING OBJECTIVES

This chapter will enable the reader to define and compare components under the following levels of evidence:

- Class I: primary (i.e., randomized, controlled clinical trials and time series research) and secondary (i.e., meta-analysis) measurement methods;
- Class II: case-control studies, cohort studies, prevalence studies, program evaluations, and quality improvement studies;
- Class III: case studies, databases, and registries; and
- Non-classified status: expert clinical opinion, consensus, and standards of practice.

INTRODUCTION

The professions of audiology and speech-language pathology are focused on documenting the efficacy of treatment protocols for communication sciences and disorders at the highest levels of evidence. In the March 14th, 2000 issue of *The ASHA Leader*, ASHA President Jeri Logemann encouraged wider membership participation in the National Outcomes Measurement System (NOMS) and clinical trial research. Clinical trials are considered the "gold standard" for efficacy research at the Class I levels of evidence. Furthermore, Logemann (2000) stated that clinicians seek to use techniques that have been proven to be effective through supporting evidence published in peer-reviewed journals. She added that individuals presenting their research at professional conferences should only report on clinical techniques and technologies whose effectiveness have been substantiated by evidence-based research. Although well intentioned, Logemann's (2000) suggestions are antithetical to the advancement of science and technology for at least two reasons. First, hypotheses tested by clinical trial research often have very humble beginnings, perhaps as an anecdotal report from a single-case study. Every big idea started as a small idea sometime, somewhere. Researchers and clinicians need the latitude to be creative in developing testable hypotheses from their observations and intuitions. Second, prohibiting presentations that do not meet Class I or II levels of evidence could be considered a form of intellectual censorship. Professionals attend conventions to hear a wide variety of presentations that span the continuum of scientific rigor. Thus, ASHA's efforts should not be aimed at censorship (even unintended), but on educating ASHA's membership and students about being informed consumers of research.

Audiologists, in particular, need to be cognizant of authors' professional affiliations that could potentially bias the information they provide at professional conferences. For example, employees of the leading hearing aid manufacturing companies often present instructional courses at the Annual Convention and Exposition of the American Academy of Audiology (AAA) that may contain biased information favoring their product lines. These presentations are often impressive and convincing while also being informative and professional. Of course, the opposite could be true; thus, audiologists need to be trained in research techniques in order to be able to judge quality and be informed consumers themselves. Moreover, audiologists must wear their thinking caps even into the wee hours of the night during dinner cruises or seminars offered by hearing aid manufacturers promoting their latest developments. Regardless of the situation, information presented must be judged based on its scientific merit and level of evidence. Similarly, graduate students attending their first AAA Convention are often "star struck" when attending lectures given by the "big names" in the field. Our students must be taught to have a healthy respect for these individuals, but that sometimes the "king has no clothes" and the information being presented by their "heroes" may lack scientific rigor. The purpose of this chapter is to present the advantages and disadvantages of the information provided by the different types of research at each of the levels of evidence. Table 3-1 shows the types of studies to be discussed for the various levels of evidence that were introduced in Chapter 2.

CLASS I LEVELS OF EVIDENCE

Class I levels of evidence involve research in which there is random assignment to intervention and control groups or phases (Fratalli, 1998a). Examples include investigations that use either primary (e.g., randomized, controlled clinical trials and times series research or single-subject design research) or secondary/synthetic methods (e.g., meta-analysis) of outcomes measurement. *Primary measurement methods* are those in which the investigator both collects and analyzes the data. *Secondary measurement methods* of data analysis involve using already available information in order to gain new insights.

Primary Measurement Methods

Randomized, Controlled Clinical Trials

The term "*randomized, controlled clinical trials*" may already be well known by some readers. However, the term is best understood after carefully defining each of its parts. The term "*randomized*" has to do with the method used to assign subjects to treatment (i.e., receives experimental protocol) and control groups (i.e., receives placebo). Random assignment to groups requires that chance is the only factor operating, such that each subject has an equal opportunity of receiving the experimental treatment. *Random assignment* ensures that subjects' characteristics of age, sex, and so on are distributed equally (except for chance variance) and cannot confound or bias the statistical significance of differences

Table 3-1. Examples of studies at various levels of evidence discussed in this chapter.

CLASS I
> Primary Measurement Methods
- Randomized, Controlled Clinical Trials
- Time Series Research
> Secondary Measurement Methods
- Meta-analysis

CLASS II
- Case-control studies
- Cohort studies
- Prevalence Studies
- Program Evaluations
- Quality Improvement Studies

CLASS III
- Case Studies
- Databases and Registries

NON-CLASSIFIED
- Expert Clinical Opinion
- Standards of Clinical Practice
- Consensus

between or among the groups (Hulley, Feigal, Martin, & Cummings, 1988). The term "*controlled*" means that investigators have ensured that the experimental and control groups are equivalent, to the greatest extent possible, with the exception of the manipulation of the independent variable through elimination of any bias or systematic error. Two major sources of bias in clinical trials are observer and subject bias. As discussed in the last chapter, *observer bias* is a consistent distortion expressed, either consciously or subconsciously, by the individual administering the experimental protocol that can affect measurement of the dependent variable (Hulley & Cummings, 1988). Similarly, *subject bias* is a consistent distortion expressed, either consciously or subconsciously, by the individual receiving the experimental protocol that can affect measurement of the dependent variable (Hulley &

Cummings, 1988). Use of "*double-blinding*" by researchers eliminates both observer and subject bias because neither the person collecting data nor the subject knows the status (i.e., treatment or placebo) of the administered condition. For example, double-blinding was easily accomplished in one of the early clinical trials of the NIDCD/VA study comparing the relative effectiveness of three commonly used single-channel hearing aid circuits (peak-clippers, compression-limiting, and wide dynamic range compression) that were all contained within the same in-the-ear hearing aid case (Larson, et al., 2000).

Randomized, controlled clinical trials satisfy the three requirements for true experimental research (Maxwell & Satake, 1997):

- subjects randomly assigned to two or more groups,

- active manipulation of independent variables, and
- one or more groups receive the treatment and another group does not (i.e., control group).

Randomized, controlled clinical trials involve the use of group designs that can differ along several dimensions, including the types of questions to be answered. Group design research can answer three types of questions (Maxwell & Satake, 1997):

- *Descriptive questions*—seek to obtain a complete inventory of observable characteristics of certain objects or events.
- *Relationship questions*—concern how the variation of one variable is predicated upon that of another variable.
- *Difference questions*—focus on determining if there is a significant difference between and/or among two or more different groups (i.e., between-subjects design) or two or more different conditions from a single group of subjects (i.e., within-subjects design) for some measured value.

Only the results of studies answering difference questions can claim causality (Maxwell & Satake, 1997). Furthermore, these studies must be well controlled. This textbook assumes that readers have basic skills to evaluate the soundness of group-design research

Time-Series Research

Times-series research involves obtaining repeated measurements of a single or small group of subjects over time (Schiavetti & Metz, 1997). Data are collected at periodic intervals between which some sort of treatment occurs (Silverman, 1998). *Single-subject designs* are a type of time-series research in which each subject serves as his/her own control. Certain types of single-subject

design research have been classified as meeting the criteria for Class I levels of evidence. However, a brief review of the basic elements of single-subject design research is required prior to any further discussion of this issue.

Single-subject designs have both independent and dependent variables. Single-subject designs include at least two segments (Schiavetti & Metz, 1997):

- *Baseline* is a period of behavioral observation during which subjects' behavior is measured at regular intervals without any application of interventions or change in environmental conditions.
- *Treatment* is a period during which the independent variable is manipulated or the treatment is applied.

Data are recorded on a graph similar to that shown in Figure 3-1.

The dependent variable is represented on the ordinate (y-axis) and time is represented on the abscissa (x-axis). Subjects' behavior is charted by placing a dot at the intersection of the behavioral value and the time interval at which the behavior was observed. Lines contiguously connect these observations to form a line that must be carefully observed for successful application of the independent variable. For example, researchers should ensure that the baseline phase of the experiment continues until a stability of the dependent variable has been achieved. *Stability* has been defined as no more than 5% variability from interval-to-interval and/or no upward or downward trends in measurement of the dependent variable (Schiavetti & Metz, 1997). Figure 3-1 shows some possible variations in measurement of a dependent variable over time.

Silverman (1998) suggested a coding scheme to describe various types of single-subject designs by representing different phases of a study by a letter:

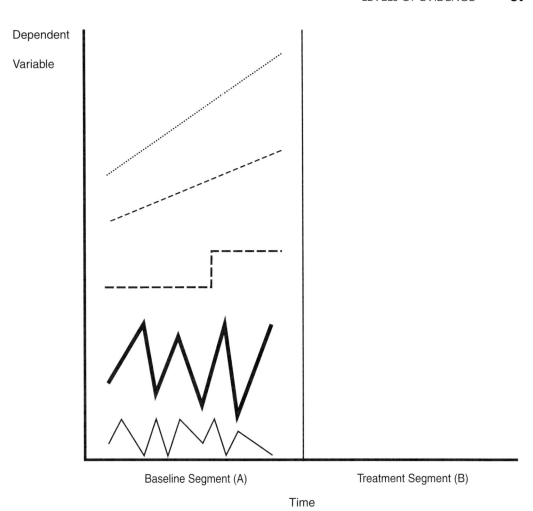

Figure 3-1. Possible performance of the dependent variable during the baseline of a single-subject design study (Schiavetti, N., & Metz, D.E. (1997). *Evaluating research in communicative disorders, 3rd edition.* Needham Heights, MA: Allyn & Bacon. Adapted with permission © Allyn & Bacon, 1997).

- A: baseline
- B: first treatment or intervention condition
- C: second treatment or intervention condition that is different from the first

He also suggested separating adjacent segments of the study with a dash (e.g., A-B) and using subscript to represent the first, second time, and so on that baseline or treatment is introduced (e.g., A_1, A_2, B_1, B_2 ...).

There are many types of single-subject designs ranging from very simple to complex. The simplest designs contain only one element. The A-only design (i.e., baseline only) is simply measuring the behavior of a subject over time without any manipulation of an independent variable. A-only designs are also known as "case studies" or "longitudinal diary studies" (Silverman, 1998) and are considered to be Class III levels of evidence (i.e., non-experimental methods) discussed below. Similarly, the B-only design (i.e., treatment only) represents a single segment that begins with intervention and represents the therapeutic model used by speech-language pathologists and audiologists (Silverman, 1998). Major limitations of the B-only design are that there is no proof of what changed patients' behavior and the lack of control of confounding variables (e.g., subject maturation). The B-only design is classified under the Class III levels of evidence.

The A-B design (i.e., baseline-treatment), also known as the "before and after" design, is a combination of the A-only and B-only designs (Silverman, 1998). Although more rigorous than the B-only design, researchers cannot claim that the independent variable (e.g., intervention) caused patients' change in behavior. The A-B design is considered to be at the Class II levels of evidence (i.e., quasi-experimental).

The A_1-B-A_2 design (i.e., baseline-treatment-baseline) is also known as the "withdrawal design" and is the simplest single-subject design that qualifies for Class I levels of evidence. The inclusion of a second baseline (i.e., removal of treatment) allows researchers to claim causality between intervention and changes in subjects' behavior if the dependent variable returns to baseline levels during this segment, as shown in Figure 3-2.

A weakness in this design is that it may be inappropriate for intervention approaches that may have longstanding effects (Silverman, 1998). In addition, in some cases, it is unethical to remove treatment from patients, even for short periods of time. However, multiple-baseline designs involving two or more functionally independent target behaviors (i.e., multiple baselines across behaviors) can be used so that patients do not need to "relapse" to demonstrate causality (Silverman, 1998). For example, Figure 3-3 shows a multiple-baseline design across two behaviors (adapted from McReynolds & Kearns, 1983) with a purpose of determining if a single treatment is effective in changing two behaviors within the same subject.

Initially, baseline measurement is made on behaviors A and B and once stability has been obtained, treatment is started on behavior A while behavior B continues in baseline (McReynolds & Kearns, 1983). If behavior B does not change while treatment is applied to behavior A, it shows that the independent variable (i.e., intervention) changes behaviors only when it is applied to dependent variables and is not affected by factors such as time, maturation, and other extraneous variables (McReynolds & Kearns, 1983). When the treatment phase for behavior A is completed, treatment then begins for behavior B and continues until a change occurs, demonstrating that the independent variable affects change in both behaviors A and B (McReynolds & Kearns, 1983). However, if behavior B does not change, then the effect of the independent variable has not been demonstrated and the design has the same status as an A-B design without experimental control (McReynolds & Kearns, 1983). Other variations of multiple

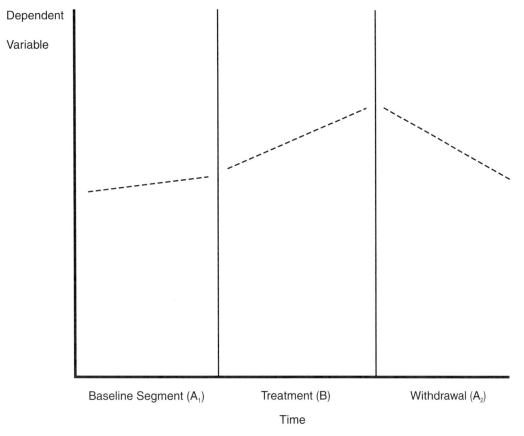

Figure 3-2. A graph of the results of an A-B-A single-subject design study in which the dependent variable significantly improved during treatment and decreased during the second baseline or reversal.

baseline designs include measuring the same behavior across several settings, subjects, and groups (McReynolds & Kearns, 1983; Schiavetti & Metz, 1997). Multiple baseline designs are the most commonly used design in the communication sciences and disorders literature (Kearns, 1986). Just as in group-design research, studies employing single-subject designs must be well controlled. Appendix III-A provides information about different evaluation strategies, clinical research questions, selected design options, and basic considerations in using single-subject experimental designs (Kearns, 1986). Furthermore, valuable resources can be found on the com-

panion CD-ROM. Appendix III-B contains a "Checklist for Evaluating Scientific Articles" (Schiavetti & Metz, 1997), and Appendix III-C contains a "Checklist for Evaluating or Designing Single-Subject Studies" (Kearns, 1986) to be used by readers for critiquing scientific investigations.

Group- or Single-Subject Designs?

Investigators disagree about the appropriateness of the classification of single-subject designs into the Class I level of evidence. Vignettes 3-1 and 3-2 contain two viewpoints by Randall R. Robey and Julie Wambaugh, one

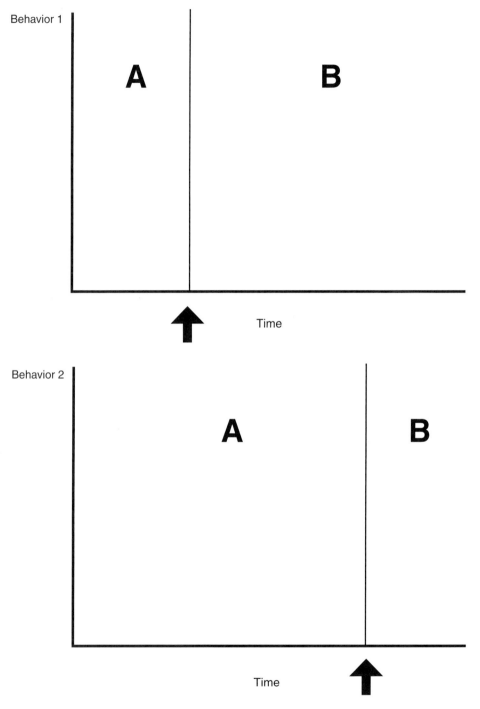

Figure 3-3. The graph of a multiple baseline single-subject design involving two behaviors (Adapted from McReynolds & Kearns, 1983).

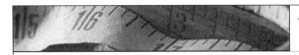

VIGNETTE 3-1

SINGLE-SUBJECT DESIGN VERSUS RANDOMIZED GROUP DESIGN

RANDOMIZED GROUP DESIGN

Randall R. Robey

Fundamental to the many serious challenges facing clinicians and clinical scientists working in the area of communication disorders is the serial testing of, first, efficacy and, then, effectiveness for each of many specific treatment protocols. Furthermore, the efficacy and effectiveness of specific treatment protocols must be examined in each of several dimensions: (a) specific impairments (e.g., observed performances regarding certain treatment objectives), (b) composite or overall impairment (e.g., a standardized test or severity index), (c) handicap or activity limitation, (d) disability or participation restriction, and (e) quality of life. Given the magnitude of the overall task, the issue for decision is not a unilateral choice between group or single-subject research designs, but rather determining which purposes each serves best.

The essence of research designs comparing group data is nomothetic inquiry (i.e., seeking to uncover universal explanations). The product of such inquiry is generalization from a representative sample of individuals drawn from a certain clinical population to the general membership of that population. That is, general explanations for large groups (populations) are obtained by studying representative small groups (samples) and the generalization, or inductive inference, from subset to set is qualified through the mathematics of probability. The statistical probability required to establish treatment efficacy (i.e., the warrant for the general expectation that a treatment will bring about desired outcomes when administered in routine clinical practice) is obtained directly through group-design research. Furthermore, group-design research can yield statistical inferences regarding constructs such as overall communication impairment, handicap, and quality of life.

A unique advantage of group research is a design characteristic termed external control (e.g., an independent no-treatment control group). Through external controls, outcomes for experimental treatments are interpreted in the context of an independent reference (e.g., no treatment, a treatment known to be efficacious) provided that subjects are randomly assigned to treatment conditions. In fact, random assignment of subjects to treatment conditions is the broadly accepted standard for examining the issue of causality which is central to establishing efficacy.

No research design intrinsically yields more potent or more valuable findings than does any other research design. Because all designs can be misused, the quality of any research finding is governed by the care and rigor with which a design is implemented. For group-design research, this means precautions such as testing focused and theory-driven null hypotheses through planned contrasts on cell or marginal means of parallel-group research designs, managing Type I error prudently, conducting a priori statistical-power analyses to determine adequate sample sizes, thoughtfully determining inclusion and exclusion criteria, examining results in terms of individual as well as group-average results, and controlling treatment in terms of protocol, schedule, and duration.

CONTINUES

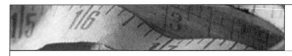

VIGNETTE 3-1

RANDOMIZED GROUP DESIGN   (CONTINUED FROM PAGE 41)

Whether an experimentalist chooses to implement a group or a single-subject research design, the fundamental responsibility is exactly the same: preserve, to the extent possible, all of construct validity, external validity, internal validity, and statistical-conclusion validity. In addition, scientific rigor demands independent replications of findings obtained through both forms of research. In that respect, the wisdom of the American Psychological Association in developing objective and apparent criteria for establishing treatment efficacy through both group and single-subject research merits our attention.

(Reprinted with permission © American Speech-Language-Hearing Association, Robey, R.R. (1999). Speaking out: Single-subject versus randomized group design. Asha, 41(6), 14–15.)

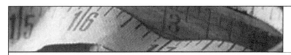

VIGNETTE 3-2

SINGLE-SUBJECT DESIGN VERSUS RANDOMIZED GROUP DESIGN

SINGLE-SUBJECT DESIGN

Julie Wambaugh

Single-case experimental designs and randomized group designs are used to reveal functional relationships between independent and dependent variables and both are recognized as appropriate methods for demonstrating treatment efficacy. The importance of understanding the relative merits of these designs is critical to the advancement of our field, both scientifically and clinically. The theoretical underpinnings of each design type are quite different, and it has been argued that single-case experimental designs are particularly useful for the study of behavior change.

The assumptions that behavior occurs at the level of the individual and that temporality is a critical aspect of behavior were central to the development of single-case experimental methodologies. Consequently, single-case designs require repeated measurement of the behavior(s) of interest over time in an individual. Single-case designs use continuous measurement to highlight and control intrasubject variability so that the effects of treatment, above and beyond that variability, can be determined.

Because of their focus on individuals and in-depth examination of behavior, single-case designs are ideally suited for developing and testing treatments. Subjects serve as their own controls, which allows the investigator flexibility in evaluating and optimizing treatment effects without sacrificing experimental control. That is, depending upon a subject's response to treatment, the investigator can make modifications in the design (e.g., extending the phase of treatment application) to facilitate or better understand treatment effects. Such flexibility is typically not an option with randomized group designs,

CONTINUES

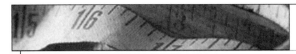

VIGNETTE 3-2

SINGLE-SUBJECT DESIGN   (CONTINUED FROM PAGE 42)

which rely on a limited number of behavioral measurements at predetermined intervals and prohibit differential treatment of subjects within experimental conditions. Continual measurements made throughout the course of a single-subject case design provide a complete depiction of a subject's response curve. Complete response curves are necessary in treatment development so that important information such as a delayed response to treatment or a declination in an initially positive treatment response can be recorded and treatment modified accordingly.

Maximizing treatment is a strength of single-case experimental research that is important with respect to two criticisms frequently leveled at single-case research: a lack of reliance on statistical analysis and possible limited generality. Visual inspection of data graphically displayed over time is the primary means of analysis in single-case designs. Statistical analysis of single-case data is superfluous if the investigator's primary interest is in the subject's achievement of a prespecified level of performance. If the focus is on determining the probability of a treatment outcome, appropriate statistical analyses are available for use with single-case designs. In contrast, inferential statistics are used routinely in randomized group designs to determine if statistically significant differences exist among groups.

Programmatic research involving direct and systematic replications is necessary with single-case designs to demonstrate the degree to which the findings of an investigation may be generalized across subjects, response classes, and settings and to different variables, methods, and processes. Although critics have argued that in-depth analysis of a limited number of individual subjects offers little basis for inferring generality, maximizing treatment effects and controlling variability enhances the probability of generality. Generalization of results from group designs can also be problematic in that it is limited by the adequacy of the random sample(s) obtained and inferences may be made only to populations and not to individuals.

Although single-case designs may be superior for developing and testing treatments, they do not provide actuarial data, as can group designs. However, the application of meta-analysis to single-case data appears to have potential for synthesizing outcomes from single-case experiments.

Single-case designs also offer some logistical advantages over group designs in the study of treatment efficacy. There has been increasing awareness that treatment effects should be measured at various levels of functioning (e.g., impairment, activity, participation) and in terms of quality of life. The repeated measurement opportunities afforded by single-case designs offer ideal conditions for identifying relationships among levels of outcomes. Repeated measurements at various levels would be possible with randomized group designs, but large numbers of subjects typically preclude such measurements.

Despite their divergent approaches to examining relationships among variables, single-case and randomized group designs are not incompatible in the study of communication disorders. The designs can be used in a complementary fashion or in combination. Both offer important contributions to the establishment of empirically supported treatments in communication disorders.

(Reprinted with permission © American Speech-Language-Hearing Association, Wambaugh, J. (1999) Speaking out: Single-subject versus randomized group design. Asha, 41(6), 14-15.)

favoring group designs and one supporting the value of single-subject designs, respectively (Robey, 1999; Wambaugh, 1999).

In addition, advantages and disadvantages of single-subject versus group-design research are summarized in Table 3-2 (adapted from Connell & Thompson, 1986; Kearns, 1986; McReynolds & Thompson, 1986; Robey, 1999; Schiavetti & Metz, 1997; Wambaugh, 1999).

Table 3-2. Advantages and disadvantages of single-subject designs versus group-design research (Adapted from Connell & Thompson, 1986; Kearns, 1986; McReynolds & Thompson, 1986; Robey, 1999; Schiavetti & Metz, 1997; Wambaugh, 1999).

Single-Subject Designs

Advantages	Disadvantages
■ Detection of individual differences	■ Difficulty in controlling for order-and-sequence effects
■ Determination of factors that do/do not contribute to behaviors	■ Generalization to a population generally not possible
■ Employment across varied behaviors, subjects, and settings	■ Statistical procedures assessing reliability of data not well-developed
■ Exploration of intra- and inter-subject variability	
■ Flexibility in design before and during an experiment	
■ Generalization to "real people" rather than an abstraction of an average group member	
■ Identification of "functional relationships" between independent and dependent variables	
■ Utilization by clinician-researchers	

Group Designs

Advantages	Disadvantages
■ Ease in controlling order-and-sequence effects	■ Application to excluded subjects (e.g., those with unusual forms of disorders, co-morbidity of conditions) or across service-delivery sites difficult
■ Execution of protocol no more than once for each subject per condition	■ Generalizations made to a theoretical "average" member of a particular population
■ Generalization from subject sample to representative population	■ Lacks flexibility of design during an experiment
■ Statistical power for making inferences between the effects of independent variables on dependent variable(s)	■ Limitation in the number of behaviors for consideration per experiment
■ Statistical procedures for assessing reliability well-developed	■ Requirement of 10 or more subjects
	■ Requirement of rigid experimental control in "ideal conditions"

Some researchers believe that randomized clinical trials are the "gold standard" for efficacy research. However, large studies may not provide information regarding the effects of treatment for excluded subjects with comorbidity or unusual forms of disorders in non-traditional service-delivery sites (Frattali, 1998a; Holland, Fromm, DeRuyter, & Stein, 1996). For example, currently the largest hearing aid clinical trial involves collaboration between the Department of Veterans Affairs (DVA) and the National Institute of Deafness and other Communication Disorders of the National Institutes of Health (NIDCD-NIH). The DVA, the largest public health-care system in the United States, permits participation of hundreds of suitable subjects meeting specific criteria from eight DVA centers across the country, providing the desired statistical power for a large-scale clinical trial (Beck, 1999; Bratt, 1999). In addition, the internal validity of these clinical trials was very high because precise system-wide experimental procedures were implemented at each center. Unfortunately, optimal circumstances for undertaking clinical trials rarely exist in the "real world," particularly for all types of patients across a wide variety of behaviors and service-delivery sites and behaviors. Moreover, efficacy studies demonstrating benefit, improvement in quality of life, and reduction of health-care costs for unserved and underserved groups of patients are needed prior to reimbursement for hearing aids by most third-party payers. For example, third-party payers may believe that purchasing hearing aids for patients with Alzheimer's disease (AD) is wasteful because they are considered to be difficult or even impossible to test (Palmer, Adams, Bourgeois, Durrant, & Rossi, 1999). Furthermore, large-scale randomized clinical trials would be difficult with this population because of the unique behavioral manifestations of the disorder within individuals and a lack of an organized health-care system to manage these patients.

Thus, benefits provided by single-subject designs (flexibility across patients, behaviors, and service-delivery sites) are needed for efficacy studies of hearing aid treatment in patients with AD. Using a multiple-baseline single-subject design, Palmer, et al., (1999) demonstrated a reduction of caregivers' report of negative behaviors (e.g., negative statements, forgetfulness, pacing) and an increase in patients' likelihood of participating in interactions, conversations, and awareness of environmental sounds in patients after being fit with hearing aids. Therefore, in some cases, single-subject design research may be more appropriate for hearing aid efficacy studies than randomized clinical trials for some patients.

Secondary Methods of Data Analysis: Meta-analysis

Meta-analysis is a means of objectively synthesizing the outcomes of many investigations, with both positive and negative outcomes, in order to weigh the scientific evidence of a particular treatment (Robey & Dalebout, 1998). Secondary methods are needed to validate efficacy research because causality between intervention strategies and positive patient outcomes cannot be substantiated on the results of a single evaluation. For example, Robey and Dalebout (1998) completed a meta-analysis of a few studies investigating the reduction of hearing handicap post-hearing aid fitting as measured by either the *Hearing Handicap for the Elderly* (HHIE; Ventry & Weinstein, 1982) and/or the *Hearing Performance Inventory* (HPI: Giolas, Owens, Lamb, & Schubert, 1979). They found that hearing aid treatment is effective when indexed as a reduction in patient-perceived hearing difficulty (Robey & Dalebout, 1998). Meta-analyses are subject to three sources of error (Robey & Dalebout, 1998):

- failure to exclude primary studies that cannot contribute a valid estimate of effect size,
- failure to include primary studies manifesting valid estimates of effect size, and
- simple procedural errors in archiving and/or calculation.

CLASS II LEVELS OF EVIDENCE

Class II levels of evidence include quasi-experimental (non-random assignment) clinical studies with prospective or retrospective data collection with reliability and generalization of the findings, including: case-control studies, cohort studies (i.e., prospective, retrospective, and double cohorts), prevalence studies, program evaluations, and quality improvement studies (Frattali, 1998a).

Case-Control Studies

Case-control studies are conducted after the outbreak of a pathologic condition (i.e., retrospective) and include identifying groups of subjects with and without a disease, measuring predictor variables, and then assessing the significance of any differences found in predictor variable to suggest potential causes of the disease (Newman, Browner, Cummings, & Hulley, 1988). The steps in designing a case-controlled study are shown in Figure 3-4 and involve (Newman, et al., 1988):

- establishing a sample of cases,
- establishing a control group, and
- measuring the predictor variables.

For example, a case-control design could be used to assess cardiovascular disease as a predictor variable for noise-induced hearing loss by assembling a sample of workers with noise-induced hearing loss, sampling from a population of workers with normal hearing, and then measuring presence of cardiovascular disease in both groups.

The strengths of case-control designs include their short duration and high yield of information from relatively few subjects, and usefulness in generating hypotheses about a large number of variables from a single study (Newman, et al., 1988). For example, other predictor variables such as high cholesterol could have been evaluated in the study. However, case-control designs have sampling and differential measurement bias whose effects can be reduced by techniques listed in Table 3-3.

Cohort Studies

There are three types of cohort studies:

1. prospective,
2. retrospective, and
3. double-cohort studies.

Prospective cohort studies are started before an outbreak of a disease to assess who does and does not develop the pathologic condition (Frattali, 1998a). Two purposes of cohort studies are to:

1. describe the *incidence* of certain outcomes over time (i.e., descriptive), and
2. analyze *associations* between and/or among risk factors and those outcomes (Cummings, Ernster, & Hulley, 1988).

Incidence is the number of new cases of a disease or pathologic condition that develops over a specified period of time per the number of individuals at risk (Newman, et al., 1988). The steps in designing a cohort study are shown in Figure 3-5 and involve (Cummings, et al., 1988):

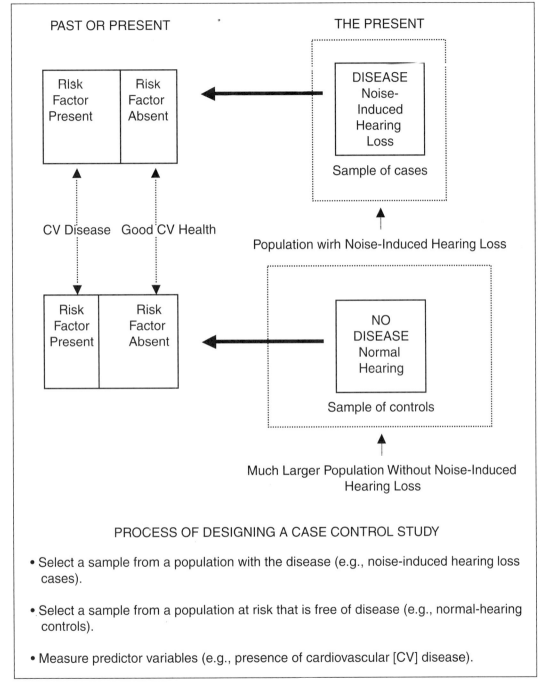

PAST OR PRESENT

THE PRESENT

Risk Factor Present	Risk Factor Absent

DISEASE Noise-Induced Hearing Loss

Sample of cases

CV Disease   Good CV Health

Population wirh Noise-Induced Hearing Loss

Risk Factor Present	Risk Factor Absent

NO DISEASE Normal Hearing

Sample of controls

Much Larger Population Without Noise-Induced Hearing Loss

PROCESS OF DESIGNING A CASE CONTROL STUDY

- Select a sample from a population with the disease (e.g., noise-induced hearing loss cases).

- Select a sample from a population at risk that is free of disease (e.g., normal-hearing controls).

- Measure predictor variables (e.g., presence of cardiovascular [CV] disease).

Figure 3-4. Design of a case-control study (Adapted with permission from T.B. Newman, W.S. Browner, S.R. Cummings, & S.B. Hulley, in *Designing clinical research*, S.B. Hulley & S.R. Cummings (Eds.) © Lippincott, Williams, & Wilkins, 1988).

Table 3-3. Ways of reducing sampling and measurement bias in case-control studies (Adapted from Newman, Browner, Cummings, & Hulley, 1988).

Reduce sampling bias by:
- Sampling the cases and controls in the same way
- Matching cases and controls on major factors related to the disease
- Using two or more control groups
- Using a population-based sample

Reduce measurement bias by:
- Using data before the outcome has occurred
- Using "blinding" techniques for the subject and observer

- assembling a cohort,
- measuring the predictor variable(s),
- following the cohort, and
- measuring the outcome.

For example, a prospective cohort design could be used to determine if a significantly higher proportion of a sample of babies who had at least one high-risk factor at birth, but who passed a newborn hearing screening and acquire a sensorineural hearing loss before age 12 years, than a proportion of a sample of babies who also passed the newborn hearing screening with no high-risk factors. Predictor variables (e.g., high-risk factors) would be measured from two samples (e.g., presence/absence of high-risk factors) drawn from the population of infants born in four metropolitan hospitals during 1999 whose hearing sensitivity would be assessed for the next 12 years.

The advantages of a prospective cohort design are: (Cummings, et al., 1988; Newman, et al., 1988):

- establishment of a sequence of events;
- avoidance of bias in measurement of predictor variables;
- avoidance of survival bias;
- assessment of several outcomes;
- growth in the number of outcome events over time; and

- provision of incidence, relative risk, and excess risk statistics.

On the other hand, cohort studies are very expensive to complete and require very large sample sizes (Cummings, et al., 1988; Newman, et al., 1988). Other types of designs in this area include retrospective and double-cohort studies. *Retrospective cohort studies* involve identification of a sample and measurement of predictor variables *after* the outcome has occurred (Cummings et al, 1988). *Double-cohort studies* involve the identification of *two or more samples* (i.e., one group with exposure to a particular risk factor and another sample of controls who have had no or a lower level of exposure to the risk factor) (Cummings, et al., 1988).

Prevalence Studies

Prevalence studies, also known as *cross-sectional studies*, determine the number of individuals having a pathologic condition at one point in time per the number of people who may be at risk (Newman, et al., 1988). The purpose of a cross-sectional study is to describe variables and their distribution patterns (Newman, et al., 1988). The steps for designing a cross-sectional study are described in Figure 3-6 and involve (Newman, et al., 1988):

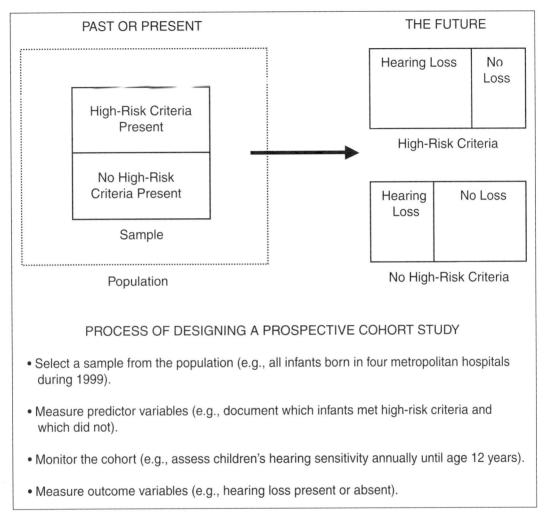

PAST OR PRESENT

THE FUTURE

High-Risk Criteria
Present

No High-Risk
Criteria Present

Sample

Population

Hearing Loss	No Loss

High-Risk Criteria

Hearing Loss	No Loss

No High-Risk Criteria

PROCESS OF DESIGNING A PROSPECTIVE COHORT STUDY

• Select a sample from the population (e.g., all infants born in four metropolitan hospitals during 1999).

• Measure predictor variables (e.g., document which infants met high-risk criteria and which did not).

• Monitor the cohort (e.g., assess children's hearing sensitivity annually until age 12 years).

• Measure outcome variables (e.g., hearing loss present or absent).

Figure 3-5. Design of a prospective cohort study (Adapted from S.R. Cummings, V. Ernster, & S.B. Hulley, in *Designing clinical research*, S.B. Hulley & S.R. Cummings (Eds.) © Lippincott, Williams, & Wilkins, 1988).

■ selecting a sample from the population
■ selecting a sample from the population without the disease, and
■ measuring the predictor and outcome variables.

For example, a cross-sectional study could be used to determine the prevalence of hearing loss in the elderly population and its association to a genetic predisposition to presbycusis. A sample of 200 elderly persons from a metropolitan area could be selected with 100 of those individuals having a member of their immediate family exhibiting presbycusis and 100 individuals with no family history of this condition. Subsequently, the number of individuals both with presbycusis and a family history of the condition could be measured from the sample. From these data, the overall prevalence of presbycusis (e.g.,

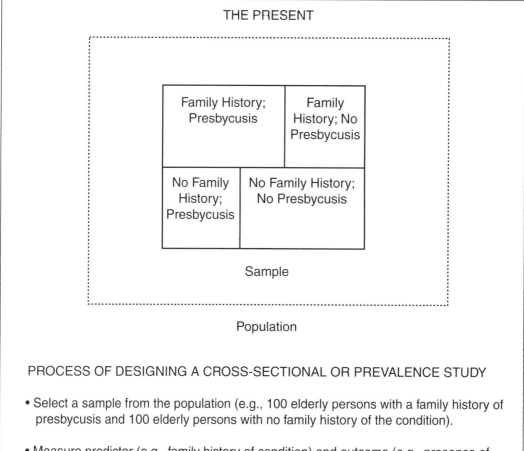

Figure 3-6. Design of a cross-sectional or prevalence study (Adapted with permission from T.B. Newman, W.S. Browner, S.R. Cummings,& S.B. Hulley, in *Designing clinical research*, S.B. Hulley & S.R. Cummings (Eds.) © Lippincott, Williams, & Wilkins, 1988).

the number of affected individuals at the time) can be estimated along with its association to a family history of the condition (e.g., the number of individuals who both have presbycusis and a family history of the condition, compared to the number of individuals who simply have the condition).

Cross-sectional studies have advantages and disadvantages. For example, an advantage of this type of study is that researchers can obtain answers to questions right now without having to wait to see who does and does not develop a disease reducing the overall cost of the investigation (Newman, et al., 1988). However, a major disadvantage of this type of research design is that researchers cannot establish a causal relationship between predictor (e.g., family history of presbycusis) and outcome variables (e.g., developing presbyscusis) (Newman, et al., 1988). Second, because cross-sectional studies can only measure prevalence and not incidence, their results can only provide limited information about the prognosis and natural history of a disease process, like presbycusis, for example (Newman, et al., 1988).

Program Evaluations

Program evaluation methods determine if a program is meeting both its clinical and administrative goals (Frattali, 1998a). Program evaluations can be either an internal requirement of the administration of a facility and/or an external requirement of an outside accrediting agency. Furthermore, program evaluations can be formative or summative. *Formative evaluation* is used when a program is ongoing; can be used to determine necessary changes in program direction or improvements in service; and includes these key steps (Wilkerson, 1998):

- Establish program goals and important outcomes
- Specify objectives to meet goals
- Select pertinent measures of objectives
- Assess program performance on those measures
- Compare performance to desired objectives
- Identify potential changes to meet objectives
- Implement program changes
- Measure performance again to assess attainment of objectives
- Re-enter the cycle

Summative evaluation is used to determine whether a completed program was successful (Wilkerson, 1998).

Formative and summative program evaluations are important for clinical service delivery, research, and training programs and are required both internally by adminis-

trators and externally by accrediting and/or funding agencies. For example, audiology departments within large hospitals may be required by hospital administrators and the Professional Services Board (discontinued nationally recognized accreditation mechanism) to engage in ongoing self-study of fulfilling program objectives, of both providing effective clinical services to current (formative) and discharged (summative) patients. Similarly, federal funding agencies, such as the National Institute of Deafness and other Communication Disorders of the National Institutes of Health (NIDCD-NIH), require principal investigators of multi-year grants to report progress toward objectives both in annual reports (formative) and then in final progress reports (summative). In addition, the Council on Academic Accreditation (CAA) requires accredited programs to assess both current students' ratings of courses (formative) and then graduates and their employers on perceived knowledge and performance in particular areas of clinical service delivery (summative). As more Au.D. programs open, both formative and summative evaluations will play a key role in program development, improvement, and long-term success. These issues are discussed further in Chapter 14.

Quality Improvement Studies

Quality improvement methods determine whether clinical services comply with "gold" standards of care, such as preferred practice patterns, practice guidelines, and critical paths (Frattali, 1998a). Quality improvement involves a three-step process of measuring current levels of performance, establishing means for improvement, and then instituting new and better methods of clinical service delivery (Berwick, Godfrey, & Roessner, 1990; Frattali, 1998b).

Audiologists involved in quality improvement efforts need to ask questions that provide direction and lead from an aim, to current knowledge, to a cycle of learning and improvement (Frattali, 1998b):

- What are we trying to accomplish? (aim or intended outcome)
- How will it be known that any changes made are an improvement? (current knowledge)
- What changes can be made that will result in improvements? (new knowledge)

The cycle is self-perpetuating, known as the Plan-Do-Study-Act (PDSA), and has four stages (Deming, 1982; Frattali, 1998b):

- Plan (A trial is developed.)
- Do (The trial is performed and data are collected.)
- Study (The data are studied and compared to previous data.)
- Act (Changes are made based on the new information.)

For example, the head audiologist at a large, metropolitan, not-for-profit speech and hearing center was concerned about relatively low patient satisfaction ratings of service during the hearing aid adjustment period. Numerous written complaints indicated that patients felt "out-of-touch," even neglected, during their hearing aid trial periods. Several specific complaints centered around being told to attend the center's open clinic hours if they had problems with hearing aids, rather than being able to speak with an audiologist. Moreover, staff audiologists took an average of two days to return patients' phone calls. Similarly, patients complained that they rarely were seen by the same audiologist for post-fitting appointments, resulting in a lack of continuity in care.

Disturbed by these outcomes, the head audiologist met with staff to *plan* what to *do* about improving patient satisfaction in this area. The group decided to address the problems in several ways. First, audiologists would see the same patients throughout the entire diagnostic and rehabilitation process. Second, audiologists would return phone calls on the day on which they were received. Third, patients would be given a variety of ways to interact with their audiologists and other patients. Busy patients might opt to communicate with their audiologists through E-mail or with other patients via the message boards on the speech and hearing center's homepage, for example. Similarly, retired patients might decide to attend a group hearing aid orientation program.

The new measures were employed for a trial period of one year with patient satisfaction data collected quarterly. At the end of the year, a *study* was conducted that found a statistically significant improvement in patient satisfaction ratings with each subsequent quarter. The quality improvement study was so successful that the head audiologist decided to *act* by incorporating the changes on a permanent basis and conducting similar quality improvement studies in other areas of service delivery.

CLASS III LEVELS OF EVIDENCE

Case studies and databases/registries are examples of non-experimental or Class III levels of evidence. Although these methods are subjective and lack experimental control, they can be used by clinicians for large groups of subjects and can provide the impetus for quasi-experimental and experimental studies (Frattali, 1998a).

Case Studies

Case-study research studies specific individuals in detail and compares the results to historical controls or non-randomized clinical trials. In-depth analysis can be of value because they: (McReynolds & Thompson, 1986; Schiavetti & Metz, 1997):

1. Investigate rare clinical occurrences
2. Aid in the development of clinical insights
3. Examine exceptions to accepted rules
4. Describe/identify potential variables for evaluation in experimental studies.

Case studies, however, have some limitations, such as low generalization of results and subjective bias of experimenters (Schiavetti & Metz, 1997).

Case studies involve a single-subject and utilize either the A-only or B-only design. Case studies have a long history in communication sciences and disorders. The A-only design is descriptive in which a behavior (or behaviors) is described as it (they) occur naturally in the environment (McReynolds & Kearns, 1983). Examples of A-only designs are diary or longitudinal studies of subjects for a relatively long period of time, perhaps years (McReynolds & Kearns, 1983; Silverman, 1998). The B-only design is the most common single-subject design employed in communication sciences and disorders (McReynolds & Kearns, 1983). Typically, procedures used in treatment are documented as carefully as possible and patients' progress is reported (McReynolds & Thompson, 1986). Although, the behavior to be treated is not measured before application of the independent variable (i.e., treatment), standardized tests are used to measure related behaviors prior to treatment (McReynolds & Kearns, 1983). For example, Spencer, Tye-Murray, Kelsay, and Teagle (1998) conducted a four-year case study (e.g., B-only design) on a young child who had made good progress with a cochlear implant, despite the presence of family

(e.g., possible unreliable reports of child's progress, limited parental interaction with the child) and school-related concerns (e.g., questionable educational programming and support services) before implantation. The case study does not imply causality between cochlear implantation and the child's success, but rather an exception to traditional expectations of failure for patients not meeting all patient selection criteria for cochlear prostheses.

Databases and Registries

National *databases* or *registries* allow clinicians and researchers to both contribute and compare their data (i.e., benchmarking) on specific clinical practices, programs, or service-delivery sites (Frattali, 1998a). One of the most successful databases and registries is the NOMS, managed by the National Center for Treatment Effectiveness in Communication Disorders (NCTECD) that coordinates all outcomes and efficacy work of ASHA. Until late 1999, NOMS primarily involved outcomes measurement in speech-language pathology. The first audiology component of NOMS involves Universal Newborn Hearing Screening (UNHS) to determine outcomes associated with audiologist-managed programs. The development of the UNHS component of NOMS included a national call for participants from the nation's UNHS programs. Candidate programs were required to submit proposals as part of the application process. Over 20 centers were selected to participate in the UNHS component of NOMS. Staff from participant programs had to undergo extensive training on how to use a customized screening information and management software designed for the project by the OZ Corporation. As more states come "on board" through mandating UNHS programs, data from the NOMS will assist others in both the development and management of start-up programs.

NON-CLASSIFIED STATUS

Non-classified status includes expert clinical opinion, standards of practice, and consensus and research studies that do not meet Class III criteria.

Expert Clinical Opinion, Standards of Clinical Practice, and Consensus

Expert clinical opinion involves the expertise of recognized leaders in the field who have established themselves through clinical work and/or scholarly activity. Both ASHA and AAA rely on expert clinical opinion in a variety of ways, including, but not limited to, the refereeing of articles submitted for publication in professional journals and presentations submitted to scientific meetings; and establishing preferred practice patterns (ASHA, 1997), consensus statements, and standards of practice.

Standards of clinical practice, for example, preferred practice patterns for audiology and speech-language pathology, are statements that define universally applicable characteristics of specific clinical activities, including definitions, which professionals perform the procedures, expected outcomes, clinical indications, clinical processes, setting and equipment specifications, and documentation (ASHA, 1997). Preferred practice patterns are not official standards, but they serve as guidelines for enhancing the quality of professional services to consumers (Grantham, 1997). Preferred practice patterns have been developed for audiology on the following topics: speech-language-hearing screenings, follow-up procedures, consultation, prevention, occupational and environmental hearing conservation, audiologic assessment (basic, pediatric, and advanced), external ear procedures (examination and cerumen management), electrodiagnostic test procedures, auditory evoked response evaluation, neurophysiologic intra-operative monitoring, audiologic (aural) rehabilitation (assessment and management), assessment/treatment of central auditory processing disorders (adults and children), counseling, balance system assessment, hearing aid fitting, product dispensing, product repair/modification, assistive listening system/device selection, and sensory device selection (ASHA, 1997).

Consensus means reaching agreement regarding important issues facing the professions. For example, the issue of the use of support personnel in audiology and speech-language pathology has been a controversial issue for at least the past 30 years. Thus, a consensus panel was formed and composed of audiologists who provided expert clinical opinion and represented various professional organizations, such as the Academy of Dispensing Audiologists, American Academy of Audiology, American Speech-Language-Hearing Association, Educational Audiology Association, Military Audiology Association, and the National Hearing Conservation Association (AAA, 1997). The charge of this panel was to reach an agreement regarding the use of support personnel in the profession of audiology. Toward this aim, the panel wrote the, "Position Statement and Guidelines of the Consensus Panel on Support Personnel in Audiology" (AAA, 1997). The position statement affirmed that the consensus panel agreed that support personnel might assist audiologists in the delivery of services. Moreover, the guidelines specifically provide definitions (support personnel and supervising audiologist), qualifications for support personnel, their training, role, and supervision. Position statements and practice guidelines are subjected to peer review by members of professional organizations and must be adopted by those memberships through elected representatives on ASHA's Legislative Council, for example.

Studies That Do Not Meet Class III Criteria

Studies that do not meet criteria for Class III levels of evidence are not necessarily inferior, but are used when other research methods are not possible. For example, our profession requires that audiologists understand the impact of hearing loss on patients from diverse cultural backgrounds and their families. To do so, researchers must employ strategies, such as ethnographic methods that are appropriate for acknowledging multi-directional perspectives (Hyter, 2000). Ethnographers conduct literature searches to understand the topography of the diverse cultural environments before observing and interviewing these individuals to gain access to their perspectives on the impact hearing loss has on their world (Hyter, 2000). Through ethnographic research methods, audiologists are able to focus on the strengths of their diverse caseloads with hearing loss and their families and jointly identify culturally relevant intervention strategies (Hyter, 2000).

SUMMARY

This chapter has reviewed the levels of evidence that provide a hierarchy of stringency of scientific rigor for the profession. Readers should use this hierarchy when judging the merit of information regarding audiologic service delivery from a seemingly endless variety of sources. However, readers should realize three important points. First, lower levels of evidence are not necessarily inferior to higher levels of evidence; they are necessary and can serve an important role in establishing the best service delivery to patients with hearing impairment. For example, case studies (i.e., Class III levels of evidence) of novel treatment approaches to communication disorders can provide impetus for a randomized, controlled clinical trial

---

LEARNING ACTIVITIES

■ Obtain the latest issues of the *American Journal of Audiology: A Journal of Clinical Practice*; *Hearing Journal*; the *Journal of Speech, Language, and Hearing Research*; and the *Journal of the American Academy of Audiology*; classify each article according to its level of evidence; and analyze the results. Based on your survey, rank-order the journals from the most stringent to the least stringent. What are your conclusions?

■ Debate the use of group designs versus single-subject designs as Class I levels of evidence. Use the viewpoints of Robey (1999) and Wambaugh (1999) as a starting point. Specify different scenarios and/or areas of practice where either one or both types of design would be appropriate.

■ Use the evaluation checklists for group and single-subject design research appearing in Appendix III-B and III-C, respectively, to critique relevant articles in a recent issue of a scientific professional journal.

at the Class I levels of evidence. Second, lower levels of evidence are influenced by information from higher levels of evidence. Preferred practice patterns and standards of practice at the lowest level of evidence must be revised according to new research findings revealed through Class I and II levels of evidence, for example. Third, audiologists must be flexible in their use of the levels of evidence hierarchy for the good of the profession and their patients. On one hand, the hierarchy provides strict guidelines for establishing causality between intervention strategies and positive patient outcomes. On the other hand, the profession needs to be flexible in encouraging investigators to develop creative experimental designs through collaboration with leading hearing aid manufacturers so that the effectiveness of the latest technology can be determined prior to dissemination to consumers.

RECOMMENDED READINGS

Connell, P.J., & Thompson, C.K. (1986). Flexibility of single-subject experimental designs. Part III: Using flexibility to design or modify experiments. *Journal of Speech and Hearing Disorders, 51,* 214–225.

Kearns, K.P. (1986). Flexibility of single-subject experimental designs. Part II: Design selection and arrangement of experimental phases. *Journal of Speech and Hearing Disorders, 51,* 204–214.

McReynolds, L.V., & Kearns, K.P. (1983). *Single-subject experimental designs in communicative disorders.* Baltimore, MD: University Park Press.

McReynolds, L.V., & Thompson, C.K. (1986). Flexibility of single-subject experimental designs. Part I: Review of the basics of single-subject designs. *Journal of Speech and Hearing Disorders, 51,* 194–203.

Schiavetti, N., & Metz, D.E. (2001). *Evaluating research in communicative disorders* (3rd ed.). Needham Heights, MA: Allyn & Bacon.

Silverman, F.H. (1998). *Research design and evaluation in speech-language pathology and audiology* (4th ed.). Needham Heights, MA: Allyn & Bacon.

REVIEW EXERCISES

Fill-in-the-Blank

Instructions: Please fill-in-the-blank with the correct term from the word bank below.

1. _____ levels of evidence involve research in which there is random assignment to intervention and control groups or phases.

2. _____ measurement methods are those in which the investigator both collects and analyzes the data.

3. _____ measurement methods of data analysis involve using already available information in order to gain new insights.

4. _____ _____ ensures that subjects' characteristics of age, sex, and so on are distributed equally (except for chance variance) and cannot confound or bias the statistical significance of differences found between or among the groups.

5. _____ bias is a consistent distortion expressed, either consciously or subconsciously, by the individual administering the experimental protocol that can affect measurement of the dependent variable.

6. _____ bias is a consistent distortion expressed, either consciously or subconsciously, by the individual receiving the experimental protocol that can affect measurement of the dependent variable.

7. "_____ - _____" means that neither the person collecting data

nor the subject knows the status (i.e., treatment or placebo) of the administered condition

8. _____ - _____ research involves obtaining repeated measurements of a single or small group of subjects over time.

9. In _____ - _____ designs, each subject serves as his/her own control.

10. _____ - _____ is a means of objectively synthesizing the outcomes of many investigations, both positive and negative, in order to weigh the scientific evidence of a particular treatment.

11. _____ - _____ studies are conducted after an outbreak of a pathologic condition (i.e., retrospective) and include identifying groups of subjects with and without a disease, and then assessing the significance of differences found in predictor variables to suggest possible causes of the disease.

12. _____ _____ studies are started before an outbreak of a disease to assess who does and does not develop the pathologic condition.

13. _____ is the number of new cases of a disease or pathologic condition that develops over a specified period of time per the number of individuals at risk.

14. _____ _____ studies involve identification of a sample and measurement of predictor variables after the outcome has occurred.

15. _____ _____ studies involve the identification of two or more samples (i.e., one group with exposure to a particular risk factor and another sample of controls who have had no or a lower level of exposure to the risk factor).

16. _____-_____ studies determine the number of individuals having a pathologic condition at one point in time per the number of people who may be at risk.

17. _____ _____ methods determine if a program is meeting both its clinical and administrative goals.

18. _____ _____ methods determine whether clinical services comply with "gold" standards of care, such as preferred practice patterns, practice guidelines, and critical paths.

19. _____ - _____ research studies specific individuals in detail and compares the results to historical controls or non-randomized clinical trials.

20. National _____ / _____ allow clinicians and researchers to both contribute and compare their data (i.e., benchmarking) on specific clinical practices, programs, or service-delivery sites.

21. _____ _____ _____ involves the expertise of recognized leaders in the field who have established themselves through clinical work and/or scholarly activity.

22. _____ means reaching agreement regarding important issues facing the professions.

Word Bank:

Case-control	Observer
Case-study	Primary
Class I	Program evaluation
Consensus	Prospective cohort
Cross-sectional	Quality improvement
Databases/registries	Random assignment
Double cohort	Retrospective cohort
Double-blinding	Secondary
Expert clinical opinion	Single-subject
Incidence	Subject
Meta-analysis	Time-series

Matching

Instructions: Please match the following items with the correct statements below.

I. True
II. False

1. ____ The A-B is the minimum acceptable single-subject design that qualifies for Class I levels of evidence.
2. ____ Results from Class III levels of evidence research (e.g., case studies) can serve as impetus for formulation of hypotheses to be tested by clinical trials.
3. ____ Cross-sectional studies are also known as incidence studies.
4. ____ Ethnographic research methods are of no real value to the profession.
5. ____ The profession needs to be flexible in encouraging investigators to develop creative experimental designs through collaboration with leading hearing aid manufacturers so that the effectiveness of the latest technology can be determined prior to dissemination to consumers.

ANSWERS

Fill-in-the-Blank:
1. Class I	12. Prospective cohort
2. Primary	13. Incidence
3. Secondary	14. Retrospective cohort
4. Random assignment	15. Double cohort
5. Observer	16. Cross-sectional
6. Subject	17. Program evaluation
7. "Double-blinding"	18. Quality improvement
8. Time-series	19. Case-study
9. Single-subject	20. Databases/registries
10. Meta-analysis	21. Expert clinical opinion
11. Case-control	22. Consensus

Matching:
1. II
2. I
3. II
4. II
5. I

REFERENCES

American Academy of Audiology (1997). Position statement and guidelines of the consensus panel on support personnel in audiology. *Audiology Today, 9*(3), 27–28.

American Speech-Language-Hearing Association (1997). *Preferred practice patterns for the profession of audiology.* Rockville, MD: Author.

Beck, L. (1999). The NIDCD/VA hearing aid clinical trial and evidence-based decision-making and the VA. Paper presented at the Annual Convention of the American Speech-Language-Hearing Association, San Francisco, CA.

Berwick, D.M., Godfrey, A.B., & Roessner, J. (1990). *Curing health care.* San Francisco, CA: Jossey-Bass Publishers.

Bratt, G.W. (1999). Electroacoustic assessment of hearing aid performance in NIDCD/VA hearing aid clinical trial. Paper presented at the Annual Convention of the American Speech-Language-Hearing Association, San Francisco, CA.

Connell, P.J., & Thompson, C.K. (1986). Flexibility of single-subject experimental designs. Part III: Using flexibility to design or modify or experiments. *Journal of Speech and Hearing Disorders, 51,* 214–225.

Cummings, S.R., Ernster, V., & Hulley, S.B. (1988). Designing a new study: I. Cohort studies. In S.B. Hulley and S.R. Cummings (Eds.) *Designing clinical research* (pp. 63–74). Baltimore, MD: Williams & Wilkins.

Deming, W.E. (1982). *Out of the crisis.* Cambridge, MA: Massachusetts Institute of Technology, Center for Advanced Engineering Study.

Frattali, C.M. (1998a). Outcomes measurement: Definitions, dimensions, and perspectives. In C.M. Frattali (Ed.), *Measuring outcomes in speech-language pathology* (pp. 1–27). New York, NY: Thieme.

Frattali, C.M. (1998b). Quality improvement. In C.M. Frattali (Ed.), *Measuring outcomes* in speech-language pathology (pp. 172–185). New York, NY: Thieme.

Giolas, T.J., Owens, E., Lamb, S.H., & Schubert, E.D. (1979). Hearing Performance Inventory. Journal of Speech and Hearing Disorders, 44, 169–195.

Grantham, R.B. (1997). ASHA and the schools. In P.F. O'Connell (Ed.), Speech, language, and hearing programs in the schools: A guide for students and practitioners (pp. 24–65). Gaithersburg, MD: Aspen Publishers, Inc.

Holland, A.L., Fromm, D.S., DeRuyter, F., & Stein, M. (1996). Efficacy of treatment for aphasia: A brief synopsis. Journal of Speech, Language, and Hearing Research, 39, S27–S36.

Hulley, S.B., & Cummings, S.R. (1988). Planning the measurements: Precision and accuracy. In S.B. Hulley and S.R. Cummings (Eds.), Designing clinical research (pp. 31–41). Baltimore, MD: Williams & Wilkins.

Hulley, S.B., Feigal, D., Martin, M., & Cummings, S.R. (1988). Designing a new study: IV. Experiments. In S.B. Hulley and S.R. Cummings (Eds.), Designing clinical research (pp. 110–127). Baltimore, MD: Williams & Wilkins.

Hyter, Y.D. (2000). Seeing purple: Using ethnographic research methods as the standard rather than the exception in clinical service delivery. ASHA Leader, 5(3), 10.

Kearns, K.P. (1986). Flexibility of single-subject experimental designs. Part II: Design selection and arrangement of experimental phases. Journal of Speech and Hearing Disorders, 51, 204–214.

Larson, V.D., Williams, D.W., Henderson, W.G., Luethke, L.E., Beck, L.B., Noffsinger, D., Wilson, R.H., Dobie, R.A., Haskell, G.B., Bratt, G.W., Shanks, J.E., Stelmachowicz, P., Studebaker, G.A., Boysen, A.E., Donahue, A., Canalis, R., Fausti, S.A., & Rappaport, B.Z. (2000). Efficacy of 3 commonly used hearing aid circuits: A crossover trial. Journal of the American Medical Association, 284, 1806–1813.

Logemann, J. A. (2000). President's column: What is evidenced based practice and why should we care? ASHA Leader, 5(5), 3.

Maxwell, D.L., & Satake, E. (1997). Research and statistical methods in communication disorders. Baltimore, MD: Williams & Wilkins.

McReynolds, L.V., & Kearns, K.P. (1983). Single-subject experimental designs in communicative disorders. Baltimore, MD: University Park Press.

McReynolds, L.V., & Thompson, C.K. (1986). Flexibility of single-subject experimental designs. Part I: Review of the basics of single-subject designs. Journal of Speech and Hearing Disorders, 51, 194–203.

Newman, T.B., Browner, W.S., Cummings, S.R., & Hulley, S.B. (1988). Designing a new study: II. Cross-sectional and case-control studies. In S.B. Hulley and S.R. Cummings (Eds.), Designing clinical research (pp. 75–86). Baltimore, MD: Williams & Wilkins.

Palmer, C.V., Adams, S. W., Bourgeois, M., Durrant, J.D., & Rossi, M. (1999). Reduction in caregiver-identified problem behaviors in patients with Alzheimer's disease after hearing aid fitting. Journal of Speech, Language, and Hearing Research, 42, 312–328.

Robey, R.R. (1999) Speaking out: Single-subject versus randomized group design. ASHA, 41(6), 14–15.

Robey, R.R., & Dalebout, S.D. (1998). A tutorial on conducting meta-analysis of clinical outcome research. Journal of Speech-Language-Hearing Research, 41(6), 1227–1241.

Schiavetti, N., & Metz, D.E. (1997). Evaluating research in communicative disorders (3rd ed.). Needham Heights, MA: Allyn & Bacon.

Silverman, F.H. (1998). Research design and evaluation in speech-language pathology *and audiology* (4th ed.). Needham Heights, MA: Allyn & Bacon.

Spencer, L.J., Tye-Murray, N., Kelsay, D.M.R., Teagle, H. (1998). Learning to use the cochlear implant: A child who beat the odds. *American Journal of Audiology: A Journal of Clinical Practice. 7,* 24–29.

Ventry, I.M., & Weinstein, B.E. (1982). The hearing handicap inventory for the elderly: A new tool. *Ear and Hearing, 3,* 128–133.

Wambaugh, J. (1999). Speaking out: Single-subject versus randomized group design. *ASHA, 41*(6), 14–15.

Wilkerson, D.L. (1998). Program evaluation. In C.M. Frattali (Ed.) *Measuring outcomes in speech-language pathology* (pp. 151–171). New York, NY: Thieme.

APPENDIX III-A

Evaluation Strategies, Research Questions, Design Options, and Considerations for Single-Subject Experimental Designs

Evaluation Strategy	Clinical Research Question	Selected Design Options	Basic Considerations
Treatment-No Treatment Comparison	Does treatment, with all of its components, result in improved performance relative to no treatment?	Withdrawal and reversal designs: • ABAB • BAB • ABA	Is the therapeutic effect likely to reverse following the withdrawal treatment?
		Multiple Baseline Designs (MB) • across behaviors • across settings • across subjects	Are functionally independent behaviors or settings available? Are homogeneous subjects available?
		Multiple Probe Technique (Variation of MB)	Are functionally independent behaviors available? Are long or continuous baselines impractical?
Component Assessment	Relative to a treatment package, to what degree do separate components of treatment contribute to improvement?	Interaction (Reduction) • BC-B-BC-B • BC-B-BC-A-BC-B-BC	Can the components be examined alone and in combination with the treatment package? Can replication be obtained across subjects?
	Does the addition of a component to a treatment package facilitate treatment effectiveness?	Interaction (Additive) • B-BC-B-BC • B-BC-B-A-B-BC-B	Can the components be examined alone and in combination with the treatment package? Can replication be obtained across subjects?
Treatment-Treatment Comparison	What is the relative effectiveness of two or more treatments?	Alternating Treatments Design	Can treatments be rapidly alternated for each subject?
		Replicated Crossover Design	Are multiple subjects or target behaviors available? Can treatment be "crossed over"? Are nearly equal phase lengths possible?

(CONTINUES)

(CONTINUED FROM PAGE 62)

Evaluation Strategy	Clinical Research Question	Selected Design Options	Basic Considerations
Successive Level Analysis	Does treatment result in acquisition of successive steps in a chaining sequence?	Multiple Probe Technique	Are steps in the treatment sequence independent? Are earlier steps prerequisite to acquiring later steps?
	Does treatment effectively modify a single, gradually acquired behavior?	Changing Criterion Design	Will changes in the dependent variable correspond to changes in the criterion level? Will the dependent variable stabilize at successively more stringent criterion levels?

Kearns (1986)

(Reprinted with permission © American Speech-Language-Hearing Association, Kearns, K.P. [1986]. Flexibility of single-subject experimental designs. Part II: Design selection and arrangement of experimental phases. *Journal of Speech and Hearing Disorders, 51,* 204-214).

APPENDIX III-B

Checklist for Evaluating Scientific Articles

(Schiavetti, N., & Metz, D.E. [1997]. *Evaluating research in communicative disorders,* 3rd edition. Needham Heights, MA: Allyn & Bacon. Adapted with permission © Allyn & Bacon, 1997)

The above-referenced Appendix can be found on the companion CD-ROM.

APPENDIX III-C

Checklist for Evaluating or Designing Single-Subject Studies

(Adapted from McReynolds & Thompson, 1986)

The above-referenced Appendix can be found on the companion CD-ROM.

CHAPTER 4
Methods of Measurement

LEARNING OBJECTIVES

This chapter will enable readers to:

- Define the four levels of measurement
- Identify the characteristics, examples, appropriate statistics, and information content/power of the four levels of measurement
- Understand the process of selecting a level of measurement
- Discuss the concepts of reliability and validity in measurements (i.e., definition, assessment, threats, and enhancement)
- Critique and develop questionnaires/interview instruments using consumer satisfaction as an example

INTRODUCTION

The title of this chapter suggests that statistics are involved. We would like to remind readers that some minimal understanding of levels of measurement is necessary for meaningful utilization of outcome data. Our purpose here is not to overwhelm, but to provide a brief, basic synopsis of and implications for using various levels of measurement in outcomes measurement.

The type, quantity, and quality of data for assessing outcomes for audiology are dependent on the tools used for data collection (Kreb & Wolf, 1997). For example, across the country, many audiologists administer the *Hearing Handicap Inventory for the Elderly—Screening Version* (HHIE—S: Newman, Jacobson, Hug, Weinstein, & Malinoff, 1991) to their patients as pre- and post-treatment measures of hearing handicap. However, do rank-and-file clinicians stop to question whether these tools are the best available? Have they been devised and tested psychometrically? Are there any other tools or instruments that measure hearing handicap more precisely and accurately? Does the method of administering the instrument affect the precision and accuracy of the results, and if so, how can the process be improved? What levels of measurement do the items on the HHIE—S represent? What types of statistical procedures can be done with the data?

Busy with the day-to-day challenges and trials of service-delivery in today's world, many audiologists may simply administer the HHIE—S because someone at an instructional course at an American Academy of Audiology meeting said something about the importance of outcome measurements. The old adage, "anything worth doing, is worth doing well" is as true for making a good ear impression as it is for outcomes measurement, which requires the ability to both ask and answer the questions posed at the beginning of this chapter. Indeed, for many clinicians, 10, 20, or even 30 years may have passed since their course in research methods in graduate school. Somewhere in the back of their minds is that lecture about levels of measurement, reliability and validity of measurement, statistical analyses, psychometrics, and so on. The purpose of this chapter is to review the levels of measurement, reliability/validity of measurements, and critical analysis of questionnaire/interview instruments.

LEVELS OF MEASUREMENT

Measurement is describing phenomena using methods in which the results can be analyzed statistically (Hulley & Cummings, 1988). Table 4-1 shows the various levels of measurement, their characteristics, examples, use of appropriate statistics, information content, and power (adapted from Hulley & Cummings, 1988; Schiavetti & Metz, 1997; Silverman, 1998).

There are two categories of measurement scales: *categorical variables* and *continuous variables*. Categorical variables classify phenomena into categories and consist of two types: nominal and ordinal (Hulley &

Cummings, 1988). *Nominal* measurement, as the name implies, involves classifying phenomena into mutually exclusive, unordered categories (Hulley & Cummings, 1988; Schiavetti & Metz, 1997; Silverman, 1998). For example, patients can be classified into mutually exclusive categories, such as male or female, or newborns can pass or fail a hearing screening. Nominal classification schemes with only two options are known as *dichotomous variables*. The types of statistical analyses that can be conducted on nominal data are counts, rates, proportions, relative risk, chi-square, Mantel-Haentzel, regression, and so on (Hulley & Cummings, 1988). Although nominal variables are straightforward and easy to measure, the statistical analyses that can be used are limited and the information content and power are low (Hulley & Cummings, 1988).

Ordinal measurements include classifying phenomena into mutually exclusive categories that are rank ordered, with intervals that are not quantifiable (Hulley & Cummings, 1988; Schiavetti & Metz, 1997; Silverman, 1998). For example, patients can be classified by degrees of hearing loss (e.g., minimal, slight, moderate, etc.), attitude types, and so on. The types of statistical analyses that can be conducted on ordinal data include those appropriate for nominal data plus medians, and rank correlations (e.g., Spearman) (Hulley & Cummings, 1988). Although providing more information power and content than nominal variables (i.e., intermediate versus low), ordinal variables require more human judgments, thus increasing the likelihood of observer bias (Hulley & Cummings, 1988). For example, Goldstein and Stephens (1981) devised four attitudinal types toward aural rehabilitation and hearing aids that assign patients to one of four categories that range from strongly positive (i.e., Type I) to strongly negative (i.e., Type IV). Although the continuum provides a way to rank order patients on the basis of attitude, audiologists must use their own judgment in assigning patients to categories, which subjects the classification scheme to observer bias.

Continuous variables have quantified intervals on an infinite arithmetic scale and include interval and ratio data. The *interval* level of measurement includes designated points on a continuum with identifiable, equal, and quantifiable intervals with no absolute zero point. For example, interval data include standard scores on subtests of the *SCAN-C: Test for Auditory Processing Disorders in Children—Revised* (Keith, 2000b) or

Table 4-1. Scales, defining characteristics, examples, appropriate statistics, advantages, and disadvantages for various levels of measurement (Adapted from Hulley & Cummings, 1988; Schiavetti & Metz, 1997; Silverman, 1998).

CATEGORICAL VARIABLES				
Type of Measurement	**Characteristics**	**Examples**	**Appropriate Statistics**	**Advantages and Disadvantages**
NOMINAL	Unordered, mutually exclusive categories Absolute/qualitative character of variables	Pass/Fail, Sex (male vs. female)	Counts, rates, proportions, relative risk, chi-square, Mantel-Haentzel, regression	Advantages • Straightforward to measure • Observer bias low Disadvantages • Limited statistical applications • Low information content and power
ORDINAL	Ranked or ordered, mutually exclusive categories or groupings with intervals that cannot be quantified	Attitude types, degrees of hearing loss, Ratings of loudness	Counts, rates, proportions, relative risk, chi-square, Mantel-Haentzel, regression, median Spearman's rho	Advantages • Contain more information than nominal variables • Intermediate information content and power Disadvantages • Limited statistical applications • Requires judgment of audiologist/patient • Subject to bias

(CONTINUES)

Table 4-1. (continued from page 65)

CONTINUOUS VARIABLES				
Type of Measurement	Characteristics	Examples	Appropriate Statistics	Advantages and Disadvantages
INTERVAL	Intervals along a scale that are equal, identifiable, and quantifiable No absolute zero point	Ratings on the scales used on the standard scores on the SCAN, SCAN-A, or SCAN-C tests	In addition to the statistics mentioned above, mean, standard deviation, t-test, analysis of variance, more powerful regression	Advantages • Variety of applicable statistical procedures • High information content and power Disadvantages • Reliability and validity of measurements subjected to bias • Cannot determine equivalence of ratios among scale values
RATIO	Intervals along a scale that are equal, identifiable, and quantifiable Specification of ratios between intervals Absolute zero point	Ear canal volume Electrophysiologic measurements Real ear insertion gain	In addition to the statistics mentioned above, mean, standard deviation, t-test, analysis of variance, more powerful regression	Advantages • Variety of applicable statistical procedures • High information content and power • Can establish equivalence of ratio among scale values Disadvantages • Reliability and validity of measurements subjected to bias

ratings on the seven, equal-appearing interval scales of the *Satisfaction with Amplification in Daily Life* (SADL: Cox & Alexander, 1999). A zero on the composite score on the SCAN-C does not mean an absence of central auditory processing abilities any more than

0 decibels sound pressure level (dB SPL) means the absence of sound, for example. Moreover, although the intervals between 1 and 2 on the SADL scales are the same as between 4 and 5, it is not possible to establish the equality of ratios between these

intervals. In addition to the types of statistical procedures that can be used with categorical data, interval data can also be subjected to obtaining means/standard deviations and to conducting t-tests, analysis of variance, more powerful regression, and so on (Hulley & Cummings, 1988). The interval level of measurement has a high degree of information content and power.

The *ratio* level of measurement, like interval data, involves the identity, magnitude, and equality of intervals; the specification of ratios between numbers; and an absolute zero point (Schiavetti & Metz, 1997), and includes most physical measurements in audiology, such as ear canal volume, real-ear insertion gain, electrophysiologic measures (e.g., wave V latencies), and so on. Behavioral measures can also be at the ratio level of measurement, such as word recognition scores (Schiavetti & Metz, 1997). The statistical analyses that can be applied to ratio data are the same as those for interval data.

RELIABILITY AND VALIDITY OF MEASUREMENTS

As discussed in Chapters 2 and 3, *reliability* is the consistency or precision of measurement, while *validity* is the truth or accuracy in measurement. In order for a measurement to be valid or accurate, it must also be reliable and precise. A measurement can be reliable, but not valid. However, for a measure to be valid, it must also be reliable. For example, in order to be valid, a newly developed measure of hearing aid benefit must *consistently* and *truthfully* measure patients' outcomes with amplification to be valid. For example, an instrument can consistently (i.e., reliably) make highly repeatable, yet completely erroneous measures of what it claims to measure.

Threats to Reliability

Reliability can be affected by random error; the greater the random error, the less precise is the measurement (Hulley & Cummings, 1988). Three sources of error in measurement involve observer, subject, and instrument variability (Hulley & Cummings, 1988). *Observer variability* is the variability introduced when either a single individual (i.e., intra-observer) administers an instrument differently from one patient to the next or when an instrument is administered differently by a group of observers (i.e., inter-observer). An audiologist may introduce intra-observer variability while using different words, when interviewing different patients, for example. Similarly, audiologists participating in a clinical trial across VA medical centers may introduce inter-observer variability by altering the manner of data collection stipulated by the standard protocol. The second source of random error is *subject* or *patient variability* that refers not only to the inherent differences within the subject/patient (i.e., intra-subject), but also across patients/subjects (i.e., inter-subject). Some elderly patients may not be as alert in responding to pure-tone stimuli in the morning, as they would be if the audiologic evaluation was scheduled in the afternoon, thus introducing a source of intra-subject variability, for example. Similarly, elderly patients, as a group, vary in their ability to complete certain tasks that can create a source of inter-subject variability. The third source of random error is *instrument variability* that refers to the inconsistency in measurement caused by variations in environmental conditions, such as background noise (Hulley & Cummings, 1988). For example, hearing aid wearers may provide more negative ratings of hearing aid benefit when completing a hearing aid satisfaction questionnaire in a noisy environment rather than in a quiet room.

Assessment of Reliability

Reliability can be assessed in at least three different ways. The first method of assessing the reliability of measurement is inter- and intra-observer reliability. *Inter-observer reliability* is the degree to which two independent observers are consistent in their measurements of the same phenomenon. For example, if two audiologists agree that the same behavior of an infant is a truly attentive response to a noisemaker, then inter-observer reliability is high. *Intra-observer* is the degree to which the same observer is consistent in obtaining the same measurements of the same phenomena. If an audiologist measures an infant's behavior in real time the same as when re-measuring the session on videotape, then the intra-observer reliability is high. Inter-observer and intra-observer reliability are calculated as the agreement between two independent observers or between two different ratings of the same event by the same observer, respectively. Figure 4-1 shows the steps in calculating the degree of inter-observer reliability.

The first step in assessing inter-observer reliability is to align the behavioral events measured by two independent observers. For example, two public school nurses may have conducted pure-tone hearing screenings of the same children during the same day. The second step is to tally the number of agreements and disagreements between the two observers. In this example, the nurses obtained the same results for eight children and disagreed for two. The third step is to input the data into the equation [(Agreements)/(Agreements + Disagreements)] x 100 to obtain the percent of inter-observer reliability. In this example, the nurses had an 80% inter-observer reliability. The same process for inter-observer reliability could be completed for intra-observer reliability using the formula in our example, if the same nurse screened the same children twice during the

same day. Generally, 90% or higher agreement is acceptable for intra- or inter-observer reliability.

Although it is not always necessary to obtain intra- and inter-observer reliability for all measurements, calculation of agreement for *at least* 5% of randomly selected data collection events should be satisfactory in most cases. Assessment of intra- and inter-observer reliability must be directly related to the type of research question being asked; in some cases, it might be required for all data, and may warrant the use of special equipment. For example, Johnson (2000) investigated the phoneme identification abilities of 80 children ages 6 years through young adults in four separate conditions: a control (no noise, no reverberation), reverberation-only, noise-only, and reverberation-plus-noise. The study aimed to: (1) identify the sensation level (SL: re. speech recognition threshold) at which even the youngest listeners achieved their maximum performance, and (2) assess phoneme (i.e., consonant and vowel) and consonant feature (i.e., voicing, manner, and place of articulation) identification at the specified SL. The speech stimuli were consonant-vowel-consonant-vowel nonsense syllables from List A of the *Edgerton-Danhauer Nonsense Syllable Test* (NST) (Edgerton & Danhauer, 1979) that requires observers to transcribe listeners' responses phonetically. Although the NST has been found to be easy to score, many young children and teenagers have a tendency to mumble their responses, especially when they are not sure as to what they heard. Only reliably transcribed responses were used in this study. Therefore, inter- and intra-observer agreement were each determined for all listeners' responses, and those data not achieving an acceptable level of reliability were omitted from the study. In addition, because percent correct identification of consonant features was a dependent variable in the study, scoring for reliability dictated that

STEP 1: Align behavioral events measured by two independent observers.

Event	1	2	3	4	5	6	7	8	9	10
Observer 1	+	+	+	+	+	+	+	+	+	+
Observer 2	+	−	+	+	+	+	−	+	+	+

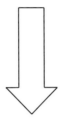

STEP 2: Tally agreements and disagreements.

Agreements   =   8

Disgreements   =   2

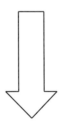

STEP 3: Input data into the equation.

Percent of Inter-observer Reliability = [(Agreements) / (Agreements + Disagreements)] x 100

= [(8) / (8 + 2)] x 100

= (8/10) x 100

= 80%

Figure 4-1. Calculation of inter-observer reliability

intra- and inter-observer agreements be calculated for the *exact* phonetic transcriptions of *all* listeners' responses, thus necessitating that all listeners' responses be videotaped for simultaneous viewing in the test room by the experimenters, and recording for reliability re-scoring at a later date. Thus, special videotape equipment and criteria were needed for determining intra- and inter-observer reliability in this study.

The second way to assess reliability of measurements is *test-retest reliability* or the *stability* of measurement. Test-retest reliability is the degree to which a procedure administered to a sample of individuals yields the same results when administered again to that sample. The individuals' scores from the first administration are correlated with each other from the second session using the coefficient of stability, and should be obtained for widely used measurement tools (Schiavetti & Metz, 1997). For example, Newman and Weinstein (1989) assessed the test-retest reliability for the *Hearing Handicap Inventory for the Elderly* and reported a high coefficient of stability for the instrument using two different administration approaches. Similarly, a weakness in test-rest reliability is the danger of the carryover or practice effects from one session to the next that can overestimate reliability and patient performance (Cordes, 1994; Pedhazur & Schmelkin, 1991; Schiavetti & Metz, 1997). Hulley and Cummings (1988) advised that the length of the period of time between test administrations might have a strong effect on the results. If the period is too short, not enough time might have elapsed to allow for random performance fluctuations, resulting in a carryover effect (Hulley & Cummings, 1988). On the other hand, if the period is too long, a lack of agreement between results can be caused by changes in the characteristics being measured (Hulley & Cummings, 1988).

Internal consistency is the third area to assess in determining the reliability of measurement. Internal consistency is the degree to which two or more items (which purport to measure the same variable) on the same instrument yield consistent results (Hulley & Cummings, 1988). Methods of assessing internal consistency have been developed to overcome the limitations of two administrations of the same test to the same sample of individuals at two different times (Schiavetti & Metz, 1997). One popular technique for assessing the internal consistency of measurement is the split-half method requiring three steps:

1. division of an instrument into two equivalent halves,
2. administration of the instrument to a group of individuals, and
3. correlation of the halves of the test with each other for determination of the reliability coefficient.

The correlation coefficient commonly used with split-half reliability is the Spearman-Brown formula (Schiavetti & Metz, 1997; Thorndike, Cunningham, Thorndike, & Hagen, 1993). The Spearman-Brown formula mathematically corrects for the split-half reduction of test items resulting in a correlation coefficient that would be expected if two versions of the same test had been administered (Schiavetti & Metz, 1997). Cronbach's alpha and the Kuder-Richardson #20 Formula (KR-20) can also be used to assess split-half reliability of dichotomous items (e.g., true/false) or for multiple-choice items (e.g., strongly agree, moderately agree, neutral, moderately disagree, strongly disagree), respectively (Schiavetti & Metz, 1997). Discussion of these statistical methods is not included here, but can be found in Maxwell and Satake (1997).

Threats to Validity

Validity can be reduced by consistent or systematic error originating from three sources:

(1) *observer bias*, (2) *subject bias*, and/or (3) *instrument bias* (Hulley & Cummings, 1988). Observer bias is a consistent distortion, either conscious or subconscious, during the collection, scoring, or reporting of data (Hulley & Cummings, 1988). For example, with knowledge of the presentation order of experimental conditions, an investigator can introduce observer bias into the scoring of listeners' responses to an open-set nonsense syllable test when assuming more errors would be made in the more difficult listening conditions than in the control condition (i.e., quiet).

Subject bias is a consistent distortion, either conscious or subconscious, of measurement by a participant in an investigation (Hulley & Cummings, 1988). A common phenomenon, known as the *Hawthorne effect*, occurs when subjects behave differently if they know that they are part of an experiment, thereby potentially affecting measurement of dependent variables (Schiavetti & Metz, 1997). Subjects may inflate self-reports of hearing aid satisfaction, if they are enrolled in a hearing aid clinical trial, for example. Instrument bias results from faulty function of a mechanical device or from measuring phenomena other than those originally intended for a particular technique (Hulley & Cummings, 1988). For example, measurement of subjects' pure-tone air-conduction thresholds may be underestimated if using an audiometer that is out of calibration from one administration of the test to the next.

Assessment of Validity

Validity of measurements can be assessed in three ways: (1) *content validity*, (2) *criterion validity*, and (3) *construct validity*. Content validity concerns how well items of an instrument measure the characteristics that they are supposed to measure (Schiavetti & Metz, 1997). In other words, the content validity of a scale, for example, is the degree to which its items represent the target domain and sample all pertinent characteristics (Hyde, 2000). Content validity, sometimes known as *face validity*, is the most desired and difficult-to-establish form of measurement validity (Maxell & Satake, 1997). Assessment of content validity of an instrument happens early in its development and requires two steps: (1) listing all possible characteristics of a behavior or phenomenon, and (2) the experimenter (author) or a group of experts deciding if the instrument measures all those characteristics (Hyde, 2000; Schiavetti & Metz, 1997). Important steps in the development of a valid measure of hearing aid benefit require listing all pertinent variables and a panel of experts ensuring that all variables are being measured on the self-assessment scale, for example.

Criterion validity is assessed through an empirical examination to determine how well a measure correlates with some outside measuring criterion (Schiavetti & Metz, 1997). There are two types of criterion validity: (1) *concurrent validity*, and (2) *predictive validity* (Schiavetti & Metz, 1997). Concurrent validity is the agreement between a particular measure under investigation and some outside validating criterion that are administered at the same time (Schiavetti & Metz, 1997). The degree of agreement is usually assessed through obtaining correlation coefficients between the results of the two measures obtained on a sample of subjects. Predictive validity is the degree to which a measure predicts future performance on some other criterion measure (Schiavetti & Metz, 1997). Predictive validity is assessed when a measure is made on a sample of subjects, time elapses, a criterion measure is administered, and then the results from the two measures are correlated to determine how well the first measure predicts subjects' performance on the second criterion measure (Schiavetti & Metz, 1997).

Construct validity (theorctical validity) is the degree with which a measure either empirically or rationally purports to measure some theoretical construct (Maxwell & Satake, 1997; Schiavetti & Metz, 1997). Recall that a construct is a model that proposes observable variables and predicts relationships (Hyde, 2000). Construct validity is difficult to determine and requires establishment of both content and predictive validity, as well as meta-analysis of the results from several investigations measuring the same phenomena (discussed in Chapters 2 and 3) (Maxwell & Satake, 1997; Robey & Dalebout, 1998). For example, construct validity can be difficult to obtain for behavioral diagnostic tests of central auditory processing disorders. First, content validity may be difficult to establish for tests of central auditory processing disorders because of the lack of agreement among experts regarding the best practices for diagnosing this pathology. Second, predictive validity for tests of central auditory processing are difficult to obtain because many measures focus on varying specific skills (e.g., pitch-pattern sequence test) that may or may not have any criterion measures for comparison. Third, meta-analysis of the results from several investigations using the same measures and the same types of subjects may be difficult to complete because of the co-morbidity of central auditory processing disorders with other behavioral disorders such as attention deficit disorder (ADD) and attention-deficit hyperactivity disorder (ADHD).

Enhancement of Reliability and Validity

There are five approaches to minimizing the variance and increasing the consistency of measurement (Hulley & Cummings, 1988):

1. Standardizing the measurement methods by including operational definitions (i.e., specific instructions for making measurements) in an operations manual
2. Training and certifying the observers
3. Refining the instruments to increase clarity and reduce ambiguity
4. Automating the instruments through developing self-response questionnaires
5. Repeating the measurement and taking the average of two or more administrations

Not only do these techniques increase reliability, but they also increase the validity of measurement. In addition, validity can be enhanced through three additional means (Hulley & Cummings, 1988). First, the blinding of both the observer and subject (i.e., "double-blinding") to the experimental protocol reduces the possibility of bias (i.e., observer and subject) and increases the validity of measurement. Second, unobtrusive measurements assess subjects' true behaviors and reduce the possibility of the Hawthorne effect. Although new hearing aid wearers may report appropriate use of assertive listening strategies learned in group therapy, direct observation of those patients during social situations may prove otherwise, for example. Third, calibrating instruments increases the likelihood of obtaining valid measurements. Audiologists usually think of "calibration" in terms of assessing the function of equipment used for measuring hearing sensitivity, performing sound surveys, or performing electroacoustic analyses of hearing aids. However, calibrating the administration of self-report scales increases the validity of measuring hearing handicap and hearing aid benefit, for example. Calibration of self-assessment tools for aural rehabilitation is discussed in Chapter 10. Calibration of self-report scales and tools begins with selecting the most appropriate measures for each clinical purpose.

SELECTING A MEASUREMENT SCALE OR TOOL

Selection of a measurement scale or tool involves several steps:

- defining the behavioral phenomena,
- considering possible measurement tools,
- evaluating the measurement tool, and
- considering methods of eliciting information from individuals.

Customer satisfaction, an important area of outcomes measurement, is used here to discuss important steps that are required to select an appropriate measurement scale or tool. This topic is discussed in greater detail again in Chapter 10 regarding the selection of self-assessment tools for aural rehabilitation.

Defining Behavioral Phenomena: Consumer Satisfaction

The rising price of health care and increased costs to consumers have heightened the demand for consumer satisfaction (Kreb & Wolf, 1997). In health care, the term "consumer" can have several meanings, including recipients of services, family members, regulators, payers, the various providers, etc., across a variety of service-delivery sites (Rao, Blosser, & Huffman, 1998). *Consumer satisfaction* is the clients'/patients' perceptions of the quality of services rendered by audiologists, the effectiveness of those services, and their outcome (ASHA, 1995). This definition sounds fairly straightforward. But, consider the meaning of the words "client" or "patient." Do these terms simply mean persons with hearing impairment? Some audiologists prefer to use the terms interchangeably. Other audiologists prefer to use

the word "patient" for those they serve with hearing impairment and use the term "client" to refer to others with whom they do business. Can the term "patient" include persons with hearing impairment and their family members as well? Indeed, audiologists may consider both elderly individuals with hearing impairment and their family members as "patients" when all are participating in group hearing aid orientation sessions, for example. In this case, measurement of patient satisfaction might involve a single measurement tool for both parties and focus on the quality of aural rehabilitation services and the reduction of hearing handicap and frustration in communicating among family members.

From time-to-time, audiologists might need to consider the satisfaction of both "clients" and "patients" from somewhat different perspectives at the same time. For example, audiologists must often be the intermediaries between management (i.e., the client) and workers (i.e., patients) when providing a mobile hearing conservation program (Balko, 1994). Successful hearing conservation programming requires audiologists' realization that although both the client and the patients are stakeholders in the program outcomes (i.e., prevention of noise-induced hearing loss), management may be focused on reducing costs while workers may want comfortable hearing protection devices and innovative educational programming. Consequently, consumer satisfaction cannot be assessed using a single measurement tool in this case.

Consumer satisfaction not only involves multiple stakeholders, but the *perceptions* of those stakeholders about the quality, effectiveness, and outcome of audiologists' services. The behavioral phenomena (i.e., perceptions) to be measured are by definition highly subjective and can potentially reduce both reliability and validity. Patients' perceptions of quality can vary from day-to-day throughout the rehabilitation process and can vary significantly across patients. In addition, patients' perceptions may involve factors (e.g., availability of parking, comfort of the waiting room) other than those directly related to the quality, effectiveness, and outcome of audiologic services, for example. Therefore, audiologists must take steps to increase the likelihood of obtaining reliable and valid measures of customer satisfaction. First, education goes a long way toward ensuring that both patients and hearing health-care professionals are "on the same page" regarding appropriate expectations. Second, audiologists can use consumer measurement tools that include features that are known to increase reliability and validity, such as providing instructions and examples to respondents about how to complete the instrument and how to respond. Third, audiologists must realize that, although consumer satisfaction is an important criterion for evaluating the value of the intervention, it is from the perspective of the patient only (Ross & Levitt, 1997). Uninformed patients, who are fond of their audiologists, but who have received less than positive aural rehabilitative outcomes may still provide favorable responses on consumer satisfaction measures because they "liked them as persons, don't like to say anything bad about anyone, were afraid that they might get them in trouble, or were afraid that future services might be negatively impacted by their true feelings," for example.

In summary, the first step in selecting measurement tools requires a careful analysis of the terminology used in defining behavioral phenomena from different points-of-view. So far, we have defined consumer satisfaction from several points-of-view. However, further discussion of the selection of tools focuses on the measurement of consumer satisfaction from the patient's perspective.

Considering and Evaluating Measurement Tools: Consumer Satisfaction

Several decisions must be made in considering the type of consumer satisfaction measurement tool to be used for a particular application. First, audiologists must determine what they want to do with the data generated from consumer satisfaction tools by asking:

- What am I trying to measure?
- What types of items do I want to use?
- What do I want to do with the data generated from these items?

There are two general types of instrument items: *open-ended* and *closed-ended* questions (Cummings, et al., 1988). Open-ended questions such as the following elicit responses from patients' own words (Cummings, et al., 1988):

1. What are the three most important benefits you believe your hearing aid should provide:

———————————————————
———————————————————
———————————————————

An advantage of using open-ended questions is that they provide patients freedom to respond without any limitations (Cummings, et al., 1988). A disadvantage of open-ended questions is that they are both difficult to code and analyze (Cummings, et al., 1988). Closed-ended questions ask patients to choose one or more pre-selected answers such as:

2. What was your most important consideration when purchasing your hearing aids?

    a. cosmetics
    b. cost

c. performance

d. other _____

Two advantages of closed-ended questions are their ease in tabulation/analysis and their clarity (Cummings, et al., 1988). Some examples of closed-response items include (Silverman, 1998):

- multiple-choice options,
- semantic differential techniques (i.e., use of bipolar opposites separated by seven, equal appearing intervals), and
- Likert scales (e.g., a series of statements that reflects a favorable or unfavorable attitude).

Multiple-choice response sets usually express ordinal amounts of some attribute, such as frequency, importance, difficulty, agreement, or attitude (Hyde, 2000). Originally, the term "Likert scale" (1952) was used for ordinal scales of agreement (e.g., strongly agree, moderately agree, neutral, etc.), but it is now used to describe many discrete and adjectival ordinal scales (Hyde, 2000). Although allowing respondents to express their opinions, open-ended items may not always be feasible or facilitate data analysis, or quality improvement. Therefore, primary use of closed-ended items with a section for comments is usually the best option for use on consumer satisfaction tools.

Audiologists must then decide on what type of closed-ended items to use, which dictates the level of measurement, the appropriate types of statistical manipulations of data, and, ultimately, the types of questions about consumer satisfaction to be investigated. Dichotomous items (e.g., yes/no questions) at the categorical level of measurement only permit audiologists to use non-parametric statistics (e.g., chi-square analyses) to determine if a significantly greater proportion of patients answer "yes" to being satisfied with services after implementation of a new patient-outreach program, for example. Use of semantic-differential items (e.g., "satisfied" and "dissatisfied" separated by seven equal-appearing intervals) at the interval level of measurements allows audiologists to conduct t-tests to determine the existence of significant improvement in the degree of consumer satisfaction after implementation of a patient-outreach program.

Second, audiologists must decide on whether to use tools that are already in existence, or to create their own. Some considerations in using existing tools are:

- Is there a standard consumer satisfaction survey used in my place of employment? Will it satisfy the needs of my department? Do published, standardized "norms" (i.e., psychometric data) exist to support the use of the survey?
- Are there any published consumer satisfaction tools used specifically in communication sciences and disorders? Will they satisfy the needs of my department? Are there norms for these tools?

Over the past 20 years, several consumer satisfaction tools have been developed and consist of standardized surveys of patients, purchasers of services, and/or practitioner satisfaction (Kreb & Wolf, 1997). For example, the American Speech-Language-Hearing Association (ASHA, 1995) has published two consumer satisfaction measures for speech-language pathology and audiology services and rehabilitation services that are available for use by clinicians and appear in Appendix IV-A. Each measure is only one-page in length and color-coded for quick identification (i.e., green for speech-language pathology and audiology services and orange for rehabilitation services). Both consumer satisfaction measures use primarily closed-ended questions (e.g., Likert-type scales) with an open-ended comments section at the end.

Any published consumer satisfaction tool should be evaluated prior to use. Appendix IV-B, found on the companion CD-ROM, contains a "Checklist for Evaluation of Tools" adapted from Cummings, Strull, Nevitt, and Hulley (1988) that assesses instruments on general factors, types of questions, format, wording, reliability, and validity. With regard to general factors, all tools should begin with a statement of purpose, why the respondent has been selected, instructions, and questions soliciting demographic information (Cummings, et al., 1988). In addition, questions on major topics should be grouped together, introduced by some sort of heading, and preceded by instructions, if the section includes new items (e.g., changing from multiple-choice questions to semantic differential items) (Cummings, et al., 1988). Audiologists should select the best tool that satisfies their needs for assessing consumer satisfaction.

Audiologists should consider the type of questions used on the instrument. Does the instrument use open-ended, closed-ended questions, or a combination? If closed-ended questions are used, the list of response choices ideally should (Cummings, et al., 1988):

■ have an option such as "other" or "none of the above" when the list of choices is not exhaustive,
■ require a "best answer" from a set of mutually exclusive options, and
■ allow selection of multiple items when questions have multiple answers.

The format of the instrument also requires evaluation. Ideal format features include (Cummings, et al., 1988):

■ Visual appearance promoting ease of completion
■ Neat, attractive, and effective use of space

■ Easy-to-read font
■ Vertical alignment of choices
■ Clear modes of selection (e.g., boxes to check, letters to circle)
■ Appropriate use of branching questions (e.g., screener questions to determine whether respondents are directed to answer additional questions or sent onward to another series of questions)

Audiologists must also consider the wording of the questions on the instrument. Wording should be clear (e.g., specific and concrete), simple (e.g., concise, use of straightforward grammatical structures, common vocabulary, and no technical terms or jargon), encourage accurate/honest responses, set the time frame, and be free of ambiguity and double-barreled questions (e.g., use of words like "or," "and," or questions that ask two questions at once) (Cummings, et al., 1988).

The most important factors in evaluating any instrument are their reliability and validity. One of the first questions for audiologists to ask is whether reliability and validity data (i.e., psychometric) have been published on the instrument (Cummings, et al., 1988). It is important to know whether any normative data have been collected on the instruments, and, if so, for what populations (Cummings, et al., 1988). For example, audiologists should not use the same norms of consumer satisfaction collected on elderly patients for young adults. Furthermore, audiologists should consider tools that are commonly used as outcome measures in the field. Use of commonly used outcome measures enables audiologists to compare their consumer satisfaction data to those of professionals in similar service-delivery sites. However, just because a particular measure is popular, it does not necessarily mean that it is a "good" instrument (i.e., reliable or valid), especially for all applications.

Audiologists face similar issues if they elect to construct their own tools and are strongly advised to evaluate available tools prior to developing a new one, however (Hyde, 2000). The decision to use an existing tool, to adapt several existing tools, or develop a completely new one requires careful consideration of several factors (Hyde, 2000). Will my employers permit use of a clinician-constructed consumer satisfaction tool? Is it possible to construct a reliable and valid tool to suit departmental needs? Appendix IV-C, found on the companion CD-ROM, contains a "Worksheet for Writing Questionnaires and Interviews" (adapted from Cummings, et al., 1988) and outlines the steps for creating an original instrument. The first step involves selecting method(s) of eliciting information from patients by considering the advantages and disadvantages of questionnaires versus interviews (Cummings, et al., 1988). Questionnaires are completed by the patients themselves and interviews are administered to the patients by clinicians and researchers (Cummings, et al., 1988). Advantages of using questionnaires include (Cummings, et al., 1988):

- economy (e.g., instruments completed by patients at home or in the waiting room reduce audiologists' time commitment in obtaining information),
- standardization (e.g., written instructions reduce the possibility of interviewers' bias in administering the instrument), and
- anonymity (e.g., patients are more likely to provide candid answers when completing a questionnaire than when interviewed by an observer).

Advantages of interviews include (Cummings, et al., 1988):

- clarity (e.g., interviewers can clarify questions to patients on the spot to reduce confusion and inaccurate responses),
- richness (e.g., interviewers can collect complex information beyond the items on

the instument),
- completeness (e.g., interviewers can ensure that no questions are omitted), and
- control (e.g., interviewers can control all aspects in the administration of an instrument).

Questionnaires are more suited than interviews for assessment of consumer satisfaction in busy audiology practices because of the advantages of economy of time, standardization of questions, and anonymity of responses, for example. However, interviews can be very appropriate in other areas of health, such as the frequent practice of conducting either face-to-face or telephone interviews with post-discharge acute-care or rehabilitation hospital patients (Rao, et al., 1998). They can also be useful to follow up on responses made on questionnaires to pursue more in-depth understanding of patients' concerns.

The second step involves composing a list of variables related to the behavioral phenomenon to be measured by the instrument. The more broad the behavioral phenomenon, the more difficult it is to write a complete list of related variables to measure. Audiologists may find it extremely difficult to identify all variables related to consumer satisfaction, for example. Audiologists must decide to use either a broad or narrow approach to consumer satisfaction. A broad approach involves considering general dimensions of consumer satisfaction. In the early 1980s, a general theory of patient satisfaction was developed with the following dimensions (e.g., variables) (Linder-Petz, 1982; Rao, et al., 1998):

- Accessibility/convenience
- Availability of resources
- Continuity of care
- Efficacy of care
- User-friendly explanations of costs/ financial services

- Humaneness
- Professionalism and respect for privacy of information gathering
- Information giving/patient education
- Pleasantness of surroundings
- Quality of care/competence of providers

Although fairly easy to write, instrument items for these dimensions are so generic that audiologists may not be able to measure important consumer satisfaction variables in situations involving complex interactions among patients, hearing instruments, the environment, and the dispenser. For example, Sandridge (1997) used the questionnaire from the MarketTrak IV (Kochkin, 1997) studies involving specific variables from four major domains focusing on satisfaction with:

- Hearing instrument features: fit/comfort, visibility, ongoing expense, warranty, ease of changing battery, packaging, and frequency of cleaning
- Performance and value: overall satisfaction, value, improvement in hearing, naturalness of sound, clearness of tone/sound, directionality, use in noisy situations, feedback, reliability, and battery life
- Specific listening situations: one-on-one, small groups, large groups, concerts/ movies, places of worship, outdoors, restaurants, riding in cars, television, and telephone
- Dispenser features: professionalism, knowledge, explanation of expectations and care of hearing aids, quality of service during fitting and post-purchase

The third step involves writing items for measuring important consumer satisfaction variables. One successful approach is to modify published instruments to suit specific needs (Cummings, et al., 1988). Johnson and Danhauer (1999) modified several features from ASHA's "*Speech-Language Pathology*

and/or Audiology Services Consumer Satisfaction Measures" (found in Appendix IV-A) in developing hearing support program questions for educational settings, rehabilitation hospitals, and long-term residential care facilities for the elderly, for example. Audiologists may obtain further ideas from reviewing the literature and contacting other clinicians and investigators regarding characteristics of effective measurement tools. When using single items or subscales from already published instruments, audiologists should be advised that those items do not retain their same psychometric properties (Hyde, 2000). Furthermore, responses on items often depend on the context in which they are presented and minor changes in the content, format, or instructions can alter patients' perceptions and responses (Hyde, 2000).

The fourth and fifth steps involve writing and revising the first draft of the instrument, respectively. The first draft should be written with the instructions presented in a clear and uncluttered manner without any consideration to length of the instrument (Cummings, et al., 1988). Topic arrangement should maintain a flow of ideas and minimize the effects of sensitive issues on respondents (Cummings, et al., 1988). Authors, their colleagues, and experts in questionnaire design should review and revise the instrument so that items will not contain confusing wording, use jargon, or ask two questions at the same time (e.g., use words like "and" or "or") (Cummings, et al., 1988).

The sixth step involves pretesting the second draft for the clarity of both the instructions and items using 2 to 5 respondents who are from diverse cultural backgrounds and generations (Cummings, et al., 1988). Audiologists practicing in southern California should attempt to pretest a consumer satisfaction instrument on a group of respondents that includes non-native speakers of English of varied ages, for example. Furthermore, audiologists should retest the instrument at different times using different interviewers/responders to increase the reliability of results (Cummings, et al., 1988). However, publishing new instruments in peer-reviewed journals for widespread acceptance and dissemination in the field requires an iterative process of scale development, with moderate (< 50) samples of subjects for pilot testing items and larger samples (> 200) for subsequent validation and norming stages (Hyde, 2000).

The seventh step involves both shortening and revising the instrument again by (Cummings, et al., 1988):

- excluding questionable items,
- rank ordering the remaining items,
- eliminating low priority items,
- arranging for an expert review, and
- then pretesting the final product on a group of respondents similar to the intended population of the instrument.

The eighth step involves precoding all closed-ended items in a consistent manner for rapid recording and entry of data (Cummings, et al., 1988). Cummings, et al., (1988) suggested developing a coding manual with explicit instructions on scoring and categorizing items for ensuring consistent and reliable coding.

SUMMARY

Assessing the value of services has become a major issue for audiologists. Outcomes measurement is about measurement. Concepts from research design courses once believed to be irrelevant by some are now important to audiologists trying to find, collect, use, and share outcome measures in improving all aspects of their practices. This chapter has reviewed and identified the psychometric characteristics, information content/power, and examples of appropriate statistics for the four levels of measurement. Readers must understand the concepts of, the threats to, and safeguards for the reliability and validity

---

LEARNING ACTIVITIES

- Identify the level of measurement, applicable statistics, and the information content/power provided for some of the leading self-assessment scales in measuring hearing aid benefit such as *Hearing Handicap Inventory for the Elderly* (HHIE) (Ventry & Weinstein, 1982), *Hearing Aid Performance Inventory* (HAPI), (Schum, 1992; Walden, Demorest, & Hepler, 1984), and the *Abbreviated Profile of Hearing Aid Benefit* (APHAB) (Cox & Alexander, 1995).

- Evaluate one of the self-assessment tools above or ASHA's consumer satisfaction measures for speech-language pathology services and/or audiology services or rehabilitation services appearing in Appendix IV-A using the "Checklist for Evaluation of Tools" (adapted from Cummings, Strull, Nevitt, & Hulley, 1988) appearing in Appendix IV-B.

- Read and critique the *Technical Report: SCAN-C: Test for Auditory Processing Disorders in Children— Revised* by Keith (2000a) that appears in Appendix IV-D. What other measures of reliability and validity would be helpful in making a decision to purchase this product? What type of reliability or validity would be the most difficult to establish for Keith (2000a)?

of measurements. We hope audiologists have learned how to select, evaluate, and even develop measures that can be used in assessing the complexity of various outcomes of service delivery.

RECOMMENDED READINGS

For details on research design and statistical procedures:

- Maxwell, D.L., & Satake, E. (1997). *Research and statistical methods in communication disorders.* Baltimore, MD: Williams & Wilkins.
- Schiavetti, N., & Metz, D.E. (2001). *Evaluating research in communicative disorders* (4th ed.). Needham Heights, MA: Allyn & Bacon.
- Silverman, F.H. (1998). *Research design and evaluation in speech-language pathology and audiology* (4th ed.). Needham Heights, MA: Allyn & Bacon.

For issues in measuring outcomes:

- Frattali, C.M. (1998). Measuring modality-specific behaviors, functional abilities, and quality of life. In C.M. Frattali (Ed.), *Measuring outcomes in speech-language pathology* (pp. 55–88). New York, NY: Thieme.
- Rao, P.R., Blosser, J., & Huffman, N.P. (1998). Measuring consumer satisfaction. In C.M. Frattali (Ed.), *Measuring outcomes in speech-language pathology* (pp. 89–110). New York, NY: Thieme.

REVIEW EXERCISES

Fill-in-the-Blank

Instructions: Please fill-in-the-blanks with the correct terms from the word bank below.

1. _____ variables classify phenomena into categories.

2. The _____ level of measurement involves classifying phenomena into mutually exclusive, unordered categories.

3. _____ variables are nominal classification schemes with only two options.

4. The _____ level of measurement involves classifying phenomena into mutually exclusive, rank-ordered categories.

5. _____ variables have quantified intervals on an infinite arithmetic scale and include interval and ratio data.

6. The _____ level of measurement involves designated points on a continuum with identifiable, equal, and quantifiable intervals with no absolute zero point.

7. The _____ level of measurement involves the identity, magnitude, and equality of intervals; the specification of ratios between numbers; and an absolute zero point.

8. _____ _____ is introduced when either a single individual observer or group of observers administers an instrument differentially from one subject/patient to the next.

9. _____/_____ _____ refers to inherent differences within and across subjects/patients.

10. _____ _____ refers to the inconsistency in measurement caused by environmental variations.

11. _____ - _____ _____ is the degree to which two independent observers are consistent in their measurement of the same phenomenon.

12. _____ _____ is the degree to which two or more items on the same instrument that measure the same variable yield consistent results.

13. _____ _____ is a consistent distortion, either conscious or subconscious, during collection,

scoring, or reporting of data by an observer.

14. _____ _____ is a consistent distortion, either conscious or subconscious, of measurement by a participant in an investigation.

15. The _____ _____ is when subjects behave differently when they know they are part of an experiment.

16. _____ _____ is the degree to which items of an instrument represent the target domain and all pertinent characteristics.

17. _____ _____ is the degree to which a measure correlates with some outside measuring criterion.

18. _____ _____ is the degree to which a measure either empirically or rationally purports to measure some theoretical construct.

19. Content validity is also known as _____ validity.

20. _____ _____ is clients'/ patients' perceptions of the quality of services rendered by audiologists, the effectiveness of those services, and their outcome.

Word Bank:
Categorical
Concurrent validity
Construct validity
Consumer satisfaction
Content validity
Continuous
Dichotomous
Face
Hawthorne effect
Instrument variability
Internal consistency
Inter-observer reliability
Interval
Nominal
Observer bias
Observer variability
Ordinal
Ratio
Subject bias
Subject/patient variability

Matching

Instructions: Please match the items with the correct statement below.

I. Nominal
II. Ordinal
III. Interval
IV. Ratio

1. ____ Frequency in hertz
2. ____ Classifications of hearing loss
3. ____ ABR wave V latencies in milliseconds
4. ____ Answers to yes/no questions
5. ____ Standard scores on subtests of the SCAN-C (Keith, 2000b).

ANSWERS

Fill-in-the-Blank:
1. Categorical
2. Nominal
3. Dichotomous
4. Ordinal
5. Continuous
6. Interval
7. Ratio
8. Observer variability
9. Subject/patient variability
10. Instrument variability

11. Inter-observer reliability
12. Internal consistency
13. Observer bias
14. Subject bias
15. Hawthorne effect
16. Content validity
17. Concurrent validity
18. Construct validity
19. Face
20. Consumer satisfaction

Matching:
1. IV
2. II
3. IV
4. I
5. III

REFERENCES

American Speech-Language-Hearing Association. (1995). *ASHA-QA: Consumer satisfaction measure.* Rockville, MD: Author.

Balko, J.P. (1994). Equipping a hearing conservation program. In D.M. Lipscomb

(Ed.), *Hearing conservation in industry, schools, and the military* (pp. 287–300). Clifton Park, NY: Delmar Thomson Learning.

Cordes, A.K. (1994). The reliability of observational data: I. Theories and methods for speech-language pathology. *Journal of Speech, Language, and Hearing Research, 37,* 264–278.

Cox, R., & Alexander, G. (1995). The Abbreviated Profile of Hearing Aid Benefit. *Ear and Hearing, 16,* 176–186.

Cox, R.M., & Alexander, G.C. (1999). Measuring satisfaction with amplification in daily life: The SADL Scale. *Ear and Hearing, 20,* 306–320.

Cummings, S.R., Strull, W., Nevitt, M.C., & Hulley, S.B. (1988). Planning the measurements: Questionnaires. In S.B. Hulley & S.R. Cummings (Eds.), *Designing clinical research* (pp. 42–52). Baltimore, MD: Williams & Wilkins.

Edgerton, B.J., & Danhauer, J.L. (1979). *Implications of speech discrimination testing using nonsense stimuli.* Baltimore, MD: University Park Press.

Goldstein, D.P., & Stephens, S.D.G. (1981). Audiological rehabilitation: Management model. *Audiology, 20,* 432–452.

Hulley, S.B., & Cummings, S.R. (1988). Planning the measurements: Precision and accuracy. In S.B. Hulley & S.R. Cummings (Eds.), *Designing clinical research* (pp. 31–52). Baltimore, MD: Williams & Wilkins.

Hyde, M.L. (2000). Reasonable psychometric standards for self-report outcome measures in audiological rehabilitation. *Ear and Hearing, 21*(Suppl. 4), 24S–36S.

Johnson, C.E. (2000). Children's phoneme identification in reverberation and noise. *Journal of Speech, Language, and Hearing Research, 43,* 144–157.

Johnson, C.E., & Danhauer, J.L. (1999). *Guidebook for support programs in aural rehabilitation.* Clifton Park, NY: Delmar Thomson Learning.

Keith, R.W. (2000a). *Technical report: SCAN-C: Test for Auditory Processing Disorders in Children—Revised.* San Antonio, TX: The Psychological Corporation.

Keith, R.W. (2000b). *SCAN-C: Test for Auditory Processing Disorders in Children—Revised.* San Antonio, TX: The Psychological Corporation.

Kochkin, S. (1997). MarkeTrak norms: Subjective measures of satisfaction & benefit: Establishing norms. *Seminars in Hearing, 18*(1), 37–48.

Kreb, R.A., & Wolf, K.E. (1997). *Clinical series 13: Successful operations in the treatment-outcomes-driven world of managed care.* Rockville, MD: American Speech-Language-Hearing Association.

Likert, R.A. (1952). A technique for the development of attitude scales. *Educational and Psychological Measurement, 12,* 313–315.

Linder-Petz, A. (1982). Towards a theory of patient satisfaction. *Social Science and Medicine, 16*(5), 577–582.

Maxwell, D.L., & Satake, E. (1997). *Research and statistical methods in communication disorders.* Baltimore, MD: Williams & Wilkins.

Newman, C.W., Jacobson, G.P., Hug, G.A., Weinstein, B.E., & Malinoff, R.L. (1991). Practical methods for quantifying hearing aid benefit in older adults. *Journal of the American Academy of Audiology, 2,* 70–75.

Newman, C.W., & Weinstein, B.E. (1989). Test-retest reliability of the Hearing Handicap Inventory for the Elderly using two administration approaches. *Ear and Hearing, 10,* 190–191.

Pedhazur, E.J., & Schmelkin, L.P. (1991). *Measurement, design, and analysis.* Hillsdale, NJ: Lawrence Erlbaum Associates.

Rao, P.R., Blosser, J., & Huffman, N.P. (1998). Measuring consumer satisfaction. In C. Frattali (Ed.), *Measuring outcomes in speech language pathology* (pp. 89–112). New York, NY: Thieme.

Robey, R.R., & Dalebout, S.D. (1998). A tutorial on conducting meta-analysis of clinical outcome research. *Journal of Speech-Language-Hearing Research, 41*, 1227–1241.

Ross, M., & Levitt, H. (1997). Consumer satisfaction is not enough: Hearing aids are still about hearing. *Seminars in Hearing, 18*(1), 7–11.

Sandridge, S.A. (1997). Consumer satisfaction with Multifocus hearing aids. *Seminars in Hearing, 18*(1), 67–72.

Schiavetti, N., & Metz, D.E. (1997). *Evaluating research in communicative disorders* (4th ed.). Needham Heights, MA: Allyn & Bacon.

Schum, D. (1992). Responses of elderly hearing aid users on the Hearing Aid Performance Inventory. *Journal of the American Academy of Audiology, 3*, 354–356.

Silverman, F.H. (1998). *Research design and evaluation in speech-language pathology and audiology* (4th ed.). Needham Heights, MA: Allyn & Bacon.

Thorndike, R.M., Cunningham, G.K., Thorndike, R.L., & Hagen, E.P. (1993). *Measurement and evaluation in psychology and education* (5th ed.). New York, NY: Macmillan.

Ventry, I.M., Weinstein, B.E. (1982). The hearing handicap inventory for the elderly: A new tool. *Ear and Hearing, 3*, 128–134.

Walden, B., Demorest, M., & Hepler, E. (1984). Self-report approach to assessing benefit derived from amplification. *Journal of Speech and Hearing Research, 27*, 49–56.

APPENDIX IV-A

Consumer Satisfaction Measure
for Speech-Language Pathology and/or Audiology

Speech-Language Pathology and/or
Audiology Services
Consumer Satisfaction Measure

After answering all items, detach here and return
READ each item carefully and CIRCLE the one answer that is best for you.

SA = Strongly Agree   **N** = Neutral   **SD** = Strongly Disagree
A = Agree   **D** = Disagree   **NA** = Not Applicable

1. It is important that we see you in a timely manner.
   A. My appointment(s) was scheduled in a reasonable period of time.   SA   A   N   D   SD   NA
   B. I was seen on time for my scheduled appointment(s).   SA   A   N   D   SD   NA

2. It is important that you benefit from Speech-Language Pathology
   and/or Audiology Service(s).
   A. I am better because I received these service(s).   SA   A   N   D   SD   NA
   B. I feel I benefited from speech-language pathology and/or audiology service(s).   SA   A   N   D   SD   NA

3. You are important to us; we are here to work with you.
   A. The support staff (e.g., secretary, transporter, receptionist, assistant)
      who served me were courteous and pleasant.   SA   A   N   D   SD   NA
   B. The clinician who served me was courteous and pleasant.   SA   A   N   D   SD   NA
   C. Staff considered my special needs (age, culture, education,
      handicapping condition, eyesight, and hearing).   SA   A   N   D   SD   NA
   D. Staff included my family or other persons important to me in the service(s) provided.   SA   A   N   D   SD   NA

4. Our Speech-Language Pathology and Audiology staff are highly trained and
   qualified to serve you.
   A. My clinician was prepared and organized.   SA   A   N   D   SD   NA
   B. The procedure(s) was explained to me in a way that I could understand.   SA   A   N   D   SD   NA
   C. My clinician was experienced and knowledgeable.   SA   A   N   D   SD   NA

5. It is important that our environment is secure, comfortable, attractive,
   distraction-free, and easy to reach.
   A. Health and safety precautions were taken when serving me.   SA   A   N   D   SD   NA
   B. The environment was clean and pleasant.   SA   A   N   D   SD   NA
   C. The environment was quiet and free of distractions.   SA   A   N   D   SD   NA
   D. The building and treatment areas were easy to get to.   SA   A   N   D   SD   NA

6. It is important that we provide you with efficient and comprehensive services.
   A. I feel that the length and frequency of my service program were appropriate.
   B. My clinician planned ahead and provided sufficient instruction and education to
      help me retain my skills after my program ended.   SA   A   N   D   SD   NA
   C. I feel that my program was well managed, involving other services when needed
      (i.e., teacher, dentist, physician).   SA   A   N   D   SD   NA

7. We respect and value your comments.
   A. Overall, the program services were satisfactory.   SA   A   N   D   SD   NA
   B. I would seek your services again if needed.   SA   A   N   D   SD   NA
   C. I would recommend your services to others.   SA   A   N   D   SD   NA
   D. Check the services you received.   ❑ Speech-Language Pathology   ❑ Audiology

8. How many times were you seen?   ❑ 1-3 times   ❑ 4 or more times

Comments: _____

_____

Thank you for your time.

CODE [   ]   Please staple/seal the questionnaire so that the Center's address is on
                the outside and return it to us.

American
Speech-Language
Hearing
Association

Quality Improvement

© 1995

(Reprinted with permission © American Speech-Language-Hearing Association, 1995)

Rehabilitation Services

Consumer Satisfaction Measure

After answering all items, detach here and return
READ each item carefully and CIRCLE the one answer that is best for you.

SA = Strongly Agree   **N** = Neutral   **SD** = Strongly Disagree
A = Agree   **D** = Disagree   **NA** = Not Applicable

1. It is important that we see you in a timely manner.
   A. My appointment(s) was scheduled in a reasonable period of time.   SA   A   N   D   SD   NA
   B. I was seen on time for my scheduled appointment(s).   SA   A   N   D   SD   NA

2. It is important that you benefit from rehabilitation services.   SA   A   N   D   SD   NA
   A. I am better because I received these service(s).   SA   A   N   D   SD   NA
   B. I feel that I have benefited from rehabilitation service(s).   SA   A   N   D   SD   NA

3. You are important to us; we are here to work with you.
   A. The support staff (e.g., secretary, transporter, receptionist, assistant)
     who served me were courteous and pleasant.   SA   A   N   D   SD   NA
   B. The clinician who served me was courteous and pleasant.   SA   A   N   D   SD   NA
   C. Staff considered my special needs (age, culture, education,
     handicapping condition, eyesight and hearing).   SA   A   N   D   SD   NA
   D. Staff included my family or other persons important to me in the service(s)
     provided.   SA   A   N   D   SD   NA

4. Our rehabilitation staff are highly trained and qualified to serve you.
   A. My clinician was prepared and organized.   SA   A   N   D   SD   NA
   B. The service(s) was explained to me in a way I could understand.   SA   A   N   D   SD   NA
   C. My clinician was experienced and knowledgeable.   SA   A   N   D   SD   NA

**5. It is important that our environment is secure, comfortable, attractive,
distraction-free, and easy to reach.**
   A. Health and safety precautions were taken when serving me.   SA   A   N   D   SD   NA
   B. The environment was clean and pleasant.   SA   A   N   D   SD   NA
   C. The environment was quiet and free of distractions.   SA   A   N   D   SD   NA
   D. The building and rehabilitation services were easy to get to.   SA   A   N   D   SD   NA

6. It is important that we provide you with efficient and comprehensive services.
   A. I feel that the length and frequency of my service program were appropriate.   SA   A   N   D   SD   NA
   B. My clinician planned ahead and provided sufficient instruction and
     education to help me retain my skills after my program ended.   SA   A   N   D   SD   NA
   C. I feel that my program was well managed, involving other services when
     needed (e.g., teacher, dentist, nursing staff, physician).   SA   A   N   D   SD   NA

7. We respect and value your comments.
   A. Overall, the program services were satisfactory.   SA   A   N   D   SD   NA
   B. I would seek your services again if needed.   SA   A   N   D   SD   NA
   C. I would recommend your services to others.   SA   A   N   D   SD   NA
   D. Check the services you received.
     ❏ Speech-Language Pathology   ❏ Audiology   ❏ Physical Therapy   ❏ Occupational Therapy

8. How many times were you seen?   ❏ 1-3 times   ❏ 4 or more times

Comments: _____

_____

Thank you for your time.

CODE [   ]   Please staple/seal the questionnaire so that the Center's
     address is on the outside and return it to us.

AMERICAN
SPEECH-LANGUAGE
HEARING
ASSOCIATION

Quality Improvement

© 1995

APPENDIX IV-B

Checklist for Evaluation of Tools

(Adapted from Cummings, Strull, Nevitt, and Hulley, 1988)

The above-referenced Appendix can be found on the companion CD-ROM.

APPENDIX IV-C

Worksheet for Writing Questionnaires and Interviews

(Adapted from Cummings, Strull, Nevitt, and Hulley, 1988)

The above-referenced Appendix can be found on the companion CD-ROM.

APPENDIX IV-D

Technical Report About the Scan-C:
Test for Auditory Processing Disorders in Children—Revised
(Keith, 2000a)

Technical Report

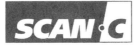

Test for Auditory Processing Disorders
in Children–Revised

Robert W. Keith

Available only from **U.S. EXCLUSIVE**
The Psychological Corporation.

Overview

The *SCAN-C Test for Auditory Processing Disorders in Children–Revised* is an individually administered test used to identify children between ages 5 years, 0 months and 11 years, 11 months who have auditory processing disorders. A revision of the original SCAN published in 1986, SCAN-C subtests were chosen to obtain information about areas that have been demonstrated to be among the most relevant to understanding auditory processing abilities.

SCAN-C assesses the perception stage of auditory processing, which is pre-cognitive. The test requires that the child repeat stimulus words or sentences, but the child is not required to understand the concept of "same or different," or to understand at a cognitive level the phonetic or phonologic differences that exist among speech sounds. This type of test avoids the cross modality and cognitive aspects of pointing to a picture in response to a word.

Revisions in the New Edition

SCAN-C provides professionals with an auditory test battery that is well-standardized and covers several areas of auditory processing. It can be administered quickly by auditory processing professionals using a portable CD player. The new CD technology eliminates noise inherent in audiocassettes and is compatible with diagnostic audiometers.

Improvements have been made to the original SCAN:

• All subtest instructions were reworded to make them easier to follow and more interesting for young children.

• The audiocassette tape was replaced with a compact disc to eliminate noise inherent in audiocassettes.
• The number of test items in the Competing Words subtest was decreased.
• A fourth subtest, Competing Sentences, was added to increase the diagnostic utility of the dichotic test battery.
• Normative data for children 5 years, 0 months to 11 years, 11 months were collected based on current U.S. Census figures.

SCAN-C Subtests

SCAN-C includes four subtests that represent functional auditory abilities in everyday listening situations:

- **Filtered Words Subtest** in which the subject is asked to repeat words that sound muffled. The test stimuli consist of monosyllabic words that have been low-pass filtered at 1000 Hz with a roll-off of 32 dB per octave. The test enables you to assess a child's ability to understand distorted speech, considered effective in identifying central auditory processing disorders.
- **Auditory Figure–Ground Subtest** which evaluates the subject's ability to understand words in the presence of background noise. Monosyllabic words were recorded in the presence of multi-talker speech babble noise at +8 dB signal-to-noise ratio. Poor performance on repeating the stimulus words may indicate a delay in development of the auditory system.
- **Competing Words Subtest** in which the subject hears two words simultaneously—one monosyllabic word presented to each ear—and is instructed to repeat the words presented in each ear. The test enables you to assess ear advantage. Poor performance may indicate a delay in maturation, underlying neurological disorganization, or damage to auditory pathways. Abnormalities shown by dichotic word test results are related to a wide range of specific disabilities, including CAPD, language disability, learning disability, and reading disorder.
- **Competing Sentences Subtest** in which pairs of sentences unrelated in topic are presented to the right and left ears. The subject is instructed to direct attention to the stimuli presented in one ear while ignoring the other. Like the Competing Words subtest, the results are used to determine levels of auditory maturation, hemispheric dominance for language, and to identify disordered or damaged central auditory pathways. The advantage of testing binaural separation with both word and sentence stimuli is to compare findings obtained with both simple and more complex linguistic levels of auditory stimuli.

Scores Reported

SCAN-C provides several important scores including subtest raw scores, subtest and composite standard scores, percentile ranks, and cumulative prevalence of ear advantage for the Competing Words subtest. Ear advantage scores are powerful indicators of hemispheric dominance for language and neurologically based language/learning disorders. The Competing Words subtest yields two ear advantage scores—one for the Right-Ear First Task and one for the Left-Ear First Task. The information presented on cumulative prevalence for ear advantage provides you with a means for examining how common or uncommon a particular child's ear advantage score is. The more extreme or atypical the ear advantage score, the greater the possibility of an auditory-based disorder such as a language or learning disability.

SCAN-C Test Design

Auditec™ of St. Louis, Missouri, produced the compact disc according to technical specifications provided by The Psychological Corporation. A male speaker, chosen for his clear articulation and Midwestern U.S. accent, recorded the test instructions and stimulus items. During the recording, the speaker was instructed to say the carrier phrase, "Say the word" or "Say" and the stimulus words in a natural manner and at the same intensity. Each word was monitored to zero with a VU meter as it was read aloud. Stimuli were recorded at approximately 4-second intervals on subtests 1 through 3 and at 5-second intervals on subtest 4. This rate allows adequate time for children to respond without prolonging the test.

Testing Environment

Standardization examiners had the option of testing in either an audiometric sound-proof test booth or a quiet room. To examine the effect that the test environment might have on a child's performance, a small study was conducted on a matched sample of 27 children. No significant differences were found on any mean subtest or composite standard scores, providing evidence that the type of testing environment does not affect the SCAN-C scores.

2

Standardization of SCAN-C

The standardization, validity, and reliability research for SCAN–C took place between June 1998 and March 1999. The test was standardized on 650 children between the ages of 5 years, 0 months and 11 years, 11 months. Data were collected on 3- and 4-year-old children; however, these data were not included in the norms due to inconsistent performance. Qualitative information obtained from 3 and 4 year olds is presented in the manual.

The SCAN–C standardization sample was representative of the general US population, stratified by age, gender, race/ethnicity, region, and parent education level, based on the 1997 U.S. Census update for children ages 5 years, 0 months to 11 years, 11 months.

Age in years and months	5.0 to 5.11	6.0 to 6.11	7.0 to 7.11	8.0 to 8.11	9.0 to 9.11	10.0 to 11.11	Total
Number	100	100	100	100	100	150	650

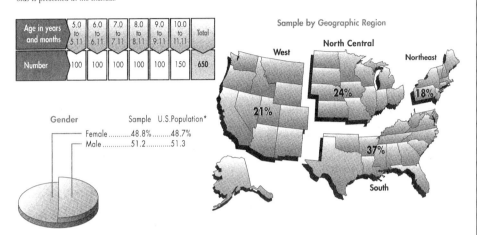

Sample by Geographic Region

West
North Central 24%
Northeast 18%
21%
37%
South

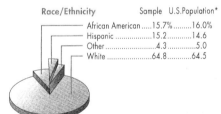

Gender   Sample   U.S.Population*

Female ....48.8%.........48.7%
Male ....51.2............51.3

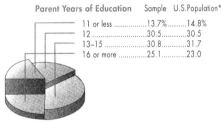

Race/Ethnicity   Sample   U.S.Population*

African American .....15.7%.........16.0%
Hispanic ....15.2............14.6
Other ....4.3..............5.0
White ....64.8...........64.5

Parent Years of Education   Sample   U.S.Population*

11 or less ....13.7%.........14.8%
12 ....30.5............30.5
13–15 ....30.8............31.7
16 or more ....25.1............23.0

The means and standard deviations of SCAN–A subtest and total raw scores confirm the original hypothesis that the auditory system of normally developing individuals is typically mature by age 12, and that results of central auditory tests are the same for individuals ages 12 through 50.

*1997 Census of Population Update, U.S. Department of Commerce, Bureau of the Census. Figures are based on the current population survey of March, 1995 for children ages 5 years, 0 months through 11 years, 11 months.

Clinical Sample

The 144 participants in the clinical study conducted during standardization ranged in age from 6 years, 0 months to 11 years, 11 months. They were required to have met the requirements for standardization as well as having been either diagnosed or suspected of having a diagnosis of Central Auditory Processing Disorder (CAPD).

Reliability

Test reliability is an indication of the degree to which a test provides you with a precise and stable score. The SCAN-C reliability coefficients for the subtests were obtained using Cronbach's coefficient alpha, and the internal consistency coefficients for the composite score were calculated with the formula recommended by Guilford. The SCAN-C composite test reliability coefficients range from .86 to .92. The reliability coefficients for the four SCAN-C subtests range from .56 to .89.

The reliability of each SCAN-C subtest and the composite score were also estimated by retesting a sample of 145 children between the ages of 5 and 11 years. The study was divided into two age groups: 65 children between 5 and 7 years old and 80 children between 8 and 11 years old. Each child was tested twice by the same examiner with a testing interval between 2 days and 6 weeks (mean testing interval was 6.5 days). SCAN-C subtest test-retest reliabilities range from .65 to .82 for the 5 to 7 year olds and from .67 to .78 for the 8 to 11 year olds.

Summary

The *SCAN—C Test for Auditory Processing Disorders in Children-Revised* enables professionals to obtain reliable central auditory test results in children between ages 5 years, 0 months and 11 years, 11 months. The test assesses the perception or pre-cognitive stage of auditory processing.

The careful, thorough procedures utilized in developing and updating this test will allow you to identify children who have auditory processing disorders and who may benefit from intervention. The results are also useful in determining levels of auditory maturation and hemispheric dominance for language.

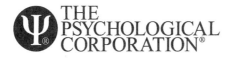

THE PSYCHOLOGICAL CORPORATION®

A Harcourt Assessment Company

555 Academic Court, San Antonio, Texas 78204-2498

1-800-211-8378
www.tpcweb.com

1 2 3 4 5 6 7 8 9 10 11 12 A B C D E

999-8900-441

CHAPTER 5
Use of Computers in Outcomes Measurement

LEARNING OBJECTIVES

This chapter will enable readers to:

- Understand the elements of computer-based data management systems (i.e., definition, components, main operations, and synergy of man versus computer)
- Describe the parts of the computer, their functions, and factors in purchasing different types of computers
- Consider the use of software for outcomes measurement (i.e., factors for purchase, user agreements, and specific programs)
- Discuss the use of the Internet (i.e., definition, access, searching, informatics, and critiquing Websites)
- Visualize the potential of personal computing and the Internet for outcomes measurement

INTRODUCTION

Desktops, laptops, palmtops (palm pilots), RAM, ROM, bytes, hard drives, zip drives, homepages, Webpages, the Internet, modems, Internet service providers ... These terms had little or no meaning to audiologists in training programs just a couple of decades ago. Many of these terms and instruments were not even blips on the technology radar screen then, so it is no wonder that seasoned practitioners have to learn a whole new jargon from their younger colleagues. It is only recently that we have seen the transition of high technology from computer shows to the daily practice of audiology. Audiologists born in

the information age adapt readily to the idea of a completely networked practice from case-history intake to outcomes measurement. Senior clinicians can learn a lot from CFY audiologists in this area. Indeed, our vocabulary from the world of personal computing is expanding each day (see Appendix V-A). Personal computing has become a necessity in almost all aspects of day-to-day life, including the hearing health-care field. Audiologists need to keep up with the technology boom or risk getting left behind.

E-mail, voice mail, instant messaging, chat rooms, and message boards are increasing our ability to communicate with our colleagues, manufacturers, professional organizations, and patients. In some cases, communication is in real time and at relatively little or no cost. Indeed, the Internet has brought the world together into an on-line global community. For example, audiologists from coast-to-coast can discuss important clinical issues via chat rooms organized through the audiology list-serves, organized by the American Academy of Audiology (AAA) and the American Speech-Language-Hearing Association (ASHA). Busy audiologists can even obtain their Doctorate of Audiology (Au.D.) degrees via distance learning programs through Nova Southeastern University, the University of Florida, and several other programs that will be available in the near future. In addition, researchers can submit their work for presentation at the annual conventions of the AAA and ASHA via the Internet. Audiologists can also find the latest hearing research on-line in ASHA's *American Journal of Audiology: A Journal of Clinical Practice*, which was one of the first to offer its articles on the Internet; others have followed. Indeed, the possibilities are endless for today's audiologists.

The Internet can offer improved service delivery for patients. For example, patients can now access information about hearing, hearing loss, and hearing aids on the Internet. A recent national survey found that most dispensers believed that consumer education is one of the most important factors for achieving positive patient outcomes (Masterson, Wynne, Kuster, & Stierwalt, 1999). Furthermore, busy patients can have their questions answered about their new hearing aids via E-mail. Patients with tinnitus and other auditory conditions can seek support from their peers via on-line support groups. However, the Internet has the potential for both positive and negative outcomes for patients. For example, unscrupulous individuals can easily use the Internet for financial gain and to provide false information, mislead, or potentially cause damage to unsuspecting consumers. Audiologists must counsel their patients about the positive and negative aspects of using the Internet.

Personal computing holds promise for outcomes measurement in audiology. The development of the modern microcomputer has changed the way data are collected, edited, stored, analyzed, and disseminated (Feigal, et al., 1988). For example, audiologists are devising creative ways of linking computer-based audiometers to the NOAH system for compiling patients' records containing diagnostic information and then tracking their progress throughout the audiologic rehabilitation process. Furthermore, a few years ago ASHA developed the Universal Newborn Hearing Screening (UNHS) component of National Outcomes Management System (NOMS) and included the training of staff from participating programs in the use of software designed by the OZ Corporation to collect and manage outcome data quality indicators (i.e., variables) toward achievement of local, state, and national benchmarks (i.e., goals) for a national study. Clearly, the use of personal computers and the Internet has great potential for outcomes measurement for the audiologist and for the profession. The purpose of this chapter is to provide readers with some basic information and skills for considering the use of personal computers for outcomes measurement.

COMPUTER-BASED DATA MANAGEMENT SYSTEMS

Outcomes measurement occurs at macro and micro levels. The micro level involves collecting, analyzing, and using outcome measures at the level of the patient. This is the level at which most audiologists think about outcomes measurement; unfortunately, most clinicians fail to see the complete power of computers for outcomes measurement. After all, elderly patients can complete consumer satisfaction questionnaires with a paper and pencil more easily than with a click of a mouse! Outcomes measurement at the macro level involves collecting, analyzing, and aggregating data on clearly defined quality indicators (i.e., measures) toward the achievement of facility, local, state, or national benchmarks (i.e., goals). Outcomes measurement at the macro level requires the use of computer-based data management systems.

What does computer-based data management systems mean? The phrase is indeed a mouthful and the whole term is best understood by defining each of its parts. "Computer-based" means that personal computers are used. "Data" is the plural form of the Latin term datum, which means "given" or "fact" (Oz, 1998). "Management" means the act of directing an enterprise (Merriam Webster OnLine, 1999). A "system" is an arrangement of components that work together toward a common goal (Oz, 1998). Therefore, a *computer-based data management system* is an arrangement of computers and their peripherals that work together in collecting, processing, and archiving data.

There are six important components in computer-based data management systems (Oz, 1998):

1. Data—important input to the system to produce information or data within a context
2. Hardware—consists of computers and their peripherals:
   ⇒ Input devices
   ⇒ Keyboard
   ⇒ Microphone
   ⇒ Hand-held computers with stylus
   ⇒ Scanner
   ⇒ Output devices
   ⇒ Monitor
   ⇒ Printer
   ⇒ Speakers
   ⇒ Storage devices
   ⇒ Disk drive
   ⇒ Hard drive
   ⇒ Zip drive
   ⇒ Data communication devices
   ⇒ Modems
   ⇒ CD-burners
3. Software—are sets of instructions that tell the computer how to:
   ⇒ Take the data in
   ⇒ Process the data
   ⇒ Display the data
   ⇒ Store the data
4. Telecommunications—hardware and software that facilitate fast transmission and reception of:
   ⇒ Animation
   ⇒ Pictures
   ⇒ Sound
5. Procedures—are rules for achieving optimal and secure operations in data processing including:
   ⇒ Priorities in running different applications
   ⇒ Security measures
6. People—are information systems professionals and users who:
   ⇒ Analyze organizational needs
   ⇒ Design and construct information systems
   ⇒ Write computer programs
   ⇒ Operate the hardware
   ⇒ Maintain the software

These six components work together to perform the four main operations of a computer-based data management system (Oz, 1998):

1. entering data (i.e., input),
2. changing and manipulating the data (i.e., data processing),
3. getting information out (i.e., output), and
4. storing data and information (i.e., storage).

Indeed people and computers must work together in a synergistic fashion, each contributing unique qualities to data management systems. Figure 5-1 illustrates this unique relationship between man and machine (adapted from Oz, 1998).

The size of the entity (e.g., solo private practice, hospital, or regional state department of health) using the data management system determines if one, two, or more computers will be needed and how the computers will communicate (network) with each other. A series of computers networked together can use the same software with managing data in compiling patients' records for electronic billing, for example. However, aggregation of outcome data at a regional, state, or national level requires the communication among computers in different geographic locations through use of the Internet. Before ending this chapter on harnessing the power of computers for outcomes measurement, readers should consider some basic properties of computers, software, and the Internet.

PERSONAL COMPUTERS

All computers regardless of size, age, or function have the same basic components (Oz, 1998):

- *Input device*—receives signals from outside the computer and sends them inside (e.g., keyboard).
- *Central processing unit* (CPU)—is a microprocessor chip that accepts instructions/data, executes those instructions, and then stores the output in memory for later use.
- *Memory*—has two types:
  ⇒ *Internal memory*—is the limit of data and information that can be stored and the speed with which stored information can be retrieved.
  ⇒ *External memory*—stores the same types of information as internal memory, but for longer periods of time.
- *Output devices*—deliver the information from the computer to the user or another computer.

Audiologists may wonder when should new computers be purchased. Basically, two questions should be asked (Dodd, 2000b): 1) Does my present computer support the needed or desired applications? 2) Would modifications to my computer be required to utilize those applications and need two or three upgrades? Unless the answer to both of those questions is "yes," then it may not be time to purchase a new computer. A computer should last three to four years because most of the software available today can be used on computers purchased a few years ago (Dodd, 2000b); however, as with new cars, stereos, and even hearing aids, technology does change rapidly and some users may elect to replace their computer systems more frequently to stay current.

Furthermore, some computer users do not feel satisfied with their computers unless they are the latest technology. Some individuals may only use a computer for a year before purchasing the next latest and greatest model. Unfortunately, the minute a computer hits the market, it is already "old news" to those on the cutting-edge of the industry. Therefore, purchasing a computer that will satisfy both personal and professional needs over the long run is a difficult choice, but still a good investment.

The first issue to consider is whether to purchase the device from a retail outlet or directly from the manufacturer. The answer to this question depends on three factors: preference, availability, and value (Dodd, 2000b). If there is a strong preference for a particular hardware brand, audiologists should investigate whether the manufacturer sells its products directly over the Internet, through retail

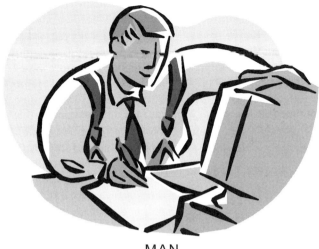

MAN

- Thinks

- Has common sense

- Makes decisions

- Instructs the computer on what to do

- Learns new methods and techniques

- Accumulates expertise

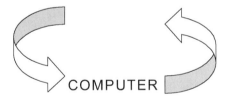

COMPUTER

- Calculates/performs programmed logical operations

- Stores/retrieves data rapidly

- Performs logical functions accurately

- Executes long, tedious operations

- Automates routine functions economically

- Is adaptable

Figure 5-1. Synergy between man and machine in computer-based management systems (Adapted from Oz, 1998).

outlets, or both (Dodd, 2000b). Companies such as Gateway (www.gateway.com) sell their products directly to consumers whereas; some manufacturers like Compaq (www.compaq.com) sell their products both directly to consumers and through retail outlets. Another issue is product availability. Retail outlets may have limited supplies of certain models that may necessitate ordering directly from the manufacturer. Manufacturers may be slightly more expensive than retail outlets when considering taxes, shipping, and handling, however (Dodd, 2000b). On the other hand, even though retail outlets may be less expensive than manufacturers, they rarely offer comparable warranties and/or technical support. Another option is local microcomputer manufacturers that build custom computers systems based on the needs and desires of the consumer. Local microcomputer manufacturers usually provide excellent on-site troubleshooting. Unfortunately, many of these firms may be "here today and gone tomorrow." Local manufacturers may decide to shift their company emphasis to Website development jeopardizing the quality of customer service provided to their computer customers, for example. Thus, it is important to check out the company thoroughly prior to purchase.

Some audiologists may desire a new computer for use "on the go," for example, and may consider purchasing a notebook or handheld computer. *Notebook computers*, also known as laptop computers, provide the power of a desktop computer that can be transported and used anywhere. Notebook computers can offer several advantages over the even smaller handheld devices (Dodd, 2000b):

■ full-sized key board,
■ support of most multi-media formats, and
■ complete data-storage capabilities.

Handheld computers (i.e., palmtops or palm pilots), provide users with easy-to-use

mobile PC companions with access to hearing health-care related activities, such as keeping up with patient schedules, running simple spreadsheets and databases, storing critical information, and loading programs addressing specific needs (Wynne, 2000). These computers now go by the acronym "PDA," which stands for "personal digital assistant" (Denton, 2000). PDAs are getting smaller (e.g., as thin a 0.4 inches), lighter (e.g., as light as 4 ounces), and more functional (Denton, 2000). The PDAs can send and receive short E-mails, "surf" the Internet, and store short verbal messages (Wynne, 2000). Generally, PDAs are not meant to be "stand alone" computers, but may be appropriate for the audiologist practicing "on the go" in various service-delivery sites who may wish to access special clinical applications such as (Dodd, 2000b; Wynne, 2000):

■ programming digital hearing aids
■ recording chart notes
■ administering the *Hearing Handicap Inventory for the Elderly* (HHIE) (Ventry & Weinstein, 1982) or the *Abbreviated Profile of Hearing Aid Benefit* (APHAB) (Cox & Alexander, 1995); and
■ creating/retrieving:
  ⇒ patients' records (e.g., names of spouses, children, hearing aids, date of warranty expiration);
  ⇒ make, model, and serial number of hearing aids; and
  ⇒ warranty expiration date.

When purchasing a PDA, one should follow these tips (Denton, 2000):

■ Consider units based on the Windows CE or Palm operating systems as they have the largest collection of third-party applications.
■ Purchase a PDA that has a long battery life, as power sources are not always available.

- Ensure that you can carry the PDA anywhere.
- Consider a grayscale display as color displays add to the size and cost of the PDA.
- Purchase enough memory to allow for some growth, but not more than you need.

Ideally, PC technology will continue to evolve, assisting audiologists in caring for the hearing health-care needs of their patients and managing outcome data across service-delivery sites.

Whether purchasing a handheld, notebook, or desktop computer, audiologists should consider doing the following:

- Assess the computer needs of your practice (e.g., hardware requirements for key software).
- Consult with staff regarding their preferences.
- Ask colleagues about the effective use of computers in their practices.
- Read the latest consumer guides for purchasing computers.
- Investigate appealing rebates (e.g., $400 rebate for committing to a three-year subscription to an Internet service provider).
- Avoid "bundle" deals that may include things that you may not need (e.g., ink jet printers).
- Wait 24 hours before making any purchase.

SOFTWARE

Software is simply sets of instructions that control the operations of a computer, whether cutting, pasting, or displaying text; mathematically manipulating numbers; running programs; copying/deleting documents; and so on. The variety of software on the market grows by the day. Software for outcomes measurement can take several forms. For example, continued development of software for computer-assisted aural rehabilitation (CAAR) for instructing and training persons with hearing impairment will improve outcomes through cost containment and 24-hour patient accessibility (Sims & Gottermeier, 2000). Furthermore, software has been developed for hearing conservation programs, UNHS programs, complex computations for hearing aid fittings, assessment of patient needs, and documentation of patient outcomes.

Prior to purchase, users should evaluate software to see if programs suit their specific needs. What should users evaluate when purchasing software? Some of the factors for consideration include (adapted from Oz, 1998):

- Fitness for purpose (Does it satisfy needs?)
- Ease of learning to use (How long will it take to learn how to use the software?)
- Ease of use (Is it easy to use? Does it require the user to memorize a lot of commands?)
- Compatibility with existing hardware (Do I have the necessary hardware to run this program such as type of computer, hard disk space for loading software, processing capability, Windows programs, and additional hard disk space for patient records?)
- Compatibility with other software (Is it compatible with related software and other operating systems? Is it easy to move the data and output it to other programs?)
- Reputation of vendor (Do professional contacts and references provide positive feedback regarding the vendor? Does the vendor deliver what it promises? Does vendor stand by its pricing?)
- Availability and quality of telephone support (Do references provide positive feedback regarding the technical support received? Is the technical support on the telephone knowledgeable?)

- Networking (Can many computers share the software?)
- Cost (Is detailed pricing information available? Is this the best price for the best quality and performance?)

Once software has been purchased, users often must agree to a software usage agreement. By clicking the "I agree" button during software installation, users are agreeing to a usage agreement that they are (Dodd, 2000a):

(*NOTE: This list is not inclusive for all applications. Users are responsible for reading and adhering to all the terms listed in each agreement they sign.*)

- cognizant that the software developer owns the copyright to all text, graphics, audio, video, design, and other unique aspects of the software;
- recognized as the licensees, not the owners, of the software;
- permitted to:
  ⇒ install and use the application on only one PC at a time,
  ⇒ sell or give the software to other users provided that they uninstall the program from their PC and keep any part of the software product (e.g., user's manual, diskettes, CD-ROMS, and bundled hardware components);
- Not permitted to:
  ⇒ rent or lease the software,
  ⇒ alter the source code or program in any way,
  ⇒ use the software for illegal purposes, or
  ⇒ export the software.

Regardless of the software used in outcomes measurement, consideration of agreements for usage is consistent.

Currently, there are two computer-based data management systems for UNHS programs. The first system, developed by Optimization Zorn (OZ), is the Screening and Information Management Solutions (SIMS) software. The OZ system states that the success of any UNHS program is dependent on its effectiveness to detect newborns with hearing loss and to connect those children with hearing health-care services. SIMS is designed to manage infant-centered information and contains the following main areas: (1) patient information, (2) data archiving and backup, (3) referral information, (4) user information, (5) program management, (6) data collection, and (7) data transfer. The second system is the HI*TRACK software available from the National Center for Hearing Assessment and Management (NCHAM) at Utah State University. The software was developed with the input from managers of dozens of hospital-based UNHS programs in order to implement an efficient system and successful detection and intervention program. The system provides audiologists with the means of tracking infants' status regarding hearing screening, diagnostic assessment, and referral to follow-up services.

With regard to software for hearing conservation, the Bertrand-Johnson Acoustics Incorporated Company has developed CORTI© software—an effective tool for hearing conservation program (HCP) management. CORTI© helps companies to identify efficiently workers subject to noise-induced hearing loss (NIHL), controls costs, and provides full compliance with government regulations. The main features of CORTI© are data accumulation and analysis, and individual and group reports. With regard to data accumulation, CORTI© allows for:

- unlimited aggregation of all HCP-related data (e.g., audiometric tests), job histories, noise measurements (e.g., dosimetry and sonometry), and hearing protective device information; use of all major audiometric microprocessors;

import or transfer of data collected by other software packages; and

- interfacing with human resource information systems.

CORTI© also analyzes accumulated data to comply with OSHA regulations for:

- identification of workers exposed to or transferred to at or above the action level or a time-weighted average of 85 dB A,
- hearing loss classification in three main categories (e.g., normal hearing, loss caused by medical pathology, and high-frequency hearing loss),
- standard threshold shift (STS) calculation with allowance made for the aging effects according to OSHA,
- baseline adjustment upon confirmation of hearing loss,
- hearing impairment calculation according to the formula selected by the user, and
- calculation of worker time-weighted average (TWA) occupational noise exposure.

In addition to automatic data analysis, CORTI© also prepares and generates a variety of individual and group reports such as:

- Company hearing profiles
- Individual employee reports
- Industrial hygiene reports
- Medical administrative reports
- Retrospective evaluation of estimated noise exposure reports
- Standard threshold shift reports

The reports are based on user-defined parameters (e.g., age group, sex, workstations, TWA, hearing protection device (HPD), years of exposure) used permitting customization for specific information requirements and for company internal coding. Additional features for outcomes measurement using CORTI© are discussed in Chapter 8, "Outcomes Measurement in Hearing Conservation."

Establishment of the Hearing Instrument Manufacturers' Software Association (HIMSA) holds great promise for industry-wide outcomes measurement for hearing instrument fitting. HIMSA has the aim of developing, marketing, and supporting an integrated hearing-care software system. HIMSA is a privately owned company, but operates much as a consortium of companies (i.e., hearing aid and equipment manufacturers) using the same software. The company's main software system is NOAH that is designed to provide hearing health-care professionals with a unified system for performing patient-related tasks. At the center of NOAH is the "integration framework" allowing hearing instrument fitting, audiologic measurement, and office management systems to share a common database. For example, audiologists can complete patients' audiologic profiles (e.g., pure-tone audiometry, speech audiometry, and loudness sensitivity) using a tool from one supplier that can be passed to the common database for use by any fitting systems from other suppliers. NOAH can also be used to record journal notes regarding patient sessions.

Software programs containing the most widely used outcomes measures for hearing handicap, hearing aid benefit, and overall satisfaction could be interfaced with NOAH. For example, Newman, Jacobson, Weinstein, and Sandridge (1997) enabled the results of the *Hearing Handicap Inventory for the Elderly* (HHIE) (Ventry & Weinstein, 1982) and *Hearing Handicap Inventory for Adults* (HHIA) (Newman, Weinstein, Jacobson, & Hug, 1990) to be reported via the use of computer-generated macro statements for use in reporting hearing disability-handicap profiling. The profile can be used to answer the following questions (Sims & Gottermeier, 2000):

- What is the patient's probability of benefiting from amplification?

- Is audiologic intervention warranted?
- What are the probabilities of patients' compliance with recommendations?

In addition, the Audiology and Speech Pathology Software Development Group in the School of Audiology and Speech Pathology at Memphis State University has developed a software program for the *Abbreviated Profile of Hearing Aid Benefit* (APHAB) (Cox & Alexander, 1995) with the following features:

- A "Clinician Entry Mode" for quick data entry of written questionnaire data
- Ability to compare results of two hearing aids
- Normative data for elderly and young populations

In addition, this group has developed software for the *Satisfaction with Amplification in Daily Life* scale (SADL) (Cox & Alexander, 1999) that evaluates the satisfaction that patients feel with their current hearing aids compared with their new hearing aids, or to other hearing aid users using four subscales: positive effect, service and cost, negative features, and personal image. Interfacing outcomes measurement software with NOAH has potential for development of a system that could establish an industry-wide system to track patient outcomes at multiple levels. For example, alterations in NOAH could enable the tracking of patient outcomes by audiologists who can then send those data for aggregation at the level of the manufacturer.

Benchmarks (i.e., goals) with corresponding quality indicators (i.e., variables) could be established for industry-wide standards for patient outcomes. As technology changes and as data are continually aggregated, standards of patient care could improve to higher and higher levels. In time, the information could be available to the public, third-party payers, and government agencies regarding the effectiveness of our services.

Audiologists may wonder why they need to become knowledgeable about software for outcomes measurement when there are so few available applications. Audiologists need to understand the power of software for outcomes measurement for at least five reasons, however. First, results of a recent random survey of members of the American Academy of Audiology by Johnson and Danhauer (2001) indicated that only 66% of the respondents were involved in any sort of outcomes measurement, fewer than 20% used computers to do so, and many questioned that, "In a busy private practice, who has time for outcomes measurement?" Consequently, audiologists need to get involved with the development of software that can streamline the outcomes measurement process. Second, expertise in computer-based information management systems is another way for audiologists to carve out their professional niches. For example, in response to a controversy about whether speech-pathologists' scope of practice included directing UNHS programs, the American Academy of Audiology (AAA, 2000) published a position statement supporting audiologists' unique ability to serve this role by providing discipline-specific services, including monitoring outcome measures for quality assurance requiring adeptness with computer-based data management systems. Third, software can automate many of the processes and tasks assigned to audiologists and support personnel. SIMS automatically prepares and prints reports to all UNHS stakeholders (e.g., parents, pediatricians, and school systems) saving audiologists' valuable time and energy, for example. Fourth, the more that software directs audiologic practice within the health-care system, the more software-savvy audiologists will not only be included in the decision-making process, but also be indispensable to hospital administrators in managing their UNHS programs. These programs are discussed in detail in later chapters of this textbook. Fifth, if the profession is to be taken to a higher level, insightful audiologists will harness the power of computers and the Internet for outcomes measurement.

INTERNET

Defining and Accessing the Internet

Until a few years ago, the Internet was just a communications network connected to the government and some researchers that could transmit text only (Oz, 1998). The U.S. Department of Defense's Advanced Research Projects Agency (ARPA) first developed an experimental computer network called the ARPA.net to serve as a communications network among the government and universities that would work when no others (e.g., radio, telephone, and television) could, such as in the event of a nuclear attack (Gralla, 1997; Oz, 1998). Today, the *Internet* is a network of communications media to which hundreds of thousands of computers have been connected (Oz, 1998). The *World Wide Web* is a system that links together vast quantities of information from all over the world using the Internet (Levine, Young, & Reinhold, 1997). The Internet is growing at a phenomenal rate and keeping up with the changes and developing the potential for our profession is a never-ending process (Masterson, et al.,1999).

How does one get connected to the Internet? Today, that is not a difficult task as all PCs come "Internet ready." The biggest decision users must make is how they will access the Internet. One way is to use an on-line service (e.g., CompuServe or America On-line) that is especially easy to use for those with little or no computer experience. These on-line services provide access to the Internet in addition to their own unique con-

tent, special areas, and services available to members only who must pay a monthly subscription varying in price according to the number of hours used per month. Various monthly pricing plans are available, ranging from a few hours a month to unlimited usage. Specific advantages to these services are (Levine, et al., 1997):

■ User-friendly interface
■ Special features unique to that provider
■ Capability to log on from most cities in the United States as well as abroad by just making a local phone call
■ Better security
■ Longevity
■ Extensive user support

Most people opt for an Internet service provider for the following reasons (Levine, et al., 1997):

■ Lower costs
■ Higher speeds
■ Choice of access tools (e.g., Netscape, Eudora, and so on)
■ Use of latest Internet services
■ Less censorship
■ Higher status on the Internet "pecking-order"

Users often have several Internet-service providers (ISPs) to choose from in their local area. Users should consider the following when selecting from several different ISPs (Levine, et al., 1997):

■ Payment options (e.g., flat fee versus hourly rate)
■ System availability
■ Availability of services (e.g., user home-pages)
■ Modem speeds
■ Reciprocal arrangements with providers at other locations

- Support for various user platforms (e.g., Macintosh)
- Customer support

Once set up with a system, the ISP should provide a quality connection or one that maintains speed and does not tend to disconnect (Henry, 2000). If experiencing poor connections, Henry (2000) suggested troubleshooting through consideration of the following factors:

- Contact the phone company to check the quality of the phone line.
- Check to see if phone lines are noisy (e.g., Pick up the telephone, dial 1 to get rid of the dial tone, and listen for noise).
- Determine if there is any external interference, such as extremely high temperatures bearing down on phone lines.
- Determine if your phone line can support your modem speed.
- Determine if slower speeds or disconnections occur during the "rush hour" on the Information Superhighway.
- Try using the local access number that is physically closest to your location.
- Ask the following questions of your ISP:
  ⇒ Does the ISP support V.90 (i.e., the current 56 kilobytes per second modem standard)?
  ⇒ Does the ISP have multiple modem pools available for use if some component of the system goes down?
  ⇒ How often does the ISP update its software?
  ⇒ What type of modem does the ISP use and what type does it recommend for subscribers to use?

A pricier alternative to ISPs is Digital Subscriber Lines (DSLs) that offer the advantages of increased speed (i.e., average cable-modem speed ranges from 500 kilobits to 3 megabits per second) and no lengthy dial-up and log-in procedures (Phelps, 2000). Internet access speeds are expected to increase in the future.

Searching the Internet

Once connected to the Internet, audiologists need to know how to access information from this vast, unorganized worldwide communication complex (Leeper & Gotthoffer, 1999). Finding specific information on the Internet can be compared to finding a needle in a haystack and is very frustrating without an organized approach (Phelps, 2000). A successful approach requires the knowledge of Web directories and search engines. *Web directories* are organized, hierarchically arranged catalogs of the World Wide Web consisting of major topic headings that are progressively broken down into more and more specific sub-topics (Levine, et al., 1997). Two popular Web directories are Yahoo! (www.yahoo.com) and Infoseek (www.infoseek.com). Search engines differ from directories in that they use "spiders" or "robots" to scour the Internet constantly for page titles, keywords, or even the entire Website textual content (Sullivan, 1998). *Search engines* are actually computer programs that collect Webpage information, index it, and make it possible to search the index (Levine, et al., 1997). There are three types of search engines differing in size and function. The first is known as an open-set engine that is usually very large; some examples are presented below along with their universal resource location (URL) or Internet address (Sullivan, 1998):

- AltaVista   www.altavista.digital.com
- Excite   www.excite.com
- Hotbot   www.hotbot.lycos.com
- Infoseek   www.infoseek.go.com
- MetaCrawler   www.metacrawler.com
- Webcrawler   www.webcrawler.com
- Yahoo   www.yahoo.com

The second type of search engine is the meta-search engine that enables the user to search more than one engine at the same time. The third type is the limited-set search engine that is limited in scope to a specific Internet protocol, medium, database, site, or personal computer (Sullivan, 1998). For example, site-specific search engines are available on the Websites of the American Academy of Audiology (www.audiology.org) and the American Speech-Language-Hearing Association (www.asha.org). Because details for effectively searching the Internet are beyond the scope of this chapter, readers are referred to sources listed here in "Recommended Readings." Appendix V-B contains some helpful tips for effectively searching the Internet (Sullivan, 1998); each search engine has a "help" page for users to consult.

Audiologyinfo, LLC was one of the world's first virtual audiologies companies, developed by Paul Dybala (1999). It ran some of the most advanced Websites related to audiology, hearing loss, and hearing aids. The Network's goal was to empower audiologists, students, and persons seeking information about hearing loss through access to information. One Website, Searchwave—an award-winning search engine devoted to the profession of audiology is now defunct. It documented nearly 2000 Websites. Searchwave's homepage had a directory with various categories (e.g., anatomy-physiology, clinics-services, conservation, disorders, assessment, manufacturers, personal pages, professionals, publishers, rehabilitation, science-research, and training-continuing education), a standard search mechanism, and a list of both new and "star sites" highly rated by users. Another Website for audiologists is Audiology Online(www.audiology .com) that provides online continuing education units (CEUs), articles, interviews, opportunities to ask experts questions, national chat rooms, classified ads, and links to important industry Websites. A glossary of Internet terms and tips for effective searching are located in Appendices V-A (Bloom, 1998; p. 128) and V-B (Sullivan, 1998), respectively.

Informatics

Another important contribution to outcomes measurement is "*informatics,*" a seamless interchange of information from person-to-person, person-to-computer, computer-to-person, and from computer-to-computer in areas of (Kreb & Wolf, 1997):

- Research and education (e.g., databases via the United States National Library of Medicine (www.nlm.nih.gov) with databases on health information; library services; research programs, and new, noteworthy, and general information
- Electronic publishing (e.g., availability of scientific journal articles for downloading such as the *American Journal of Audiology: A Journal of Clinical Practice* (www.professional.asha.org)
- Telemedicine (e.g., development of manufacturer assessment of hearing instrument function via the Internet, face-to-face counseling via computer video-conferencing)
- E-mail (e.g., fast communication from patient to clinician, accessibility to bulletin boards and listservs)
- Patient access (e.g., information regarding hearing loss, hearing aids, and aural rehabilitation; support groups, bulletin boards, and chat groups with others having hearing loss)

Audiologists interested in positive patient outcomes must be fluent in informatics. Information is powerful!

Evaluating Websites

Audiologists should critically evaluate Websites before recommending them to colleagues, students, and patients. So, how do you evaluate a Website? Appendix V-C, found on the companion CD-ROM, contains a *"Checklist for Evaluating Websites."* Evaluation of Websites requires consideration of the dimensions of currency, content/information, accuracy, authority, navigation, experience, multimedia, treatment, and miscellaneous factors. Currency of a Website is determined by how up-to-date it is. For example, has the last revision date been posted on the homepage? Has it been updated recently? Has the frequency of planned revisions been posted? A Website may not contain the most current information even though it may have been updated, however. It is best to crosscheck the currency of information with multiple sources.

The content/information of Websites must also be evaluated. For example, is the purpose of the site clearly stated? While it is fairly easy for audiologists to determine the purpose of a particular Website, the task may be difficult for patients who may not be critical consumers of information regarding hearing health care. Will the information provided be useful for undergraduate students, graduate students, audiologists, researchers, and/or patients? Some Websites are specific with regard to the targeted audience, while others have something for everyone. For example, the Websites of the American Speech-Language-Hearing Association (www.professional.asha.org) and the American Academy of Audiology (www.audiology.org) have specific pages for professionals and for consumers.

Websites must also be evaluated regarding the accuracy of the posted information. Audiologists must realize that even though information appears on the Internet, this does not guarantee that it is accurate. Internet users must be more critical when on the Internet than when considering the accuracy of information in trade journals, for example. Although generally not peer reviewed, the contents of trade journals at least undergo an editorial review prior to publication, whereas it is "surfer beware" on the Internet. The sources of information should be clearly stated on the Website and should be scrutinized according to the levels of evidence mentioned in Chapter 3. Another indication of adequate quality control of a Website is the use of proper grammar, correct spelling, and the absence of typographical errors. Furthermore, a credible Website should post the person(s) or organization(s) responsible for the accuracy of the information and means for contacting those individuals via E-mail or message boards. Lastly, the ultimate test of validity is if a panel of experts or authorities in the field favorably evaluates the Website.

The Website authors, managers, or organizations should be clearly identified and their reputations carefully scrutinized. Are those responsible for the Website authorities in the field? Are they accessible through E-mail, regular mail, or telephone? Does inspection of the domain name reveal the site's origin? The last three letters after the dot indicate the origin of the site. For example, ".com" is a commercial site, ".edu" is an educational site (e.g., college or university), and ".gov" is a government site. In general, educational and government sites should not be considered superior to commercial sites, but approached differently. Users should approach information presented by commercial sites with caution as it may be somewhat biased toward their products.

The basis of the navigation through a Website should be evident in its organization. Are the site's options clear on its homepage? Are the links easy to identify, logically grouped, and relevant to the overall subject matter? For example, links to all permanent supporting pages are easily identified in a column on the left-hand side of ASHA's homepage and are listed in alphabetical order. In addition, the homepage lay out should be consistent on all supporting pages with a link back to the homepage. All the ASHA Website's supporting pages have the same logical layout as the homepage with a link back to the homepage at their top, for example. Finally, the icons on the page should clearly represent what they intend. Links can be presented through icons, a picture, or through words. Many Websites, like ASHA's, use words to represent links rather than icons that are more easily misinterpreted.

Each Website should provide a unique experience to a user justifying the time spent during its exploration. The quality of the experience depends on the perspective of users and their purpose for visiting the Website. Thus, is the site worth the time and does it satisfy the general needs of students (e.g., undergraduate and graduate), audiologists, researchers, and/or patients? Furthermore, the Website should provide a visual and auditory pleasing experience through its layout (e.g., tasteful use of colors, fonts, and spacing) and use of multimedia (e.g., use of sounds, graphics, animation, and video). Engaging Websites use a "Goldilocks" approach to design, not too busy, not too plain, but just right.

Users must also carefully consider the Website's treatment of various subject matters and other miscellaneous factors. Is the site free from stereotyping? Are there any obvious biases toward the information presented in the Website? If so, audiologists should seek additional information on the topic and/or contrasting points-of-views from other sites. In addition, Websites should be evaluated on loading time, download options, per-use costs, security of private information, ease of printing, and availability of site-specific search engines. For example, Websites should load fairly quickly. After all, time is money especially if subscribing to an Internet service provider is based on the number of hours used per month. Websites should also provide a variety of download options, such as smaller images, text only, or non-frame versions. Top Websites can also be recognized by the type and number of commendations awarded, which are usually posted on their homepages. Users tend to prefer Websites that can be used either free-of-charge or require small fees for use or specific functions. Users need to be confident that the information provided on-line will be kept secure from third-party theft. Furthermore, users should be wary of Websites that innocuously ask for their name and E-mail address as a requirement for using the Website. Why is the information needed? Who will have access to that information and what will it be used for? Finally, users should be able to print information without having to reconfigure their systems, and, in short enough segments, to prevent a system-wide backup for others.

ACCESSING THE POTENTIAL OF COMPUTER TECHNOLOGY FOR OUTCOMES MEASUREMENT

This chapter has been difficult to write because the promise of personal computing for outcomes measurement, a recent focus for the profession, has yet to be realized. At first glance, it seems as if few are using personal computers for outcomes measurement. For example, only a few software programs are dedicated to or show potential for use in outcomes measurement in limited areas of audiologic practice. As discussed earlier and in greater detail in Chapter 6, UNHS programs are developing systems for aggregating data on quality indicators for local, state, and national benchmarks. We hope at this point that readers are taking issue with this point-of-view and can see the influence of personal computing at multiple levels affecting patient outcomes. Indeed, every patient who searches the Internet for information about hearing loss and hearing aids prior to seeking help from professionals has already formed some expectations regarding the possibilities of a positive outcome. Patients may then select a hearing health-care professional, but only from those audiologists who have created a Webpage advertising their private practices. The quality of services rendered may depend on whether that audiologist accesses the latest information on the Internet and considers the levels of evidence supporting the use of various audiologic procedures and products. Few hearing aid manufacturers post the results of the latest clinical trials supporting the efficacy of high-technology hearing aids over more conventional circuitry, however. Moreover, the hearing health-care industry, the American Speech-Language-Hearing Association, and the American Academy of Audiology should collaborate in aggregating efficacy data in a central database accessible to the public, government officials, and third-party payers on the World Wide Web.

Obviously, several steps must occur before the potential of personal computing can be realized for outcomes measurement. Readers may be thinking that, of course, all it takes is for software manufacturers to develop the outcomes measurement software for audiologists' use. Poof, problem solved! Unfortunately, the solution is not that easy. The process for developing software and computer-based data management systems actually begins with the rank-and-file audiologists' knowledge of outcomes measurement and a commitment to excellence in service delivery. To many audiologists, outcomes measurement is simply administering consumer satisfaction questionnaires to patients, eyeballing the data, and filing the results in a cabinet. However, what good are those data if they are not analyzed, used, and

shared with others? Therefore, the second step involves appropriate use of outcomes measurement of quality indicators at multiple interconnected levels toward system-wide benchmarks of hearing health-care excellence. HI-TRACK and SIMS software (discussed earlier) assist UNHS programs use outcomes measurement of quality indicators appropriately to achieve local, state, and national mandated benchmarks. Unfortunately, clearly defined quality indicators and benchmarks have not been established in other areas of practice. Thus, the third step involves identification of profession-wide outcomes at multiple levels throughout the various continua of patient hearing health care. For example, the hearing health-care industry needs to develop benchmarks and quality indicators for patient care from the point-of-entry at diagnosis of hearing loss to discharge from the rehabilitation process. What are the best measures of hearing handicap? What is a significant decrease in hearing handicap on those measures? Do different hearing instruments and circuitry result in a greater reduction of handicap? Answers to those questions are necessary prior to developing new or using existing software such as NOAH for an industry-wide data management and outcome measures aggregation system, for example. Finally, audiologists must believe in the "power of one" in providing feedback to software manufacturers. Software manufacturers need input for developing and modifying their products to suit the needs of practicing audiologists to meet their patients' needs in the new millennium.

SUMMARY

This chapter has considered the use of computers in outcomes measurement. Readers should understand the elements of computer-based data management systems; be able to describe the parts of a computer, their functions, and factors in purchasing different types of computers; consider the use and evaluation of software for outcomes measurement; and discuss the use of the Internet. These basic skills are necessary to visualize the potential of personal computing and the World Wide Web for creating efficient outcomes measurement systems that collect, analyze, aggregate, and disseminate data for quality indicators in the achievement of benchmarks across specific areas of audiologic practice and service-delivery sites.

LEARNING ACTIVITIES

- Draft a detailed letter to HIMSA suggesting use of software, such as NOAH 3.0 for use in an industry-wide hearing instrument outcomes measurement system.

- Visit the Websites of leading hearing aid and equipment manufacturing companies and determine the percentage that provide outcome data for their latest products.

- Develop a Web Guide for patients to use in critically evaluating information obtained on the Internet.

RECOMMENDED READINGS

Gralla, P., Ishida, S., Reimer, M., & Adams, S. (1999). *How the Internet works: Millennium edition.* Indianapolis, IN: Que Education and Training.

White, R., Downs, T., & Adams, S. (1999). *How computers work: Millennium edition.* Indianapolis, IN: MacMillan Computer Publishers.

REVIEW EXERCISES

Fill-in-the-Blank

Instructions: Please fill-in the blank below with the correct term from the word bank.

1. _____ _____ receive signals from outside the computer and send them inside.

2. _____ _____ _____ are microprocessor chips that accept instructions/data, execute those instructions, and then store the output in memory for later use.

3. _____ _____ is the limit of data and information that can be stored and the speed with which stored information can be retrieved.

4. _____ _____ stores the same types of information as internal memory, but for longer periods of time.

5. _____ _____ deliver the information from the computer to the user or another computer.

6. _____ _____ provide the power of a desktop computer that can be transported and used anywhere.

7. _____ _____ provide users with easy-to-use mobile personal-computing companions.

8. _____ is simply sets of instructions that control the operations of a computer, whether cutting, pasting, or displaying text; mathematically manipulating numbers; copying /editing documents, and so on.

9. The _____ is a network of communications media to which thousands of computers have been connected.

10. The _____ _____ _____ is a system that links together vast quantities of information from all over the world via the Internet.

11. _____ _____ are organized, hierarchically arranged catalogs of the World Wide Web consisting of major topic headings that are progressively broken down into more and more specific sub-topics.

12. _____ _____ are actually computer programs that collect Webpage information, index it, and make it possible to search the index.

Word Bank:

Central processing units
External memory
Handheld computers
Input devices
Internal memory
Internet
Notebook computers
Output devices
Search engines
Software
Web directories
World Wide Web

Matching\

Instructions: Please match the following items with the correct statements below.

I. Computer
II. Man

1. ____ Makes decisions
2. ____ Is adaptable
3. ____ Performs logical functions accurately
4. ____ Has common sense
5. ____ Automates routine functions economically
6. ____ Learns new methods and techniques

7. ____ Accumulates expertise
8. ____ Thinks
9. ____ Stores/retrieves data rapidly
10. ____ Calculates/performs programmed logical operations

ANSWERS

Fill-in-the-Blank:	Matching:
1. Input devices	1. II
2. Central processing units	2. I
3. Internal memory	3. I
4. External memory	4. II
5. Output devices	5. I
6. Notebook computers	6. II
7. Handheld computers	7. II
8. Software	8. II
9. Internet	9. I
10. World Wide Web	10. I
11. Web directories	
12. Search engines	

REFERENCES

American Academy od Audiology. (2000). Posiiton statement: Role of the audiologist in the newborn hearing screening program. *Audiology Today, 12*(3), 39.

Bloom, S. (1998). Hearing healthcare practitioners take a practical look at the Internet. *The Hearing Journal, 51*(6), 19–20, 22, 24–28.

Cox, R.M., & Alexander, G.C. (1995). The Abbreviated Profile of Hearing Aid Benefit (APHAB). *Ear and Hearing, 16,* 176–186.

Cox, R.M., & Alexander, G.C. (1999). Measuring satisfaction with amplification in daily life. The SADL scale. *Ear and Hearing, 20,* 306–320.

Denton, C. (2000). It's a small, small world: Size matters in the world of portable digital assistant. *Smart Computing in Plain English: Tough Questions and Straight Answers, 11(5),* 12–14.

Dodd, J. (2000a). Software: Questions and answers. *Smart Computing in Plain English: Tough Questions and Straight Answers, 11*(5), 42–46.

Dodd, J. (2000b). Hardware: Questions and answers. *Smart Computing in Plain English: Tough Questions and Straight Answers, 11*(5), 49–53.

Dybala, P. (1999). FYI: Building an audiology clinic/practice Web site. *Audiology Today, 11*(5), 16.

Feigal, D., Black, D., Hearst, N., Grady, D., Fox, C., Newman, T.B., & Hulley, S.B. (1988). Planning for data management and analysis. In S.B. Hulley & S.R. Cummings (Eds.), *Designing clinical research* (pp. 159–171). Baltimore, MD: Williams & Wilkins.

Gralla, P. (1997). *How the Internet works.* Emeryville, CA: Ziff-Davis Press.

Henry, H. (2000). Find the sources of online mysteries: Tracking down problems and solving them. *Smart computing reference series: Troubleshooting* (3rd ed., pp. 192–196). Lincoln, NE: Sandhills Publishing.

Johnson, C.E., & Danhauer, J.L. (2001). *A survey of audiologists on outcomes measurement.* Paper presented at the 13th Annual Convention and Exposition of the American Academy of Audiology, San Diego, CA.

Kreb, R.A., & Wolf, K.E. (1997). *NSSHLA clinical series 13: Successful operations in the treatment-outcomes-driven world of managed care.* Rockville, MD: National Student Speech-Language-Hearing Association.

Leeper, L.H., & Gotthoffer, D. (1999). *Quick guide to the Internet for speech-language pathology and audiology.* Boston, MA: Allyn & Bacon.

Levine, J., Young, M.L., & Reinhold, A. (1997). *The Internet for dummies: Quick reference.* Foster City, CA: IDG Books Worldwide.

Masterson, J.J., Wynne, M.K., Kuster, J.M., & Stierwalt, J.A.G. (1999). New and emerging technologies: Going where we've never gone before. *ASHA, 41*(3), 16–20.

Newman, C.W., Weinstein, B.E., Jacobson, G.P., & Hug, G.A. (1990). The Hearing Handicap Inventory for Adults: Psychometric adequacy and audiometric correlates. *Ear and Hearing, 11,* 430–433.

Newman, C.W., Jacobson, G.P., Weinstein, B.E., & Sandridge, S.A. (1997). Computer-generated hearing disability/handicap profiles. *American Journal of Audiology: A Journal of Clinical Practice, 6*(1), 17–21.

Oz, E. (1998). *Management information systems.* Cambridge, MA: Course Technology an International Thompson Publishing Company.

Phelps, A. (2000). Internet: Questions and answers. *Smart Computing in Plain English: Tough Questions and Straight Answers, 11*(5), 56–58.

Sims, D.G., & Gottermeier, L. (2000). Computer applications in audiologic rehabilitation. In J.G. Alpiner & P.A. McCarthy (Eds.), *Rehabilitative audiology: Children and adults* (3rd ed., pp. 556–571). Baltimore, MD: Lippincott Williams, & Wilkins.

Sullivan, R.F. (1998). Searching for information on the World Wide Web: Has an infinitude of monkeys created www.kinglear.com? *The Hearing Journal, 51*(6), 34, 36, 38–39.

Ventry, I.M., Weinstein, B.E. (1982). The hearing handicap inventory for the elderly: A new tool. *Ear and Hearing, 3,* 128–134.

Wynne, M.K. (2000). Page ten: An introduction to hand-held PCs. *The Hearing Journal, 53*(2), 10, 12,14, & 16.

APPENDIX V-A

Glossary of Useful Internet Terms

(Bloom, S. [1998]. Hearing healthcare practitioners take a practical look at the Internet. *The Hearing Journal, 51*[6], 19-20, 22, 24–28. Adapted with permission © Lippincott, Williams, & Wilkins, 1999)

The following list, while not exhaustive, will provide the average Internet user with a working vocabulary in the language of cyberspace.

ACCESS: . . . . to locate information electronically.

BOOKMARK: . . . . listing of an Internet location, for quick access.

BROWSER (also WEB BROWSER): . . . . . software that allows a computer to find and retrieve information on the Internet.

CHAT: . . . . interactive Internet "talk" by typing and sending messages.

CYBERSPACE: . . . . the realm of the Internet.

DATA: . . . . information stored in a computer, which can be accessed.

DATABASE: . . . . collection of information on a particular subject.

DOMAIN: . . . . title that identifies an Internet address, such as "wwilkins" for *The Hearing Journal.*

DOWNLOAD: . . . . to bring data from another computer to yours.

E-MAIL: . . . . electronic mail; sending messages via computer.

E-MAIL ADDRESS: . . . . user's location, such as dkirkwood@wwilkins.com (for the editor of *The Hearing Journal*).

EMOTICONS: . . . . emotion icons that e-mailers can use to express their feelings, such as smiles :) or frowns :(or winks ;-).

FAQ: . . . . frequently asked questions.

FREEWARE: . . . . software that can be downloaded without cost.

HACKER: . . . . experienced, knowledgeable computer user.

HARDWARE: . . . . keyboard, monitor, circuitry, and other elements that make up a computer.

HOMEPAGE: . . . . primary page of a Web site.

HTML: . . . . HyperText Markup Language, used to create electronic documents on the World Wide Web.

HTTP: . . . . HyperText Transport Protocol: protocol used to transport data on the Web.

HYPERLINK: . . . . icon or word a user can select to open a file.

ICON: . . . . picture or graphic that represents a program or file.

INTERNET: . . . . Worldwide collection of computer networks that can communicate with each other.

LINK: . . . . icon or word in a document or on a homepage that allows user to jump to another document that is related.

LISTSERV: . . . . mailing program on a particular topic that automatically e-mails relevant materials.

LOG ON (also SIGN ON): . . . . connect to the Internet.

LOG OFF (also SIGN OFF): . . . . disconnect from the Internet.

LURK: . . . . eavesdrop on "discussions" without participating.

MAILBOX: . . . . place where e-mail messages are stored; once read, they can be saved, deleted, forwarded, and/or answered.

MODEM: . . . . piece of electronic equipment that enables computer to transmit data over telephone line.

OFF-LINE: . . . . not logged on to the Internet.

ON-LINE: . . . . logged on to the Internet.

PROTOCOL: . . . . rules that govern the exchange of data between or among computers.

RECEIPT NOTIFICATION: . . . . message telling user that e-mail was delivered.

SEARCH ENGINE: . . . . program that searches for data on the Internet, prompted by insertion of a keyword.

SERVICE PROVIDER: . . . . organization that for a fee will provide a gateway to the Internet, such as America Online, MSN, CompuServe, and so forth.

SHAREWARE: . . . . software that can be downloaded and tried before being purchased.

SOFTWARE: . . . . programs or applications for wordprocessing, formatting, spreadsheets, games, and so forth.

SUFFIX: . . . . designation of origin of domain, such as ".com" for commercial, ".gov" for government, ".edu" for educational, or ".org" for organization.

URL: . . . . Uniform Resource Locator, a standard format in a World Wide Web address, such as http://www.anycompany.com.

USENET: . . . . giant bulletin board for information, postings, discussions.

WEBMASTER: . . . . a person who develops, builds, and maintains a Website.

WEBSITE: . . . . address on the Internet.

WWW: . . . . World Wide Web, written as www in an Internet address; a section of the Internet for text, graphics, and sound.

APPENDIX V-B

Helpful Tips for Effective Searching

(Sullivan, R.F. [1998]. Searching for information on the World Wide Web: Has an infinitude of monkeys created www.kinglear.com? *The Hearing Journal, 51*[6], 34, 36, 38–39. Adapted with permission © Lippinott, William, & Wilkins, 1999)

- Use search directories if you want to find information on a general topic. Search engines are best for gathering a universe of information on a highly circumscribed topic.
- Specialized directories with smaller, subject-oriented databases, tend to produce more valid, up-to-date samples of information.
- Make sure your spelling is correct for search engines.
- Be as specific as possible in your search request.
- Use quotations marks for phrases and names. Use capital letters to specify proper names and locations.
- Learn Boolean Operators described in the table on the next page to refine searches as used by different engines. Consult the engine or directory's HELP resource for details.
- Use multiple browser windows, one for the engine and one to explore sites.
- Don't look beyond the first page or two of results. Search again with different key words.
- Bookmark sites that look promising.
- Print out pages on-line for reference or reading when you are not at a computer. Make sure the URL prints on each page for reacquisition. If available as a feature on your search directory or engine, request notification of changes to sites of interest.

OPERATOR	EXAMPLE	APPLICATION
AND	ear AND infection	Requires both terms in the document, not necessarily adjacent.
+	+ear +infection	Same as above
"..."	"ear infection"	Requires adjacency of terms in phrase.
NOT	+"hearing aid battery" +zinc NOT mercury	Will require zinc and exclude documents mentioning mercury hearing aid batteries.
−	+ "hearing aid battery" +zinc −mercury	Same as above
OR	sensorineural OR "sensory neural"	Acquires documents with EITHER or BOTH terms.
[no operator]	recruitment "loudness growth"	Same as OR, above
NEAR	recruitment NEAR compression	Acquires documents where (in AltaVista) one term is within 10 words of the other.
[Nesting]	(analog OR digital) AND programmable AND "hearing aid"	Without parentheses, the search would be: Analog OR digital AND programmable AND "hearing aid"
[Wildcard]	Audiolog*	Acquires documents with audiology, audiologist, audiological
[Stopwords]	Portland NEAR "OR" AND Portland NEAR ME	Without quotes, engines may ignore OR or consider it an operator.
[Case sensitivity]	AuD OR Au.D.	Forces exact match, ignores auD, AUD, aud, AU.D., etc.

APPENDIX V-C
Checklist for Evaluating Webpages

The above-mentioned Appendix can be found on the companion CD-ROM.

C H A P T E R   6

Outcomes Measurement in Early Hearing Detection and Intervention (EHDI) Programs

L E A R N I N G   O B J E C T I V E S

This chapter will enable readers to:

- Discuss the current status of early hearing detection and intervention (EHDI) programs in the United States
- Contact centers that assist in implementation of EHDI programs
- Use checklists in completing important outcomes in the implementation of hospital and state EHDI programs (White & Maxon, 1999)
- Understand the importance of outcomes measurement in EHDI programs
- Know the important principles and benchmarks/quality indicators mentioned by the Joint Committee on Infant Hearing's Year 2000 Position Statement
- Consider the use of computer-based data management systems
- Understand the importance of state and national data management systems
- Use a worksheet in the achievement of EHDI program benchmarks

INTRODUCTION

"You've come a long way baby!" ... Yes, this catchy phrase can be applied to our profession's long fight for mandatory universal newborn hearing screening programs in the United States. Students in training often snicker at some of the early infant hearing screening procedures used in the 1960s and 1970s. But, we had to start somewhere. And some audiologists, such as Marion Downs, have been fighting for the establishment of such programs for their entire careers, which in Marion's case alone has spanned 6 decades. Some of the major milestones within the past two decades have included

the Healthy People 2000 statement (e.g., reducing the average age of identification of hearing loss to no more than 12 months), development of the automated auditory brainstem response unit (AABR) (Peters, 1986), proven effectiveness of transient-evoked otoacoustic emissions (Johnsen, Bagi, & Elberling, 1983), the NIH Consensus Statement, the Joint Committee on Infant Hearing Position Statement (JCIH, 1994), and so forth (Robinette & White, 1998).

On March 18, 1999, United States Congressman James T. Walsh (R-NY) introduced, the "Early Hearing Loss Detection, Diagnosis, and Intervention Act of 1999" (H.R. 2923) to the U.S. House of Representatives. The bill supported early detection, diagnosis, and intervention for newborns and infants with hearing loss. Specifically, the Walsh bill provides federal funding for state grants to develop early hearing detection and intervention (EHDI) programs. The bill also directed the Health Resources and Services Administration (HRSA), the Centers for Disease Control and Prevention (CDC), and the National Institute on Deafness and other Communicative Disorders (NIDCD) of the National Institutes of Health (NIH) to network in linking screening programs with community-based intervention programs, monitor the impact of EHDI activities, and provide technical assistance on data management and applied research.

In May of 2000, the "Joint Committee on Infant Hearing (JCIH) Position Statement 2000: Principles and Guidelines for Early Hearing Detection and Intervention Programs" was adopted unanimously by the American Speech-Language-Hearing Association's (ASHA) Legislative Council as well as by 5 of 6 organizations that comprise the JCIH: ASHA, the American Academy of Audiology (AAA), the American Academy of Pediatrics, the Council on Education of the Deaf, and the Directors of Speech and Hearing Programs in the State Health and Welfare Agencies (DSHPSHWA) (Boswell, 2000). Vignette 6-1 includes important portions of an article written by Susan Boswell with statements from Terese Finitzo, Ph.D., chair, and Allan O. Diefendorf, Ph.D., past chair of the JCIH.

What victories our profession has achieved. However, the founding fathers of Audiology would say,"Whoa! Stay the course! The battle is not yet over!" But, wait. Isn't recognition on Capitol Hill and victories in state legislatures enough? No. EHDI programs will not be known by those accomplishments. They will be known by their data.

In other words, destiny lies in the data and proving EHDI programs' worth through outcomes measurement, especially considering the recent statement made by the United States Preventative Service Task Force (USPSTF) that the efficacy of UNHS to improve long-term language outcomes remains uncertain (Thompson, et al., 2001). Therefore, the purpose of this chapter is to discuss methods of outcomes measurement for EHDI programs at local, state, and national levels. Although implementation of EHDI programs is not within the scope of this textbook, and thus will not be discussed in detail here, supplementary information for establishing EHDI programs is provided at the end of the chapter: (1) Appendix VI-A: "Contact Information for Centers Assisting in the Implementation of Early Hearing Detection and Intervention Programs," (2) Appendix VI-B: "Factors Predictive of Successful Outcome of Deaf and Hard-of-Hearing Children of Hearing Parents" (Yoshinaga-Itano, 1999), and (3) Appendix VI-C: "Outcome Checklist for Implementing Early Hearing Detection and Intervention (EHDI) Programs (Adapted from White & Maxon, 1999)." Appendix VI-C can be found on the companion CD-ROM.

JOINT COMMITTEE ON INFANT HEARING YEAR 2000 POSITION STATEMENT

Many of the current recommendations for the implementation of EHDI programs have resulted from the efforts of the American Academy of Pediatrics and the Joint Committee on Infant Hearing (JCIH). For example, in 1999, the "American Academy of Pediatrics Task Force on Newborn and Infant Hearing Statement on Newborn and Infant Hearing Loss: Detection and Intervention" endorsed the implementation of EHDI by reviewing the primary objectives and impor-

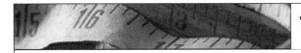

VIGNETTE 6-1

SOME STATEMENTS REGARDING EHDI PROGRAMS

Susan Boswell

... The JCIH position statement supports identification of hearing loss before age 3 months of age using physiologic tests, and intervention before 6 months.

"At the core of the EHDI lies the commitment to improving language development for children who are deaf and hard of hearing," said audiologist Terese Finitzo, JCIH chair.

"Research has shown that children who were identified and are receiving intervention before 6 months of age are functioning at a language level at age 5 on par with hearing peers," Finitzo said.

"The position statement is about accountability to our babies and families and to the state and federal governments," Finitzo said. Bolstered by data demonstrating the success of EHDI systems that have led to the passage of universal newborn hearing screening laws in 30 states, the position statement supports programs that include three core components: birth admission screening, follow-up medical and audiologic evaluation, and family-centered early intervention.

The statement, which updates the 1994 JCIH guidance on the establishment of EHDI systems, is used nationally and internationally as guidance in establishing preferred practices.

"EHDI systems should assure a seamless transition for infant and family from screening through intervention," Finitzo said.

The principles outlined in the position statement are designed to be used by clinicians who provide services to families in the process of early detection and intervention of hearing loss, as well as by administrators in health care and school systems.

"It's important that programs that are involved in intervention closely follow guidelines for Part C of the Individuals with Disabilities Education Act," said Allan Diefendorf, past chair of the JCIH and one of three ASHA representatives to the JCIH with Judith Gravel and Richard Folsom.

"The document may also be used by policymakers and third-party payers to look at what is the state of the art and science in EHDII," Diefendorf continued.

The JCIH position statement also links to the Healthy People 2010 national health objective 28-11 in the vision and hearing chapter (Vol. 11). That objective recommends increasing the proportion of newborns who are screened for hearing loss by 1 month of age, have audiologic evaluation by 3 months, and are enrolled in appropriate intervention services by 6 months.

(Reprinted with permission © American Speech-Language-Hearing Association, Boswell, S. (2000). Nurturing Newborns' Hearing: Joint Committee Statement Guides EHDI Programs. ASHA Leader, 5(12), 1, 7.)

tant components; it recommended screening parameters that define effective programs. A summary of the outcomes of that meeting is provided in Table 6-1 (Hall, 2000).

The Joint Committee on Infant Hearing (JCIH) supports early detection of, and intervention for, infants with hearing loss through integrated, interdisciplinary state and

Table 6-1. Summary of the American Academy of Pediatrics Task Force on Newborn and Infant Hearing, Statement on Newborn and Infant Hearing Loss: Detection and Intervention

Criteria to justify universal screening (for any disorder):
- A test with high sensitivity and specificity (to keep referrals to a minimum) that is easy to perform.
- No other clinical parameters can be used to detect the disorder.
- Early screening, diagnosis, and intervention improves outcome.
- Screening programs are acceptably cost-effective.

Guidelines for the *screening* portion of a universal newborn hearing screening program (UNHSP):
- At least 95% of newborns must be screened using a physiologic measure in both ears (the goal is 100% of the target populations).
- Screening must detect bilateral hearing loss > or = 35 dB HL.
- The false-positive rate for the screening technique (the percent of infants without hearing loss who fail the screening) should be < or = 3%, and the referral rate for subsequent formal audiologic assessment should be 4% or less.
- The screening technique should not miss any babies with hearing loss (a false-negative rate of 0%).
- OAEs and ABR, either alone or together, are acceptable screening methods, as both techniques "are non-invasive, quick (< 5 minutes), and easy to perform" (p. 527).
- Hospitals where babies are born should set up a UNHSP, designate a medical (physician) director, and assemble an adequate staff (the statement includes a listing of 10 detailed guidelines on the objectives and activities included in the screening program).

Guidelines for the *tracking and follow-up* portion of a UNHSP:
- For a program to be considered effective, at least 95% of all babies with a refer screening outcome initially should undergo follow-up diagnostic audiologic assessment (the goal is 100%). The same guideline applies for those infants who are not screened in the hospital and whose parents agreed to the screening.
- In agreement with programs required in Part C of the Individuals with Disabilities Education Act (IDEA), state departments of health should (see article for details):
  ⇒ Develop and maintain a centralized system for monitoring hearing screening programs (in the state)
  ⇒ Track all referral and miss outcomes (see above)
  ⇒ Communicate follow-up findings to the child's parents, physicians, audiologists, and speech-language pathologists
  ⇒ Verify hearing screening of babies not born in hospitals
  ⇒ Provide reports of the screening performance for each hospital
  ⇒ Provide reports of individual UNHSPs performance to the Centers for Disease Control and Prevention (CDC) Early Hearing Detection and Intervention Program

Guidelines for the *identification and intervention* portion of a UNHSP:
- The goal of universal screening is to identify all (100%) of infants who are born with hearing loss (see above criteria) by 3 months after birth, and to intervene appropriately by 6 months.
- The child's physician should direct and coordinate care for the child with hearing impairment, with appropriate support from others.

continues

Table 6-1. *(continued)*

- To provide expert services to infants with hearing loss, a regionalized approach to identification and intervention is necessary.
- Training and education of additional expert care providers will be needed due to the increased demand associated with the implementation of UNHSPs.

Guidelines for the *evaluation* portion of a UNHSP:
- Quality control should be maintained for each UNHSP by the state monitoring system.
- This system should also evaluate regularly the tracking and follow-up components of UNHSPs.
- In addition, state departments of health should evaluate regularly the intervention services within UNHSPs.

(American Academy of Pediatrics Task Force on Newborn and Infant Hearing, 1999)

national systems of EHDI programs, evaluation, and family-centered intervention (JCIH, 2000). The JCIH Year 2000 Position Statement is based on the following eight principles:

- "All infants have access to hearing screening using a physiologic measure. Newborns who receive routine care have access to hearing screening during their hospital birth admission. Newborns in alternative birthing facilities, including home births, have access to and are referred for screening before one month of age. All newborns or infants who require neonatal intensive care receive hearing screening before discharge from the hospital. These components constitute universal newborn hearing screening (UNHS).
- All infants who do not pass the birth admission screening and any subsequent rescreening begin appropriate audiologic and medical evaluations to confirm the presence of hearing loss before 3 months of age.
- All infants with confirmed permanent hearing loss receive services before 6 months of age in interdisciplinary intervention programs that recognize and build on strengths, informed choice, traditions, and cultural beliefs of the family.

- All infants who pass newborn hearing screening but who have risk indicators for other auditory disorders and/or speech and language delay receive ongoing audiologic and medical surveillance and monitoring for communication development. Infants with indicators associated with late-onset, progressive, or fluctuating hearing loss as well as auditory neural conduction disorders and/or brainstem auditory pathway dysfunction should be monitored.
- Infant and family rights are guaranteed through informed choice, decision-making, and consent.
- Infant hearing screening and evaluation results are afforded the same protection as all other health care and educational information. As new standards for privacy and confidentiality are proposed, they must balance the needs of society and the rights of the infant and family, without compromising the ability of health and education to provide care (American Academy of Pediatrics, 1999).
- Information systems are used to measure and report the effectiveness of EHDI services. While state registries measure and track screening, evaluation, and intervention outcomes for infants and families, efforts should be made to honor

a family's privacy by removing identifying information wherever possible. Aggregate state and national data may also be used to measure and track the impact of EHDI programs on public health and education while maintaining the confidentiality of individual infant and family information.

- EHDI programs provide data to monitor quality, demonstrate compliance with legislation and regulations, determine fiscal accountability and cost effectiveness, support reimbursement for services, and mobilize and maintain community support."

In addition, the position statement introduced, defined, and enumerated important benchmarks and quality indicators for birth admission hearing screening, confirmation of hearing loss, and early intervention. *Benchmarks* are quantifiable goals or targets for monitoring and evaluation. *Quality indicators* reflect a result in relation to stated benchmarks that are monitored using well-established practices of statistical process control to assess program consistency and stability (JCIH, 2000; Wheeler & Chambers, 1986). Figure 6-1 shows a child and parent who have benefited from EHDI programming.

Tables 6-2, 6-3, and 6-4 show those benchmarks and their respective quality indicators for birth admission hearing screening, confirmation of hearing loss, and early intervention, respectively. The benchmarks and quality indicators for birth admission hearing screening are clearly defined, but are not for confirmation of hearing loss and early intervention due to the lack of published data to provide targets (JCIH, 2000). Until such data are available, the JCIH recommends that programs should strive to provide care to 100% of infants needing services. Computer-based

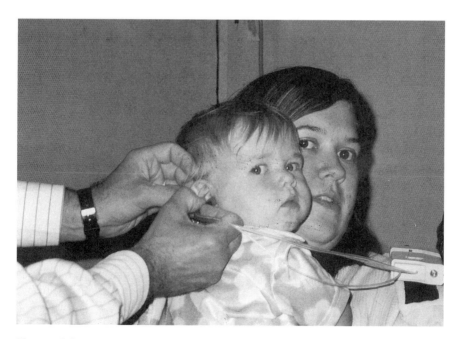

Figure 6-1. A young child and his mother who have benefited from early hearing detection and intervention (EHDI) efforts.

Table 6-2. Benchmarks and quality indicators for birth admission hearing screening

BENCHMARKS
- Within 6 months of program initiation, hospitals or birthing centers screen a minimum of 95% of infants during their birth admission or before 1 month of age.
- The referral rate for audiologic and medical evaluation following the screening process (in-hospital during birth admission or during both birth admission and outpatient follow-up screening) should be 4% or less within 1 year of program initiation.
- The agency within the EHDI program with defined responsibility for follow-up (often a state department of health) documents efforts to obtain follow-up on a minimum of 95% of infants who do not pass the hearing screening. Ideally, a program should achieve a return-for-follow-up of 70% of infants or more.

QUALITY INDICATORS
- Percentage of infants screened during the birth admission.
- Percentage of infants screened before 1 month of age.
- Percentage of infants who do not pass the birth admission screening.
- Percentage of infants who do not pass the birth admission screening who return for follow-up services (either outpatient screening and/or audiologic and medical intervention).
- Percentage of infants who do not pass the birth admission/outpatient screening(s) who are referred for audiologic and medical intervention.
- Percentage of families who refuse hearing screening on birth admission.

(Joint Committee on Infant Hearing, 2000).

Table 6-3. Benchmarks and quality indicators for confirmation of hearing loss

BENCHMARKS
Note: There are few published data available to provide targets for programs involved in confirmation of hearing loss. Until benchmark data that provide a goal are published, programs should strive to provide care to 100% of infants needing services.
- Comprehensive services for infants and families referred following screening are coordinated between the infant's medical home, family, and related professionals with expertise in hearing loss and the state and local agencies responsible for provision of services to children with hearing loss.
- Infants referred from UNHS begin audiologic and medical evaluations before 3 months of age or 3 months after discharge for neonatal intensive care unit infants.
- Infants with evidence of hearing loss on audiologic assessment receive an otologic evaluation.
- Families and professionals perceive the medical and audiologic evaluation process as positive and supportive.
- Families receive referral to Part C coordinating agencies, appropriate intervention programs, parent/consumer and professional organizations, and child-find coordinators if necessary.

QUALITY INDICATORS
- Percentage of infants and families whose care is coordinated between the medical home and related professionals.

continues

Table 6-3. *(continued)*

- Percentage of infants whose audiologic and medical evaluations are obtained before an infant is 3 months of age.
- Percentage of infants with confirmed hearing loss referred for otologic evaluation.
- Percentage of families who accept audiologic and medical evaluation services.
- Percentage of families of infants with confirmed hearing loss that have a signed Individual Family Services Plan (IFSP) by the time the infant reaches 6 months of age.

(Joint Committee on Infant Hearing, 2000).

Table 6-4. Benchmarks and quality indicators for early intervention

BENCHMARKS
Note: It should be the goal of the intervention component of an EHDI program that all infants be served as described below. Since specific benchmarks for early intervention have yet to be reported, target percentages are not noted here. The JCIH strongly recommended that these data be obtained so that benchmarks may be made available.

- Infants with hearing loss are enrolled in a family-centered early intervention program before 6 months of age.
- Infants with hearing loss are enrolled in a family-centered early intervention program with professional personnel who are knowledgeable about the communication needs of infants with hearing loss.
- Infants with hearing loss and no medical contraindication begin use of amplification when appropriate and agreed upon by the family within 1 month of confirmation of the hearing loss.
- Infants with amplification receive ongoing audiologic monitoring at intervals not to exceed 3 months.
- Infants enrolled in early intervention achieve language development in the family's chosen communication mode that is commensurate with the infant's developmental level as documented in the IFSP and that is similar to that for hearing peers of a comparable developmental age.
- Families participate in and express satisfaction with self-advocacy.

QUALITY INDICATORS
- Percentage of infants with hearing loss who are enrolled in a family-centered early intervention program before 6 months of age.
- Percentage of infants with hearing loss who are enrolled in an early intervention program with professional personnel who are knowledgeable about overall child development as well as the communication needs and intervention options for infants with hearing loss.
- Percentage of infants in early intervention who receive language evaluations at 6-month intervals.
- Percentage of infants and toddlers whose language levels, whether spoken or signed, are commensurate with those of their hearing peers.
- Percentage of infants and families who achieve the outcomes identified on their IFSP.
- Percentage of infants with hearing loss and no medical contraindication who begin use of amplification when agreed upon by the family within one month of confirmation of the hearing loss.
- Percentage of infants with amplification who receive ongoing audiologic monitoring at intervals not to exceed 3 months.

continues

Table 6-4. *(continued)*

- Number of follow-up visits for amplification monitoring and adjustment within the first year following amplification fitting.
- Percentage of families who refuse early intervention services
- Percentage of families who participate in and express satisfaction with self-advocacy.

(Joint Committee on Infant Hearing, 2000).

data management systems can facilitate the measurement and reporting of the effectiveness of EHDI services.

COMPUTER-BASED DATA MANAGEMENT SYSTEMS

Currently, there are two commercially available computer-based data management systems: (1) HI*TRACK, and (2) Screening Information Management Systems (SIMS) that are described below.

HI*TRACK Data Management Software (National Center for Hearing Assessment and Management, 2000:
Internet: www.infanthearing.org/software /index/html)

HI*TRACK is a computer-based data management system available from the National Center for Hearing Assessment and Management (NCHAM) at Utah State University. Recall that information about contacting the center appears in Appendix VI-A. HI*TRACK software is utilized by over 200 hospitals that use a wide variety of equipment including Clarity, AuDX, Algo, and IL088 screeners. The software was designed with input from dozens of hospital-based EHDI program managers to assist audiologists in directing successful programs. HI*TRACK can be used by a UNHS program that relies on otoacoustic emissions

(OAEs) or auditory brainstem responses (ABRs) to screen infants for hearing loss. Depending on the screening equipment used, the software can be linked directly to the screening software or it can function as a stand-alone system. HI*TRACK system requirements are:

- IBM compatible computer
- 15 megabytes (MB) of free hard disk space
- At least 486-33 processing capabilities
- 16 MB of RAM
- Windows 95, 98, or 2000 operating systems
- Additional hard disk space if more than 5,000 patients in the database

The HI*TRACK modules:

- Facilitate comprehensive data collection
- Generate letters to patients and physicians
- Compile data that can be used to improve screener performance
- Deliver a variety of essential tracking, follow-up, and administrative reports
- Electronically archive data where it can be retrieved when needed

HI*TRACK has three plug-in modules: (1) INFOLINK, (2) HI*SCREEN, and (3) HI*DATA.

INFOLINK and HI*SCREEN are both information collection modules that require a one-time-only recording of babies' identifying background information and screening results. INFOLINK is a Windows-based program that collects a wide range of critical variables at the onset of screening that is electronically transferred to the HI*TRACK module for essential patient tracking and data management. The use of the Windows-screen format with drop-down menus and user-friendly "click and fill" data-entry fields decreases user time and increases program accuracy. INFOLINK is a self-sufficient program that is useful for all currently available screening equipment. HI*SCREEN, on the other hand, is a DOS-based program designed for use by Otodynamics IL088 screeners. Similar to INFOLINK, the HI*SCREEN module facilitates accurate and efficient data recording and transfer on a wide variety of variables to HI*TRACK.

HI*DATA is a program within HI*TRACK that allows audiologists to transfer electronically hospitals' data to regional and administrative centers and state agencies. Hospitals are assigned a unique identifying code. With a simple keystroke, all new records and existing hospital records, updated since the last transfer, are extracted for transfer to the regional or state HI*TRACK database. Depending on the needs of the agency, the program has the flexibility to either include or exclude patients' identifying information. The electronic linking of HI*TRACK databases through the use of HI*DATA unifies separate efforts of hospitals, regional, and state agencies ensuring appropriate follow-up and outcomes measurement.

Special features in HI*TRACK enable EHDI personnel at the hospital or state level to:

- Customize the software through user-defined codes and definitions to reflect preferences of a program's participating hospitals, audiologists, screeners, and physicians.
- Establish a basic information database on all newborns screened, as well as expanded tracking databases (e.g., including diagnostic data and referral status) for infants receiving assessment or follow-up services.
- Produce both standardized and customized reports that communicate infant

screening/re-screening outcomes to parents and physicians.
- Generate timely reports on outcome data, including numbers and percentage of infants screened, missed or lost, or referred for further audiologic assessment and intervention for those found to have confirmed hearing loss.
- Create reports on user-selected variables of interest, such as infant birth weight or length of stay in the intensive-care nursery.
- Develop an archive of epidemiologic data specific to pediatric hearing loss, including risk indicators often associated with hearing loss and other disabilities.

As a non-profit organization, NCHAM's goal is to help audiologists meet the challenge of patient information and data management by offering HI*TRACK at the absolutely lowest, non-commercial price with different purchasing options. As time goes on, HI*TRACK will evolve into newer versions and purchasing options will change. Readers are encouraged to contact NCHAM (i.e., See Appendix VI-A) for information on the current version of HI*TRACK and purchasing options.

Information from Optimization-Zorn (OZ) Website (Optimization-Zorn Corporation, 2001:
Available Internet: www.oz-systems.com)

The Optimization Zorn (OZ) Corporation, based out of Dallas TX, has developed the Screening and Information Management Solutions (SIMS) © Windows-based software to help audiologists track important data in EHDI programs, from screening, to diagnosis, to intervention. Several states have selected SIMS for their state-wide computer-based data management system. OZ states that the success of any program is determined by its ability to detect newborns with hearing loss and to connect those children and their families to hearing health-care services. Contact information (i.e., address, phone number, and Website URL) can be found in Appendix VI-A.

SIMS is designed to manage information centered on the infant and contains the following components:

- Patient information
- Data archiving and backup
- Referral information
- User information
- Program management
- Data collection
- Transferring data

For example, Figure 6-2 shows the patient information page with seven levels of patient status identification: birth screening status, follow-up screening status, diagnostic status, status related to incidence based, delayed or progressive loss indicators, early intervention status, high-risk indicators, and the status of patient contact. Patient status identifier ensures that no children "fall through the cracks" (Johnson, 2000).

The system requirements for SIMS are as follows:

- Pentium processor or equivalent
- Windows 9x, Windows NT, Windows 2000, or Windows Millennium Edition (WINDOWS ME) operating system
- Minimum 32 MB RAM (64 MB RAM or higher is recommended)
- FAT 32 or NTFS file structure
- More than 10 MB of hard disk space for program files
- Hard drive capacity of 10 GB or more
- Modem

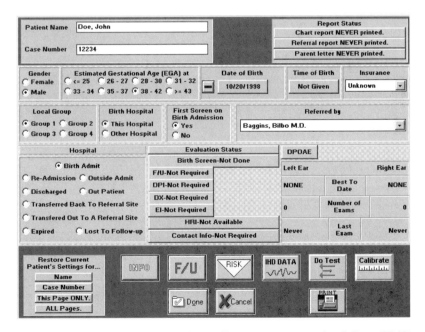

Figure 6-2. Screening and information management solution (SIMS) from OZ System's patients' information page with seven levels of patient status identification (Reproduced with permission © OZ Corporation, 2001).

- Internal ZIP drive
- Printer
- Configuration of hard drive (CPU) appropriate for UNHS volume and technology

SIMS is able to acquire data electronically from most testing technologies and incorporates screening results into the baby's record. SIMS Care Status enables audiologists to identify services that patients have received, the outcome of those services, and future tracking, follow-up, and diagnosis. SIMS is focused on enabling audiologists to overcome the follow-up and reporting challenges encountered in EHDI programs. SIMS generates user-defined reports automatically for stakeholders involved in an infant's care: parents, hospital staff, audiologists, physicians, insurers, educators, and so forth. Information may be imported or exported to hospital information systems to reduce data entry requirements further (Johnson, 2000). SIMS also notifies program personnel when a baby's next evaluation is past due, missed, or not scheduled. SIMS maintains comprehensive and integrated records for the life of the patient in a secure manner. SIMS transfer function permits the warehousing of patients' records in a central location from all test sites using a variety of media (e.g., floppy disk, Zip disk, etc.), modems, or secure Internet document transfer via E-mail (Johnson, 2000). SIMS data consolidation capability is critical to large hospitals with multiple screening sites and state programs wishing to maintain a secure, aggregated database (Johnson, 2000).

SIMS has some unique security features that ensure secure, efficient, and cost-effective patient data management. The specific security features include the following safeguards:

- Program managers can assign access limitations to screening support personnel
- Key patient information changes are not lost, creating a permanent audit trail

- Original, deleted, and merged patient files are maintained in the "background" for retrieval, if necessary
- During a transfer function, patient files are encrypted and compressed to ensure confidentiality
- Transferred patient files can have limited access to only a specified receiving location, at the sender's option
- ID "passwords" are assigned to each screener
- Automatic log-off and system "time-out" requires re-entry of ID code
- Loss of patient information is virtually impossible once saved to the hard drive.

The OZ has extensive program support services (PSS) consisting of experts and insiders in each of the areas of care. In-house experts are closely aligned with system users working in partnership with professionals in hospital, audiologic, medical, and educational sectors and public health arenas. PSS establish relationships that produce results for SIMS users through problem solving and achievement of goals. For example, OZ Systems' Help Desk/Technical Support Packages provide the security and convenience of knowing knowledgeable individuals (e.g., clinical audiologists) are available to answer questions and assist with screening program problems. Furthermore, PSS is focused on performance improvement through the use of features, such as "Just in Time Job Aid" (e.g., step-by-step instructions for hundreds of functions right at users' fingertips) and the SIMS comprehensive user's manual.

OZ systems provides focused training to hospitals when and where they want it either through "Detect and Connect" or Web-based training. "Detect and Connect" involves use of a training CD-ROM that accommodates instruction for one program manager and as many as 10 staff members (i.e., screeners). Training for program managers and staff members requires approximately 5 to 7 hours and 2 to 2 $1/2$ hours, respectively. Responding to the increased demand for accountability, OZ has included examinations for program managers and screeners on the CD-ROM that can be valuable in documenting performance.

Johnson (2000) stated that SIMS maintains an extensive series of performance indicators on all screeners and all screening equipment. For example, key information is maintained for individual support personnel and separate screening equipment within a facility, separate screening facilities or nurseries within a hospital, hospital aggregate population, and additional populations beyond the hospital, such as state departments of health (Johnson, 2000). These performance indicators assist programs exceed the Joint Committee on the Accreditation of Healthcare Organizations (JCAHO) and the National Committee on Quality Assurance (NCQA) requirements for quality control and program management (Johnson, 2000).

In summary, HI*TRACK and SIMS contain all six components of the computer-based data management systems introduced in Chapter 5 (Oz, 1998): (1) data (e.g., demographic and screening results), (2) hardware (e.g., screening equipment, computers/peripherals, and communication devices), (3) software (e.g., HI*TRACK and SIMS), (4) telecommunications (e.g., networking among computers within hospitals, modems connecting hospital databases to local, state, and national databases), (5) people (e.g., audiologists, UNHS screening personnel, physicians, patients, and their families), and (6) procedures (e.g., timetable for data analysis and program review). Furthermore, the interaction of these components determines the achievement of local, state, and national benchmarks. Directors of smaller EHDI programs may question whether the purchase of expensive software is needed to accomplish hospital goals. Furthermore, the question may be complicated by

audiologists' relationship with the particular hospital. Larger hospitals may have audiologists on staff who are in a much more advantageous position to convince administrators to purchase software than audiologists who are under contract to manage EHDI programs in smaller hospitals, whose administrators prefer to use "in-house" patient-information or "homemade" data management systems. Moreover, audiologists may be required to use software designated at the state level.

Hundreds of audiologists who may have fought long and hard to convince the medical establishment to establish EHDI programs in smaller regional hospitals from coast-to-coast are utilizing "homemade" data management systems. These heroic audiologists may believe that the purchase of HI*TRACK or SIMS software may be a luxury item and they should not "press their luck." However, by not advocating for a state-of-the-art computer-based data management system, these audiologists are putting their patients, their families, the hospitals, and themselves at risk. Risks management is now more commonly referred to as continuing quality assurance, ensuring that the performance of programs and services meet the needs of consumers (Marlowe, 1997). What are the major risks associated with not using a computer-based data management system? The inherent risks lie in patient-notification and follow-up (Marlowe, 1996). EHDI programs are useless unless results are documented, parents are notified, and follow-up services are implemented. Considerable liability might be lurking in audiologists' futures if errors and/or omissions occur. Thus, audiologists should ensure that their liability insurance is current, especially if they attempt to collect, disseminate, and archive large amounts of patient data by hand or non-standard programs.

Audiologists might remember a classic scene from the *I Love Lucy* series from the 1950s in which Lucy and Ethel were employed at a candy factory to wrap candies as they passed by on a conveyor belt. At first, the speed was nice and slow and Lucy and Ethel had no problem with their task. As the speed increased, however, Lucy and Ethel could not keep up, stuffing the unwrappable candies into their hats, clothes, and mouths. When using homemade "paper-and-pencil" data management systems, busy hospital-based audiologists may have a similar experience as more and more infants are born. What percent of babies born have had their hearing screened within one month of birth? What percent of babies were referred? Have all physicians been notified of screening results? Have those physicians informed parents of the results? What percent of the infants who were referred had their hearing evaluated by age three months? How do these statistics compare from month-to-month, from quarter-to-quarter, or year-to-year? Such questions are but a few that must be considered in evaluating the effectiveness of meeting program goals of universal screening, prompt evaluation, and early and effective intervention (JCIH, 2000). Reports from computer-based information management systems can assist individual program managers and direct the coordinating agency in measuring quality indicators associated with specific screening, evaluation, or intervention services (JCIH, 2000). Documenting patient outcomes and calculating statistics by hand can consume enormous amounts of valuable time and increase the likelihood of errors and omissions resulting in possible lawsuits.

The transfer of data for assessing quality indicators at hospital, health networks, and at state levels poses risks to the confidentiality of patients' records (Marlowe, 1996; 1997). The JCIH's Position 2000 Statement (JCIH) states that information systems that report the effectiveness of UNHS programs to state registries for measuring and tracking evaluation and intervention outcomes should do so and honor the privacy of infants and their families. Fur-

thermore, the Health Insurance Portability and Accountability Act (HIPAA), Public Law 104-191, requires use of a standard format for the electronic transmission of patient related information and further mandates compliance with patient privacy rules enacted to maintain the confidentiality of medical information (ASHA, 2001). The Health Care Financing Administration (HCFA) published standards for the Electronic Data Interchange (EDI) Rule, which would eliminate some 400 different formats for electronic health-care claims (ASHA, 2001). Audiologists who transmit health information electronically become "covered entities" and must comply with HIPAA and its EDI rule (ASHA, 2001). The Office of the Assistant Secretary (OAS) of the Department of Health and Human Services (DHHS) established, for the first time, a set of national Standards for Privacy that provides patients access to and protection of their personal information (e.g., name, address, social security number, or other data communicated either orally, on paper, or electronically) requiring a series of regulatory permissions for use and transmission (ASHA, 2001). The standards create new compliance issues for health-care professionals who engage in HIPAA standard electronic transmission of information including that involved in EHDI programs.

As stated earlier, both HI*TRACK and SIMS have mechanisms for protecting the confidentiality of patients and their families when reporting data for aggregation at state and national levels that homemade systems do not. Homemade systems rely on primitive data summary techniques, possibly gathered by clerical staff who may either not have access to records or may unknowingly release confidential data to third-parties without patient consent. Furthermore, computer-based data management systems have demonstrated efficacy in meeting the needs of large EHDI programs (Harrison, et al., 2000). Considering the liability risks in UNHS programs, audiologists will find that purchasing computer-based data management systems are wise expenditures in the long run and may be mandatory for participation in a data management system at the state level.

EHDI DATA MANAGEMENT SYSTEMS AT THE STATE LEVEL

Managing EHDI data is difficult at the local level, but even more so at the state level. Despite the passage of state laws mandating EHDI programs, creation of a state outcomes measurement system is time consuming. Currently, only a handful of statewide data management systems is in place for Texas, Colorado, Louisiana, and Utah (Marion Downs National Center [MDNC], 2000). For example, Colorado has long had a manual data management program for the Colorado Department of Public Health and Environment to aggregate data and calculate monthly statistics (e.g., the number of births, number screened, number referred at discharge, number missed, number refused, and number transferred), but it has recently taken the first step in developing a computer-based system by implementing an Electronic Birth Certificate (EBC) program (MDNC, 2000). In the past, the manual system was voluntary and dependent on the compliance of the audiologist or nursery coordinator to submit the monthly reports (MDNC, 2000). However, legislation now mandates monthly reporting of data and Colorado is utilizing data reporting systems already in place so hospitals are not implementing separate tracking and data management systems (MDNC, 2000). Currently, Colorado keeps track of children diagnosed with hearing loss in two ways. First, audiologists are requested to submit voluntarily a

Confirmed Hearing Loss Report for every infant diagnosed with hearing loss (MDNC, 2000). Second, most infants enrolled in early intervention in Colorado participate in the National Institutes of Health Grant, Family Assessment Program, awarded to the University of Colorado in 1994 (MDNC, 2000). The grant has enabled the accurate tracking of the date of intervention and the methods used for each infant.

Until centralized statewide tracking, reporting, and coordination of EHDI programs are mandatory, patients' and their families' rapid progression from screening, to diagnosis, to intervention will be an ongoing problem (Diefendorf & Finitzo, 1997; JCIH, 2000). States must work through the long and complicated process of devising efficient systems for collecting and managing data on critical quality indicators in the achievement of benchmarks (JCIH, 2000). Furthermore, outcome measures are required to justify the expenditure of taxpayers' money on EHDI programs. Moreover, advisory boards composed of key players (e.g., Maternal and Child Health (MCH) director, health department birth defects Registry Representative, Commission of the Deaf representative, Part H coordinator, department of education representative, pediatric audiologists, interventionists, and so forth) can be instrumental toward developing all aspects of a successful statewide system, including data management (NCHAM, 2000). Ultimately, states' data should be aggregated in a national database for benchmarking.

EHDI DATA MANAGEMENT AT THE NATIONAL LEVEL

Health care in the United States varies greatly from state to state and it is unlikely that the federal government will fund and manage a single permanent national EHDI outcomes measurement center. EHDI outcomes measurement at the national level is necessary if multi-state data are to be aggregated in such a way as to permit documentation of neonatal hearing loss, including prevalence and etiology across the United States (JCIH, 2000). Moreover, national professional organizations, such as ASHA and AAA, must assume leadership roles in outcomes measurement if data on quality indicators are to be aggregated toward achievement of national benchmarks for EHDI programs.

Why are national benchmarks important? National benchmarks are needed for several reasons. First, performance on quality indicators in the achievement of national benchmarks are necessary because the quality of health care, including audiologic service delivery, varies significantly from state-to-state, requiring a mechanism for comparison. Second, average national performances on quality indicators serve as a report card to audiologists regarding the status of hearing health care to the youngest citizens of this country. Third, collection of outcome data via national databases will assist in identifying benchmarks for diagnosis of hearing loss and early intervention services for young children diagnosed with hearing loss through establishment of national data sets. Recall that the JCIH Year 2000 Position Statement stated that further research was needed prior to establishing benchmarks in these areas. Fourth, outcomes measurement at the national level would generate data to examine the prevalence of hearing loss by state and region (JCIH, 2000). Fifth, these data could be used to support legislation for services to infants who are hard-of-hearing and deaf and their families (JCIH, 2000).

Currently, two federal agencies collect outcome measures pertaining to EHDI programs: 1) the Bureau of Maternal and Child Health (MCHB), and 2) Centers for Disease Control and Prevention (CDC) in conjunction with the Directors of Speech and Hearing

Programs in State Health and Welfare Agencies (DSHPSHWA) (JCIH, 2000). Currently, the CDC has a cooperative agreement with 15 states to promote state-based surveillance and tracking for EDHI. The MCHB requires that each state report the number of live births and the number of newborns screened for hearing loss during the birth admission (JCIH, 2000). Clearly, these data are not sufficient to satisfy data management needs at the national level. In 1999, a more comprehensive, but preliminary effort between the CDC and DSHPSHWA involved developing and reporting a national EHDI data set on variables, such as (JCIH, 2000):

- Number of birthing hospitals
- Number of birthing hospitals with UNHS programs
- The number of live births in the state
- The number of infants screened for hearing loss before discharge from the hospitals
- The number of infants referred for audiologic evaluation before one month of age
- The number of infants with an audiologic evaluation before three months of age
- The number of infants with permanent congenital hearing loss
- The mean, median, and minimum age of diagnosis of hearing loss for infants identified through UNHS programs
- The number of infants with permanent hearing loss receiving intervention by 6 months

Current results for this data set are available on the Internet on the CDC Website under EHDI National Database (Available Internet: www.cdc.gov/ncbddd/ehdi/home).

Several other potential mechanisms for a permanent national outcomes measurement currently exist. Besides the CDC, the most obvious is ASHA's National Center for Treatment Effectiveness in Communication Disorders (NCTECD) that operates the

National Outcomes Measurement System (NOMS). Recall that NOMS evolved from the development of the Task Force on Treatment Outcomes and Cost Effectiveness that was formed in 1993. One charge of that group was to review existing national databases, but the Task Force did not believe that any of them could meet the needs of the professions. During 1994–1996, the Task Force worked to begin development of a national database for the professions. Recognizing the extent of the task, the National Center for Treatment Effectiveness in Communication Disorders (NCTED) was formed to coordinate all outcomes and efficacy related work for the Association. Since 1997, most of the emphasis of the Center has been focused on the development of NOMS. Until late 1999, NOMS primarily involved outcomes measurement in speech-language pathology. The first audiology component of NOMS involved UNHS to determine outcomes associated with audiologist-managed programs. The development of the UNHS component of NOMS included a national call for participants from the nation's UNHS programs to participate in the initial development of the registry. Over 20 centers were selected to participate in NOMS and staff had to undergo extensive training on how to use SIMS. Readers are encouraged to watch for further news from ASHA regarding the UNHS component of NOMS.

Multicenter research projects provide another instance of establishment of national databases such as through a recent project sponsored by the National Institutes of Health entitled, "Identification of Neonatal Hearing Impairment" (Norton, et al., 2000a). The purpose of that study was to determine the accuracy of three measures of peripheral auditory system status (transient evoked otoacoustic emissions, distortion product otoacoustic emissions, and auditory brainstem response) (Norton, et al., 2000a) used in seven institutions from around the country

(e.g., Nebraska, Washington, Kansas, California, and Rhode Island), involving more than 7,179 infants from neonatal intensive care nurseries and well-baby nurseries (Norton, et al., 2000b). Not only was a large amount of data collected on each infant, monthly reports were generated to monitor subject enrollment, check for data completion, and perform data integrity checks necessitating the need for an overall, large central database at a core site (Harrison, et al., 2000). The national computer-based data management system assisted in ensuring the quality of the data collection process and analyzing the data (Harrison, et al., 2000). Unfortunately, such databases often cease operation after completion of the investigations.

Other possible permanent mechanisms for outcomes measurement at the national level include the American Academy of Audiology, the National Center for Hearing Assessment and Management (NCHAM), and the Marion Downs National Center for Infant Hearing. The authors believe that both AAA and ASHA should collaborate in developing a national UNHS database and registry. Unfortunately, many AAA members feel alienated by ASHA even going so far as resigning their memberships from the organization and seeking board certification through AAA. A unified approach is essential because the early intervention component of UNHS programs requires a team effort of professionals, including audiologists and speech-language pathologists. At this time, AAA has not been involved in working with ASHA in the development of the UNHS component of NOMS. NCHAM (www.infanthearing.org) was established at Utah State University and has been instrumental in assisting hundreds of hospitals to implement UNHS programs utilizing operational programs, disseminating information, and refining screening technology, and managing data. NCHAM developed the HI*TRACK data management software package used in hundreds of hospitals. The center may be an excellent mechanism for the aggregating and tracking outcome data at the national level. Similarly, the Marion Downs National Center for Infant Hearing was established by a federal grant from the U.S. Public Health Service to serve as a hub for the coordination of statewide systems for screening, diagnosis, and intervention for 17 states: Alabama, Arizona, Arkansas, Colorado, Hawaii, Kansas, Louisiana, Massachusetts, Michigan, Minnesota, New Mexico, Oklahoma, Rhode Island, Tennessee, Texas, Virginia, and Wyoming. A primary goal of the Center was to establish EHDI programs in those 17 states by the year 2000 and nationwide efforts of data aggregation involving those participants are underway.

WHERE DO WE GO FROM HERE?

The JCIH's Year 2000 Position Statement provides guidelines for audiologists involved in UNHS programs. Audiologists managing EHDI programs in small regional hospitals can get overwhelmed wading through all the information available on Websites, reading the literature in scientific journals, and monitoring state and federal legislation. Outcomes measurement is a small, but very important, part of EHDI programs.

What are some steps that audiologists out there in the trenches can take to get some perspective? First, audiologists must be able to visualize the "big picture" of state and national EHDI programs and their program's place within it. For example, questions to consider are what is the status of EHDI programs in my state? What types of data management systems, if any, are in place? How is my hospital linked to local agencies and school systems responsible for intervention services? How do I fit in and what is my role in outcomes management? Figure 6-3 shows a schematic of the interconnections between local, state, and national data management systems.

Second, audiologists must understand both the "top-down" and "bottom-up" interrelationships between and among these components. For example, "top-down" communication involves requests for information flowing from the national level, to the state level, to the local hospital and the practitioner. Alternatively, "bottom-up" communication includes the flow of that information from the hospital and the practitioner, to the state level, and to the national level. Third, practitioners need to realize that leadership and direction in data management systems flows not only from the top-down, but also from the bottom-up, within a dynamic relationship. For example, EHDI teams cannot afford to take a "wait and see" attitude and look for directives from above. EHDI teams at local levels may need to "lead the way" by adopting the "gold standard" of outcomes measurement in achieving the JCIH (2000) benchmarks. Fourth, audiologists must lead the way in quality assurance by participating in outcomes measurement according to the principles of continuous quality improvement (CQI) (Hosford-Dunn, Dunn, & Harford, 1995; Reisberg & Frattali, 1990; Walton, 1986). For example, managers and other EHDI team members should schedule monthly coordination meetings to review program performance on quality indicators toward achievement of JCIH (2000) benchmarks through the use of the "Worksheet for Evaluating Performance on Quality Indicators in Early Hearing Detection and Intervention (EHDI) Programs" found in Appendix VI-D. Column one on the worksheet has the benchmarks (i.e., goals) along with their respective quality indicators. Using computer-based data management programs like HI*TRACK or SIMS, program managers can calculate current and prior performances on key quality indicators and highlight those areas not "up to par" with respective bench-

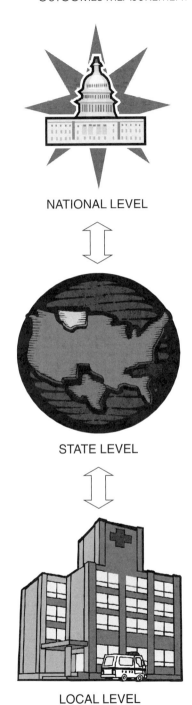

NATIONAL LEVEL

STATE LEVEL

LOCAL LEVEL

Figure 6-3. Interrelationships between and among local, state, and national data management systems.

marks to be addressed during EHDI team meetings. The third and fourth columns can be used to record notes from team discussions and specific courses of action to be taken to improve program performance, respectively. Fifth, audiologists should obtain outcome measures from a variety of stakeholders in EHDI programs. For example, collecting outcome data from parents' perceptions of EHDI programs can be extremely valuable regarding improvement in streamlining the process for patients and their families in transitioning from screening, to diagnosis, to intervention. In summary, audiologists and other practitioners must not wait for answers to come from higher levels, but can plot a course for local excellence now and advocate for implementation of higher standards at state and federal levels.

interrelationships within and among the local, state, and federal components of data management systems. In previous chapters, we mentioned the need for clinicians to recognize the "power of one" and that they can and do make a difference in their individual spheres of influence. Individual leadership can go a long way in the establishment of excellence at higher and higher levels. In spite of all the progress made in mandating EHDI programs in more than 30 states, all but a few have fallen short of "universal reimbursement," leaving audiologists to lobby for funds to establish adequate resources to implement the legislation they have supported for so long (Jacobson, 2000). The best way of lobbying for funds is through outcomes measurement demonstrating the efficacy of these programs. Indeed, our destiny is in the data.

SUMMARY

Outcomes measurement through computer-based data management systems is the barometer of performance for EDHI programs. Audiologists and other practitioners must understand the mechanisms for and

RECOMMENDED READINGS

Bess, F.H. (1998). *Children with hearing impairment: Contemporary trends.* Nashville, TN: Vanderbilt Bill Wilkerson Press.
Joint Committee on Infant Hearing (2000). Year 2000 position statement: Principles

---

LEARNING ACTIVITIES

■ Visit the Websites of the National Center for Hearing Assessment and Management (NCHAM: www.infanthearing.org) and the Marion Downs National Infant Hearing Center (www.colorado.edu/slhs/mdnc), download and print out all available information to create a guide for the implementation of EHDI programs.

■ Write a proposal to hospital administrators justifying purchase of a computer-based data management system for a UHNS program.

■ Compare both HI*TRACK and SIMS, state their advantages/disadvantages, and decide which you prefer.

■ For each benchmark in the JCIH's Year 2000 Position Statement, list possible causes of poor performance in EHDI programs.

and guidelines for early hearing detection and intervention programs. *American Journal of Audiology: A Journal of Clinical Practice, 9*(1), 9–29.

National Institute on Deafness and Other Communication Disorders. (1997). *Recommendations of the NIDCD Working Group on Early Identification of Hearing Impairment on acceptable protocols for use in state-wide universal newborn hearing screening programs.* Bethesda, MD: NIDCD Clearinghouse .

White, K.R., & Maxon, A.B. (1999). *Early identification of hearing loss: Implementing universal newborn hearing screening programs (MCHK125).* Vienna, VA: National Maternal and Child Health Clearinghouse.

REVIEW EXERCISES

Multiple Choice

Instructions: Please select the best answer for each item below.

1. Which are components in early hearing detection and intervention programs?
   A. Screening
   B. Diagnosis
   C. Intervention
   D. All of the above

2. What are "benchmarks?"
   A. Results in relation to a target
   B. Quantifiable goals
   C. Both A and B
   D. None of the above

3. What are "quality indicators?"
   A. Results in relation to a target
   B. Quantifiable goals
   C. Both A and B
   D. None of the above

`4. The Joint Committee on Infant Hearing Year 2000 Position Statement (JCIH, 2000) has clearly defined values for benchmarks for what components of EHDI programs?
   A. Screening
   B. Diagnosis
   C. Intervention
   D. B and C
   E. All of the above

5. In what direction(s) can the communication flow in multi-component data management systems (i.e., local hospitals, state, and national levels)?
   A. Top-down
   B. Bottom-up
   C. A and B
   D. None of the above

ANSWERS

1. D
2. B
3. A
4. A
5. C

REFERENCES

American Academy of Pediatrics Task Force on Newborn and Infant Hearing. (1999). Newborn and infant hearing: Diagnosis and intervention. *Pediatrics, 103,* 527–529.

American Speech-Language-Hearing Association. (2001). *An introduction to the Health Insurance Portability and Accountability Act for speech-language pathologists and audiologists.* Available Internet: www.professional.asha.org/governmental_affairs/hipaa.

Boswell, S. (2000). Nurturing newborns' hearing: Joint committee statement guides EHDI programs. *The Asha Leader, 5*(12), 1,7.

Diefendorf, A.O., & Finitzo, T. (1997). The state of information. *American Journal of Audiology: A Journal of Clinical Practice, 6*(3), 91.

Hall, J.W. (2000). *Handbook of otoacoustic emissions.* Clifton Park, NY: Delmar Thomson Learning.

Harrison, W.A., Dunnell, J.J., Mascher, K., Fletcher, K., Vohr, B.R., Gorga, M.P., Widen, J.E., Cone-Wesson, B., Foslom, R.C., Sininger, Y.S., Norton, S.J. (2000). Identification of neonatal hearing impairment: Experimental protocol and database management. *Ear and Hearing, 21,* 357–372.

Hosford-Dunn, H., Dunn, D.R., & Harford, E.R. (1995). *Audiology business and practice management.* San Diego, CA: Singular Publishing Group.

Jacobson, G. (2000). "Universal reimbursement" for "universal newborn hearing screening?" *American Journal of Audiology: A Journal of Clinical Practice, 9*(2), 2.

Johnsen, N.J., Bagi, P., & Elberling, C. (1983). Evoked otoacoustic emissions from the human ear. III. Findings in neonates. *Scandinavian Audiology, 12,* 17-24.

Johnson, M.L. (2000). OZ systems. In J.W. Hall, *Handbook of otoacoustic emissions* (pp. 362–366). Clifton Park, NY: Delmar Thomson Learning.

Joint Committee on Infant Hearing. (1994). Joint Committee on Infant Hearing year 1994 position statement. *ASHA, 36*(12), 38–41.

Joint Committee on Infant Hearing. (2000). Joint Committee on Infant Hearing year 2000 position statement: Principles and guidelines for early hearing detection and intervention programs. *American Journal of Audiology: A Journal of Clinical Practice, 9*(1), 9–29.

Marion Downs National Center for Infant Hearing. (2001). *Marion Downs National Center for Infant Hearing.* Available Internet: www.colorado.edu/slhs/mdnc.

Marlowe, J.A. (1996). Legal and risk management issues in newborn hearing screening. *Seminars in Hearing, 17*(2), 153–163.

Marlowe, J.A. (1997). The risk management perspective of the universal detection of hearing loss in newborns. *American Journal of Audiology: A Journal of Clinical Practice, 6*(3), 100–102.

Merriam-Webster-Online. (1999). Available Internet: www.merriamwebster.com.

National Center for Hearing Assessment and Management. (2000a,b, & c). *HI*TRACK data management software.* Available Internet: www.infanthearing.org.

Norton, S.J., Gorga, M.P., Widen, J.E., Folsom, R.C., Sininger, Y., Cone-Wesson, B., Vohr, B.R., & Fletcher, K.A. (2000a). Identification of neonatal hearing impairment: A multicenter investigation. *Ear and Hearing, 21,* 348–356.

Norton, S.J., Gorga, M.P., Widen, J.E., Folsom, R.C., Sininger, Y., Cone-Wesson, B., Vohr, B.R., & Fletcher, K.A. (2000b). Identification of neonatal hearing impairment: Summary and recommendations. *Ear and Hearing, 21,* 529–535.

Optimization Zorn Corporation. (2000). Newborn hearing screening. Available Internet: www.oz-systems.com.

Peters, J.G. (1986). An automated infant screener using advanced evoked response technology. *The Hearing Journal, 39,* 25–30.

Reisberg, M., & Frattali, C. (1990). Toward total quality management. *Quality Assurance Digest,* 1–5.

Robinette, M.S., & White, K.R. (1998). The state of newborn hearing screening. In F. Bess (Ed.), *Children with hearing impairment: Contemporary trends* (pp. 54–67). Nashville, TN: Vanderbilt Bill Wilkerson Press.

Thompson, D.C., McPhillips, H., Davis R.L., Lieu, T.A., Homer, C.J., & Helfand, M. (2001). Universal newborn hearing screening programs: Summary of evidence. *Journal of American Medical Association, 286,* 2000–2001.

Walton, M. (1986). *The Deming management method.* New York, NY: Pedigree/Putnam.

Wheeler, D.J., & Chambers, D.S. (1986). *Understanding statistical process control.* Knoxville, TN: SPC Press, Inc.

White, K.R., & Maxon, A.B. (1999). *Early identification of hearing loss: Implementing universal newborn hearing screening programs (MCHK125)*. Vienna, VA: National Maternal and Child Health Clearinghouse.

Yoshinaga-Itano, C. (1997). Rationale for and outcomes from the establishment and implementation of UNHS: The Marion Downs Program. In T. Finitzo, C. Yoshinaga-Itano, Y. Sininger, & E. Cherow (Eds.), *From advocacy to intervention: Steps for successful establishment of universal newborn hearing screening (UNHS) programs* (pp. 1–34). Rockville, MD: American Speech-Language-Hearing Association.

APPENDIX VI-A

Contact Information for Centers Assisting in Implemention (EHDI) Programs

MARION DOWNS NATIONAL CENTER FOR INFANT HEARING

Address: Marion Downs National Center for Infant Hearing
                University of Colorado at Boulder
                Department of Speech, Language, and Hearing Science
                Campus Box 409
                Boulder, CO 80309-0409

Phone: (303)492-6283

Website URL: http://www.colorado.edu/slhs/mdnc/

Site Contents: • An Overview
                • Program Goals
                • Technologies
                • State Programs
                • Non-funded States
                • Grant Members
                • Resources and Research
                • Statewide Systems
                • Staff
                • Upcoming Events
                • Marion Downs Profile
                • Internet Links

NATIONAL CENTER FOR HEARING ASSESSMENT AND MANAGEMENT (NCHAM) AT UTAH STATE UNIVERSITY

Address: National Center for Hearing Assessment and Management
                Utah State University
                2880 Old Main Hill
                Logan, UT 84322-2880

Phone: (435)797-3584

APPENDIX VI-A continued from page 137

Website URL: http://www.infanthearing.org/

Site Contents: Site Guide
- Our Background
- National EHDI Technical Assistance System
- Research Projects
- Sound Ideas Newsletter
- Bulletin Board
- Search Site

The Basics
- EHDI Information and Resource Center
- Newborn Hearing Screening
- Diagnostic Audiology
- Early Intervention
- Data Management
- Family Support
- Medical Home
- Program Evaluation Tools

In the USA
- Status of EHDI in USA
- Legislative Activities
- What's Happening in My State?
- State EHDI Grants
- JCIH 2000

More
- Screening Equipment Loan Program
- Frequently Asked Questions
- Issues and Evidence
- Slideshows and Videos
- Abstracts and Citations
- On the Calendar
- Links

OPTIMIZATION-ZORN CORPORATION— SCREENING INFORMATION MANAGEMENT SOLUTIONS (SIMS)

Address: Optimization-Zorn Corporation
                    2515 McKinney Avenue
                    Suite 850
                    Dallas, TX 75201

Phone: TOLL FREE 1-(888)-SCREENME
                               1-(888)-727-3366

FAX: (214)-631-4231

Website URL: http://www.oz-systems.com/

APPENDIX VI-B

Factors Predictive of Successful Outcome of Deaf and Hard-of-Hearing Children of Hearing Parents
Christine Yoshinaga-Itano (1997)

- Children whose hearing losses are identified before 6 months of age have expressive and receptive language developmental quotients (DQs) significantly higher (an average 20 DQ points) than children whose hearing losses are identified after 6 months of age. Both early and later identified children received immediate (within an average of 2 months post-identification of hearing loss) intervention services which were individually tailored by developmental assessment data.

- Children with either normal cognitive development or with impaired cognitive development whose hearing losses are identified by 6 months of age have significantly better language development than children whose hearing losses are identified after 6 months of age.

- Children with normal cognitive development whose hearing losses are identified before 6 months have language development within the normal range.

- Children with mild, moderate, moderate-severe, severe and profound sensorineural hearing losses demonstrate this effect of identification of hearing loss by 6 months of age.

- Children educated primarily through spoken language and children educated predominantly through a combination of sign language and spoken language evidence this effect of identification of hearing loss by 6 months of age.

- The impact of identification of hearing loss by 6 months of age is present regardless of gender, presence of secondary disability, level of socioeconomic status or age at testing (from 12 months through 36 months).

- Children with normal cognitive development and hearing loss identified before 6 months of age have significantly more words in their vocabulary than children identified after 6 months of age.

- Children with normal cognitive development and hearing loss identified after 6 months of age have vocabulary size which is not significantly different from children with impaired cognitive development and hearing loss identified before 6 months of age.

- Children with normal cognitive development and hearing loss identified before 6 months of age have vocabulary sizes at 31-36 months which are significantly larger than children with normal cognitive development and hearing loss identified after 6 months of age.

APPENDIX VI-C

Outcome Checklist for Implementing Early Hearing Detection and Intervention (EHDI) Programs

(Adapted from White & Maxon, 1999)

The above-referenced Appendix can be found on the companion CD-ROM.

APPENDIX VI-D

Worksheet for Evaluating Quality Early Hearing Detection and Intervention (EHDI) Programs

(Adapted from the Joint Committee on Infant Hearing Year 2000 Position Statement)

The above-referenced Appendix can be found on the companion CD-ROM.

CHAPTER 7

Outcomes Measurement in Diagnostic Audiology

LEARNING OBJECTIVES

This chapter will enable readers to:

- Acknowledge the role of outcomes measurement in diagnostic audiology
- Assess the performance of diagnostic tests and protocols
- Take necessary steps toward a proper perspective of outcomes measurement in diagnostic audiology

INTRODUCTION

In Chapter 2, we defined an outcome as a result of an intervention (Frattali, 1996). Doesn't intervention imply rehabilitation, treatment, and/or management? What are some outcomes for diagnostic audiology? Are there important outcomes for patients, their families, practitioners, and for society in general? Readers may be surprised to find that the answer to all these questions is an unqualified, yes! Positive outcomes for patients and their families include valid diagnostic testing that identifies hearing impairment when present and also suggests a course of management and rehabilitation.

Consider Cynthia's and Margaret's story in Vignette 7-1.

We will return to their story a bit later. However, Cynthia's question is a valid one. How can there not be a good diagnostic test for Alzheimer's disease? What is meant by a "good" diagnostic test in audiology? How does it differ from a "bad" diagnostic test? How do audiologists determine whether a test is good or bad? Does it depend on its validity and reliability? How are the reliability and validity of diagnostic measures determined? The purposes of this chapter are to: (1) acknowledge the role of outcomes

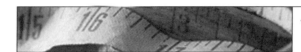

VIGNETTE 7-1

CYNTHIA AND MARGARET'S STORY

PART I

Honk! "Hey lady, move it!" yelled an irate motorist out his window at Cynthia, a forty-something soccer mom, who let her attention drift one warm September day as she was stuck in the late afternoon traffic. She had just left work staying longer than she had wanted to help a co-worker install some new software. Six months ago, Cynthia would have been angered by being caught in traffic, yelled at, and hopelessly late picking her two children up from daycare. However, Cynthia had bigger problems keeping her occupied.

In just six months, Cynthia's entire world had changed—a nasty divorce, the death of her father, and the recent decline of her mother who lived nearby in the old family home. Cynthia was numb. Feeling abandoned by her forty-something ex-husband, who suddenly expressed a need to "find himself," and grief from the loss of her father from a massive stroke, Cynthia had little time for self-pity. She knew she was the only one who could help her mother, Margaret, cope with her loss, and to assure her children that they were still loved and that, somehow, everything would be all right.

Cynthia was a survivor, but even the smallest decisions were difficult at first. Could she afford to stay in her family home? Money was tight and even with child support she couldn't manage the mortgage on what was once her "dream home" on her salary only. Soon, she found a child-friendly condominium close to her children's school. Of even more concern was how could she and her ex-husband minimize the amount of stress on the children? She soon discovered that her children took the situation quite well and viewed it as an adventure. Either they were more resilient than she had expected or were too young to realize that life, as they had known it, was changed forever. Of bigger concern was, what was wrong with her mother? She felt comfortable taking care of her children's needs, because she was their mom, but the role of caretaker to her mother seemed strange. Cynthia realized that she had been in denial and just assumed that her parents would always be there. Well, Dad was gone and her mom seemed to need her more and more each day. She called her mother twice each day, but she only answered about half the time, necessitating daily visits across town. Cynthia noticed that although her mother was dressed and the house was clean, her mother's spark was gone, she often misunderstood what she was saying, and was losing weight. Cynthia was afraid that her mother had early-Alzheimer's disease. She had visions of her mother slipping away day-by-day. From what she read, there were no definitive tests for the disease. How can there not be a good diagnostic test for this disease that is so devastating to both victims and their families?

Cynthia had been so preoccupied, that she was surprised to find herself in the parking lot of the daycare center. At least she had resolved that evening she would call her mother's long-time physician, an old family friend, to discuss her fears.

measurement in diagnostic audiology, (2) review methods for determining the validity and reliability for diagnostic tests and protocols, and (3) discuss the necessary steps toward a proper perspective of outcomes measurement in diagnostic audiology.

OUTCOMES MEASUREMENT AND DIAGNOSTIC AUDIOLOGY

Johnson and Danhauer (2001) found that only 22% of respondents in a recent nationwide survey collected outcome data in diagnostic audiology. Do audiologists, such as the individual depicted in Figure 7-1, consider diagnostic audiology an important area for outcomes measurement?

As already stated, this is probably because outcomes are most often associated with the end of the rehabilitation process. Diagnosis is an intermediate point in a three-step process of screening, determination of hearing loss (i.e., diagnosis), and intervention. There are four possible outcomes for diagnostic testing: (1) *true positives* or *hits*, (2) *true negatives* (i.e., *correct rejection*), (3) *false positives* (i.e., *false alarms*), and (4) *false negatives* (i.e., *incorrect rejections*). True positives are accurate test results that identify individuals with a condition who actually have the condition. True negatives are accurate test results that dismiss "normal" individuals as being condition-free. False positives are inaccurate test results that identify "normal" individuals as having a condition. False negatives are inaccurate test results that dismiss individuals as not having a condition when they actually do have the condition. Ideally, effective diagnostic tests have more true positives and true negatives, and few or no false positive or false negatives. In other words, true positives and true negatives have positive outcomes and false positives and false negatives have negative outcomes.

Positive diagnostic outcomes for patients result in either accurate confirmation that they have a particular condition or assurance that they do not have a particular condition. Therefore, both accurate positive and

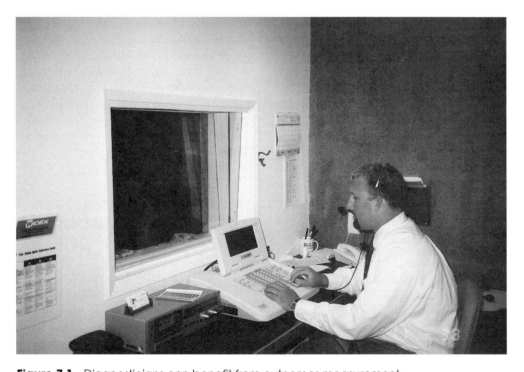

Figure 7-1. Diagnosticians can benefit from outcomes measurement.

negative test results are considered positive diagnostic outcomes. Alternatively, negative diagnostic outcomes for patients occur when they receive an erroneous diagnosis of a particular condition or false assurance that they do not have a particular condition when they actually do. Obviously, the more life-threatening a particular condition or disease, the higher are the stakes for negative patient outcomes. For example, a false positive test for cancer can cause unnecessary treatment and undo stress on patients and their significant others. False negatives on a test for cancer can be a death sentence for patients having the disease, but who do not receive treatment that could save their lives. Regarding hearing loss, negative diagnostic outcomes for patients can be serious too. Undiagnosed hearing loss in young children can have serious consequences for speech/language development and for patients' families. For example, recent data show that children whose hearing loss is identified after 6 months of age are significantly more delayed in speech and language development than those children identified before 6 months of age (Yoshinaga-Itano, 1997). A delay in identifying infants with hearing impairment denies those patients and their families access to critical intervention. Moreover, from a legal standpoint, audiologists are not immune from lawsuits from patients who believe that they have received poor treatment.

Positive and negative diagnostic outcomes for practitioners, the profession, and society have consequences on our healthcare system. Positive diagnostic outcomes are good for audiologists who feel satisfaction of having helped their patients, the profession that receives favorable press from satisfied consumers and their families, and society that benefits from the improved quality of life for its citizens. Some negative diagnostic outcomes for audiologists include loss of credibility and possible lawsuits. Negative diagnostic outcomes for the profession include a decreased likelihood of reimbursement for services from third-party payers. Negative diagnostic outcomes for society can include the increased medical and educational costs for and loss of productivity of citizens with hearing loss.

Browner, Newman, and Cummings (1988) stated that an ideal diagnostic test is: (1) valid, (2) reliable, (3) safe, (4) simple, and (5) painless. Valid tests are ones that identify those individuals with a certain condition with a positive result and persons who do not have the condition with a negative result. Reliable tests are those that produce the same results when administered multiple times to the same individual and by different examiners. As stated in Chapters 2 and 3, valid tests must also be reliable. However, reliable tests are not necessarily valid. Reliable tests can consistently provide erroneous results. Safe, simple, and painless testing is important, because dangerous, overly complicated, and/or painful, yet potentially life-saving diagnostic procedures may be avoided by some patients. For example, every year, many older women avoid having a mammogram because it can be very painful, even though it may detect the presence of cancer in its earliest, most treatable stages. Therefore, good tests may not result in positive diagnostic factors because of outcomes other than validity and reliability.

OUTCOME MEASURES FOR DETERMINING THE VALIDITY AND RELIABILITY OF DIAGNOSTIC TESTS

Validity Measures

Validity of diagnostic tests is often measured through analyzing the relationship between two variables: (1) a *predictor variable*, and (2) the *outcome variable* via a decision matrix. Because the purpose of a diagnostic procedure is to identify (i.e., predict) which individuals have or do not have a particular condition (i.e., outcome), the predictor variable is the diagnostic test and the particular condition is the outcome variable. The decision matrix used is a simple two dimensional, 2 × 2 square with the predictor variable shown on the vertical axis and the outcome variable on the horizontal axis as in Figure 7-2.

Note that each dimension has two distinct possibilities. For the predictor variable or diagnostic procedure, the two possibilities are either a patient tests positive or negative on the test. For the outcome variable, either the patient has the condition or does not have the condition based on some type

of "gold standard" of diagnosis for the condition. A *gold standard* for an outcome variable is a recognized, highly valid test for a condition. For example, predictor variables for hearing loss (e.g., OAE screening tests) are compared to the "gold standard" measurement of hearing loss (e.g., pure-tone air- and bone-conduction and/or auditory brainstem response [ABR] testing). The four squares compose all possible combinations of predictor variable levels and outcome variable levels.

Predictor variables with positive patient outcomes are those that produce accurate results of "true positives" or "true negatives." For example, box A represents "true positives"

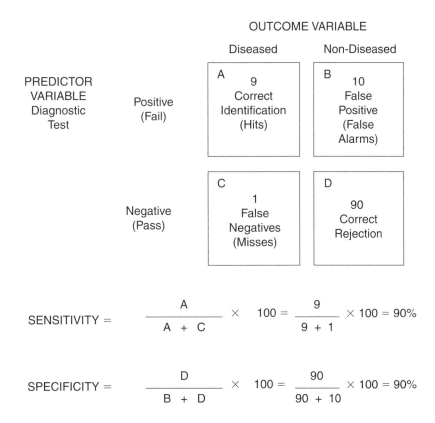

Figure 7-2. Decision matrix.

or "hits" in which a positive result on a predictor variable (e.g., screening test) results in an outcome of diagnosis of the condition by the "gold standard." Similarly, box "D" represents "true negatives" or "correct rejections" in which a negative result on a predictor variable (e.g., diagnostic test) accurately dismisses an individual as having a condition by the "gold standard." Alternatively, predictor variables with negative diagnostic outcomes are those that produce inaccurate results. For example, box "B" represents "false positives" or "false alarms" in which positive results on a predictor variable incorrectly identify a patient as having a condition, who actually does not have it. Similarly, box "C" represents "false negatives" or "misses," in which negative results on the predictor variable incorrectly dismiss a patient as not having a condition, but who actually does have it.

Decision-matrix analysis assists audiologists and clinical researchers in determining the validity of a screening or diagnostic procedure. Good or valid screening and/or diagnostic tests should have most of their patient outcomes in boxes A (i.e., hits) and D (i.e., correct rejection), such that results on the predictor variable match those of the outcomes variable. However, no screening or diagnostic procedure is perfect and some patient outcomes will fall into boxes B (i.e., false alarms) or C (i.e., misses). The distribution of patient outcomes into the four boxes helps to determine the degree of validity of predictor variables through the outcome measures of *sensitivity* and *specificity*. Sensitivity is the percentage of patients who test positive on the predictor variable and actually do have the condition. The more "hits" in relation to "false negatives," the higher the sensitivity. Specificity is the percentage of patients who test negative on the predictor variable and actually do not have the condition. The more "correct rejections" in relation to "false positives," the higher the specificity. Both indices of validity are computed using

equations representing the relationships of the four parameters in the matrix.

Sensitivity is computed by dividing "A" (i.e., the total number of "hits") by the sum of "A + C" (i.e., the number of "hits" plus "misses"). For example, Figure 7-2 shows the equation and an example for computing sensitivity. Therefore, in this case, sensitivity of the predictor variable is 90% (i.e., A / [A + C] × 100 = 9/[9 + 1] × 100 = 9/10 × 100 or 90%). Similarly, Figure 7-2 also shows the equation and an example for computing specificity. Specificity is computed by dividing "D" (i.e., the total number of "correct rejections") by the sum of "B + D" (i.e., the "false positives" plus "correct rejections"). Therefore, in this case, specificity of the predictor variable is also 90% (i.e., D/[B + D] × 100 = 90/[90 + 10] × 100 = 90/100 × 100 or 90%). Valid predictor variables are those with both high sensitivity and high specificity of greater than 90%. Sometimes, however, it is more difficult to obtain measures of specificity than sensitivity, depending on the pervasiveness of the condition. With a relatively low prevalence for hearing loss, it is easier to demonstrate specificity than sensitivity. For example, Hall (2000) stated that it may take only one day to demonstrate specificity of an OAE protocol with 100 ears, but much longer to do the same for sensitivity requiring the screening and follow-up of 100,000 low-risk infants.

Which is more important—sensitivity or specificity? Are they related to each other? The answers to these questions are "it depends" and "yes," respectively. Both sensitivity and specificity are equally important and related to each other. For example, what would be the value of a test that was supersensitive, but was not very specific? Such a test would identify most persons with a particular condition, but it would also result in a lot of false alarms or positive results for those who actually did not have the condition. Conversely, what value would a test have if it were not very sensitive, but were very specific? Such a test would dismiss most persons without the condition, but it would also miss some persons who actually had the condition. Therefore, the best testing condition is one that produces the highest sensitivity given the highest specificity and vice-versa.

Audiologists must not only select tests with good sensitivity and specificity, but also appropriate *cut-off points* or criteria for performance, separating positive from negative test results. Setting these values must be done carefully to ensure the best combination of sensitivity and specificity, costs and benefits. Our readers have done this hundreds of times when screening in environments with high ambient noise levels. What happens if the standard 20 dB HL screening level is used in these conditions? Clinicians realize that using this level will result in a benefit of identifying all those with a hearing loss, but at the cost of a high false alarm rate or positive results for those with normal hearing. Similarly, using a screening level of 40 dB HL in such conditions will result in a benefit of dismissing all those with normal hearing, but at

a cost of many misses by dismissing many patients who actually have hearing loss. Costs and benefits of varying cut-off points of diagnostic tests can extend beyond assessment of their performance. For example, Martin and Champlin (2000) recently recommended that 15 dB HL, rather than 25 dB HL, be considered as the upper limit of normal hearing sensitivity. One benefit of this proposal is that the many patients with hearing levels that average less (i.e., better) than 25 dB HL report hearing difficulties that would be dignified by the changing of these criteria (Martin & Champlin, 2000). This benefit, however, must be evaluated against the costs of medico-legal issues and changes in determination of patient disability.

Clinical researchers know that selection of a cut-off point or fence (e.g., screening level) is a balancing act between sensitivity and specificity, which is illustrated on the curve in Figure 7-3. *Receiver-operating characteristic* (ROC) *curves* are graphs of how sensitivity and specificity of tests vary based on the use of various cut-off points. Sensitivity is plotted on the vertical axis of the graph with

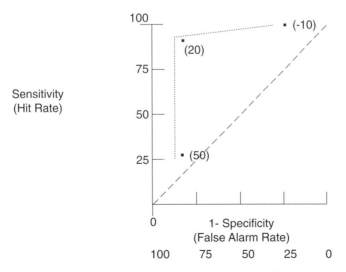

Figure 7-3. Receiver-operating characteristic (ROC) curve.

values ranging from 0 to 100%. However, specificity is labeled "1 – specificity" (in an inverse manner to that of sensitivity) on the horizontal axis. Thus, a value of "0" on this axis is actually 100% specificity. In selecting an appropriate cut-off point for a test, researchers must compute sensitivity and specificity for a range of cut-off points for a representative sample of the test population. Each cut-off point is plotted on a graph similar to that pictured in Figure 7-3 with a dot placed at the intersection of the appropriate sensitivity and specificity rates. The dots are then connected with a line resulting in the ROC curve. For example, the screening cut-off point of –10 dB HL has nearly 100% sensitivity, but less than 25% specificity, meaning that all the individuals with hearing loss would test positive on the test, but so would the vast majority of persons with normal hearing. On the other extreme, a cut-off point of 50 dB HL has a specificity of nearly 90%, but a sensitivity of about 25%, meaning that a majority of those individuals with normal hearing would test negative on the test, but only about a quarter of the persons with hearing loss would test positive on the test. Hypothetical values for the screening example discussed above show how sensitivity and specificity vary for different screening criteria. The best cut-off points are those that maximize sensitivity/specificity and are found in the upper left-hand corner of the graph. For example, the cut-off point or screening level of 20 dB HL produces a sensitivity of over 90% and specificity of nearly 80%. Diagnostic tests having an indirect relationship between sensitivity and specificity with cut-off points that produce ROC curves starting in the lower left corner and end in the upper right corner of the graph as depicted by the dashed line in Figure 7-3 are relatively worthless. An indirect relationship between sensitivity and specificity for various cut-off points is of little value for two reasons. First, sensitivity, in most cases, is just as important as specificity and vice versa. Second, any increase in sensitivity is a direct and proportional decrease in specificity and vice versa. Thus, the best cut-off point (i.e., maximum sensitivity and specificity) for a diagnostic test is one that is as close as possible to the dot appearing in the upper left corner of the graph in Figure 7-3.

Other measures that affect the validity of a test are the prevalence of a disease and the prior probability of a disease. It was just stated that sensitivity and specificity have similar importance. However, specificity is more important than sensitivity for diagnostic tests of disease with low prevalence. Recall that in Chapter 3, prevalence was defined as the number of individuals having a pathological condition at one point in time per the number of people who may be at risk (Browner, Newman, et al., 1988). Therefore, it is more important for diagnostic tests of rare diseases to be specific (i.e., dismissing persons without the disease through a negative result) than it is to be sensitive (i.e., identifying persons with the disease through a positive result). Conversely, the more prevalent a disease, the more important it is for the test to be sensitive than it is to be specific. *Prior probability* is the prevalence of a disease for a particular individual based on the demographic and clinical characteristics estimated before performing a test (Browner, Newman, et al., 1988). Prior probability is used to calculate additional measures assessing the validity of a test: the *predictive value of a positive test* and the *predictive value of a negative test* (Browner, Newman, et al., 1988; Turner, et al., 1999). The predictive value of a positive test (PV+) is the likelihood that a patient with a positive test result actually has the disease and is obtained with the equation below (Browner, Newman, et al., 1988):

$$PV+ = \frac{\text{Sensitivity} \times \text{Prior probability}}{(\text{Sensitivity} \times \text{Prior probability}) + (1 - \text{Specificity} \times 1 - \text{Prior probability}])}$$

$$PV- = \frac{\text{Sensitivity} \times (1 - \text{Prior probability})}{(\text{Specificity} \times [1 - \text{Prior probability}]) + ([1 - \text{Sensitivity}] \times \text{Prior probability})}$$

Conversely, the predictive value of a negative test (PV-) is the likelihood that a patient with a negative test result is actually free of the disease and is obtained with the equation above.

In case audiologists do not have these data, Turner, et al. (1999) provided two other equations (shown at the bottom of the page) for obtaining these values based on the hit and false alarm rates for a particular test. Browner, Newman, et al. (1988) considered both of these measures as posterior probability measures as they are determined after knowing if a test result was positive or negative. For example, Turner, et al. (1999) calculated the PV+ values for retrocochlear disease for ABR testing based on a hit rate of 99% (i.e., sensitivity = 99%) and a false alarm rate of 11% (i.e., specificity = 89%) for three disease prevalences of:

1. 2%: PV+ = 15%,
2. 5%: PV+ = 31%, and
3. 50%: PV+ = 90%.

As can be seen, the higher the prevalence, the greater the predictive value of a positive result. Unfortunately, with the prevalence ranging between 2 to 5% for retrocochlear disease, ABR has between a 15 to 31% chance of being correct with a positive result. How can this be if ABR is one of the best diagnostic procedures in the clinicians' armamentarium? Does this mean that the ABR test is useless? No, not exactly, but there are several things that audiologists can do to improve test performance by increasing the prevalence of a disease by using a screening test prior to testing or by evaluating those patients that present with symptoms of retrocochlear pathology (e.g., unsymmetric hearing loss, tinnitus, a sense of aural fullness, and/or dizziness and vertigo) or test positive on tests such as abnormal reflex decay, for example.

Reliability Measures

Two reliability measures for test procedures are *co-positivity* and *co-negativity*. Co-positivity is the extent to which two tests agree on identifying those patients with a condition (Roeser, 1995). Co-negativity, on the other hand, is the extent to which two tests agree on dismissing those patients without a condition (Roeser, 1995). Even though both definitions state that the measures are assessing the agreement of two tests, both can assess the reliability of numerous aspects of the testing situation, such as the agreement of 2 tests, 2 pieces of diagnostic equipment, or 2 screeners, for example.

In order to assess agreement, all aspects of the testing situation should be consistent except for the components under consideration. For example, a contract-for-service audiologist had noticed an increase in the false alarm rate from hearing screenings performed at the schools in the northwest part of the district assigned to Nurse Neophyte, who was new and had to leave the hearing screening inservice before the supervised practicum

1. $$PV+ = \frac{1}{1 + \dfrac{(\text{False Alarm Rate}) \times (1 - \text{Prevalence})}{(\text{Hit Rate}) \times (\text{Prevalence})}}$$

2. $$PV- = \frac{1}{1 + \dfrac{(1 - \text{Hit Rate}) \times (\text{Prevalence})}{(1 - \text{False Alarm Rate}) \times (1 - \text{Prevalence})}}$$

was completed. Nurse Neophyte had taken her audiometer with her to practice at home that evening. How difficult could it be? By October however, the audiologist knew she needed to intervene with the assistance of Nurse Bessie, an experienced hearing screener, who was known for producing the most accurate screening results in the school district. Nurse Neophyte was contacted and told to come to the school with the hearing-impaired program to screen hearing with Nurse Bessie. The audiologist wanted to assess the agreement between both nurses in screening 20 children (10 with normal hearing and 10 with known hearing loss). Figure 7-4 shows the process in determining the co-positivity and co-negativity between the two nurses.

The first step in the process was to arrange for the two nurses to screen the hearing of all 20 children using the same portable audiometer, in the same room, and on the same day. The second step was to align the results for the two screeners in a table. The third step was to put the results within a decision-matrix with the results of Nurse Bessie (i.e., the "gold standard") on the horizontal axis and those of Nurse Neophyte on the vertical axis. Box A represents cases in which both Nurses Bessie and Neophyte found positive results. Similarly, Box B is where Nurse Bessie achieved negative results and Nurse Neophyte positive results, and so on. The fourth step was to compute co-positivity and co-negativity for the two nurses by using the numbers within the decision-matrix in the appropriate equations. Co-positivity is computed by dividing "A" (i.e., the total number of "agreements on positive tests") by the sum of "A + C" (i.e., the number of "agreements on positive tests" plus "disagreements on positive tests") and multiplying by 100. Co-negativity is computed by dividing "D" (i.e., the total number of "agreements on negative tests") by the sum of "D + B" (i.e., the number of "agreements on negative tests" plus "disagreements on negative

tests") and multiplying by 100. Nurses Bessie and Neophyte had a co-positivity of 70% and a co-negativity of 90%. In other words, Nurses Bessie and Neophyte had good agreement on the achievement of positive results, but good agreement in achieving negative results, thereby explaining the reason for the high false positive rate. Nurse Bessie was able to provide Nurse Neophyte with some screening tips that resulted in a reduction of the false positive rate. It is important to remember, however, that co-positivity and co-negativity are measures of reliability, not validity. For example, two nurses could have high co-positivity and co-negativity, but poor validity if they were both instructed incorrectly on screening procedures.

TEST PROTOCOLS

Types of Protocols

Because no single diagnostic test is perfectly valid, test protocols have been developed to increase accuracy. A *protocol* is simply a testing process that consists of conducting two or more tests. Tests can be combined in two different ways: (1) in *series*, and (2) in *parallel*. Tests combined in series are performed one right after another, and, depending on the results, a decision is made after the first test based on the results either to continue on to the second test (e.g., after a positive result) or to terminate the testing process (e.g., after a negative result). Alternatively, tests combined in parallel are conducted at the same time with a decision made based on the results of two or more tests using a protocol criterion. A *protocol criterion* defines how many tests must be positive for the protocol to be positive (Turner, et al., 1999). A criterion may be strict or lax and is relative to the specific protocols under consideration. The more the number of tests that need to be positive for a protocol to be positive, the more

STEP 1: ARRANGE FOR BOTH NURSES TO SCREEN THE HEARING OF THE SAME 20 CHILDREN.

STEP 2: ALIGN SCREENING RESULTS

Children

Nurse	1	2	3	4	5	6	7	8	9	10	11	12	13	14	15	16	17	18	19	20
Bessie (Gold Standard)	+	+	+	+	+	+	+	+	+	+	−	−	−	−	−	−	−	−	−	−
Neophyte	+	+	−	+	+	−	+	−	+	+	−	−	−	−	+	−	−	−	−	−

STEP 3: PLACE RESULTS INTO THE DECISION MATRIX

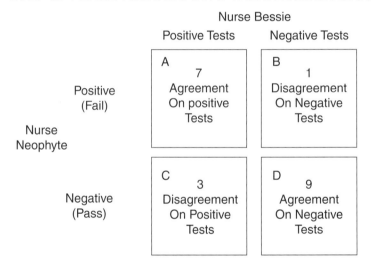

Nurse Bessie

Positive Tests   Negative Tests

Nurse Neophyte

Positive (Fail)

A   7
Agreement On positive Tests

B   1
Disagreement On Negative Tests

Negative (Pass)

C   3
Disagreement On Positive Tests

D   9
Agreement On Negative Tests

STEP 4: COMPUTE CO-POSITIVITY AND CO-NEGATIVITY

$$\text{CO-POSITIVITY} = \frac{A}{A + C} \times 100 = \frac{7}{7 + 3} \times 100 = 70\%$$

$$\text{CO-NEGATIVITY} = \frac{D}{B + D} \times 100 = \frac{9}{9 + 1} \times 100 = 90\%$$

Figure 7-4. Step-by-step approach for calculating co-positivity and co-negativity.

strict is the criterion. However, the fewer the number of tests needed for a protocol to be positive, the more lax is the criterion. Using a very strict criterion increases the sensitivity of a protocol, but it may decrease its specificity. Conversely, using a very lax criterion increases the specificity of a protocol, but it may decrease its sensitivity. In other words, a strict criterion may increase the false positive rate and a lax criterion may increase the miss rate for a protocol.

Series protocols can combine tests in one of two ways: (1) *series-positive protocol*, or (2) *series-negative protocol* (Turner, Frazer, & Shepard, 1984). Series-positive protocols consist of two tests conducted in sequence, requiring both tests to be positive for the protocol to be positive. If a negative result is obtained on the first test, the patient is dismissed. However, if a positive result is obtained on the first test, then a second test is conducted with two possible outcomes. If a positive result is obtained on the second test, then the patient is referred on for treatment. However, if a negative result is obtained, the patient is also dismissed as with the first test. Series-negative protocols consist of two tests conducted, one right after the other, pending negative results on the first test. If positive results are obtained on the first test, the patient is referred on for treatment. However, if negative results are obtained on the first test, then a second test is conducted. If negative results are obtained on the second test, the patient is dismissed. However, if a positive result is obtained, the patient is referred on for treatment. For example, the Joint Committee on Infant Hearing has recommended series-negative protocols in the 1994 Position Statements (Diefendorf, 1998; JCIH, 1994) in which positive test results on the neonatal high-risk register results in a positive outcome and referral for physiologic testing. However, if negative results are obtained on the neonatal high-risk register, then the high-risk register for infants is administered to the child. If the results on the second high-risk register are negative, the patient is dismissed. However, if the second high-risk register produces a positive outcome, then the patient is referred on for physiologic testing. The series-positive protocol has a stricter

criterion than the series-negative protocol, which needs two positive test results for the former to have a positive outcome on the protocol, whereas the latter requires only one. The Joint Committee on Infant Hearing (Diefendorf, 1998; JCIH, 1982) recommended a series-positive protocol in their 1982 Position Statement in which a positive result on the high-risk register and physiologic testing were required for a positive patient outcome leading to a referral.

Parallel protocols can be either strict or lax. *Strict parallel protocols* are those in which positive results must be obtained on two tests performed at the same time in order for a protocol to be positive leading to referral for treatment (Turner, et al., 1999). A strict parallel protocol is similar to a series-positive protocol with both requiring two positive test results for referral (Turner, et al., 1999). *Lax parallel protocols* are those that require a positive result only on one of two tests for a positive protocol leading to referral for treatment (Turner, et al., 1999). A lax parallel protocol is similar to the series-negative protocol with both requiring a positive test on only one of two tests for a positive patient outcome leading to referral (Turner, et al., 1999).

Assessment of Validity

The performance of protocols can be assessed in terms of their hit and false alarm rates in much the same way as for individual tests using clinical data (Turner, et al., 1999). Protocol hit rate, sometimes called sensitivity, is the total number of hits divided by the total number of diseased patients (Diefendorf, 1998; Turner, et al., 1999). Protocol false alarm rate is the total number of infants incorrectly identified as having a disease divided by the total number of normal patients (Diefendorf, 1998; Turner, et al., 1999). Specificity for the protocol can then be computed through the equation "1 – the false alarm rate" (Diefendorf, 1998). For example, Table 7-1 shows the hypothetical results for 20 patients, 10 with hearing loss, and 10 without hearing loss submitted to a protocol consisting of two tests.

For the 10 patients with hearing loss, test 1 has a hit rate of 90% (i.e., sensitivity) and test 2 has a hit rate or sensitivity of 80%. Using a loose criterion (i.e., positive results needed on one of two tests only), the protocol has a hit rate of 100%. However, using a

Table 7-1. Computing percentage of hits (i.e., sensitivity) and correct rejections (i.e., specificity) for parallel protocols.

Patients with Hearing Loss												
Patient #	1	2	3	4	5	6	7	8	9	10	#Positive	Hit* %
Test 1	+	+	+	+	+	−	+	+	+	+	9	90
Test 2	−	−	+	+	+	+	+	+	+	+	8	80
*Sensitivity												
Patient #	1	2	3	4	5	6	7	8	9	10	# Positive	Hit* %
Loose Criterion	+	+	+	+	+	+	+	+	+	+	10	100
Strict Criterion	−	−	+	+	+	−	+	+	+	+	7	70
*Sensitivity												

Patients with Normal Hearing												
Patient #	1	2	3	4	5	6	7	8	9	10	# Negative	Correct Rejection** %
Test 1	−	−	−	+	−	−	−	−	−	−	9	90
Test 2	−	−	−	−	−	+	−	+	−	−	8	80
**Specificity												
Patient #	1	2	3	4	5	6	7	8	9	10	# Negative	Correct Rejection** %
Loose Criterion	−	−	−	−	−	−	−	−	−	−	10	100
Strict Criterion	−	−	−	+	−	+	−	+	−	−	7	70
**Specificity												

strict criterion (i.e., positive results required on both tests), the protocol has a hit rate of 70%. For the 10 patients with normal hearing, test 1 has a correct rejection rate of 90% (i.e., specificity) and test 2 has a correct rejection rate of 80%. Using a loose criterion, the protocol has a correct rejection rate (i.e., specificity) of 100%. However, using a strict criterion, the protocol has a correct rejection rate of 70%. Thus, the same principles for assessing single test performance are the same when assessing those of protocols. In addition, selection of an appropriate cut-off value for individual tests has the same trade-offs as does determining strict versus lax criteria for test protocols involving a delicate balance between sensitivity and specificity. The readers are referred to Turner, et al., (1999) for additional details regarding the assessment of test and protocol performance.

CURRENT PERSPECTIVES OF OUTCOMES MEASUREMENT IN DIAGNOSTIC AUDIOLOGY

So far, this chapter has presented a brief overview of the empirical assessment of diagnostic test performance. At this point, some readers may be glassy-eyed and wondering, "So, what is a good diagnostic test?" Unfortunately, there is no easy answer to this question. The answer is not only in the sensitivity, specificity, and predictive value of positive results, and so forth of diagnostic tests, but also with audiologists' skills in using those

tests in clinical practice—requiring a current perspective in outcomes measurement in diagnostic audiology. Audiologists can invalidate otherwise valid tests, for example. Unfortunately, no diagnostic procedure is perfect, but audiologists can maintain a proper perspective for outcomes measurement in diagnostic audiology by taking the steps presented in Table 7-2.

First, audiologists should evaluate the studies assessing the efficacy of new and current diagnostic tests of various auditory disorders by using the checklist in Appendix VII-A, "Checklist for Evaluating Investigations of Diagnostic Tests," found on the companion CD-ROM. Studies of the tests should be evaluated on value, general factors, subject selection, treatment of bias (i.e., random error and systematic error), and validity. Regarding the general diagnostic value of a screening/test procedure for a particular auditory disorder, the following questions should be asked (Bess, Hedley-Williams, & Lichtenstein, 1999; Cadman, Chambers, Scakett, & Feldman, 1984):

- Has the effectiveness of the procedure been demonstrated previously in a randomized trial?
- Are efficacious treatments of the auditory disorder available?z
- Does the burden of suffering warrant a new screening/diagnostic test?
- Is there an already existing valid diagnostic test?
- Could the proposed diagnostic procedure reach all those who could benefit?

Table 7-2. Steps to a proper perspective for outcomes measurement in diagnostic audiology.

- Evaluate investigations of diagnostic tests
- Recall the difference between test efficacy versus test effectiveness
- Remember that diagnostic audiology is as much an art, as a science
- Understand that the best laboratory tests are not necessarily the best in the "real world"
- Acknowledge the current emphasis on managed care
- Realize that the value of diagnostic outcomes is from the perspective of the stakeholder

■ Would patients with positive test results comply with advice and interventions from audiologists?

Regarding general factors, audiologists should consider whether the new procedure fills a need in diagnostic audiology, how it improves on the shortcomings of previous tests, and if it offers any new benefits to patients. If a new test really does not improve on already existing procedures or provide any new benefits to patients, why use it? For example, nearly 100 speech discrimination tests have been developed over the past 30 years and presently new tests come on-line all the time. Many audiologists do not obtain speech discrimination measures anymore, and if they do, they use the same measures used for the last 50 years. Furthermore, audiologists need to know if those assessing the test have any vested interest in its degree of validity. Even the most scrupulous clinicians may have some bias in investigating the validity of their own test, for example.

Regarding subject selection, all studies of diagnostic tests should clearly describe the subject selection criteria and their rationale. Unless audiologists know the types of subjects used, performance values for tests reported in the literature cannot be generalized when applied to various clinical populations. In addition, the sample size must be large enough to achieve 95% confidence intervals for the test's sensitivity and specificity to reduce the effect of random error on the results (Browner, Newman, et al., 1988). For example, audiologists assessing the outcome of an inservice training program need to know the percentage of improvement in sensitivity and specificity needed to be statistically significant at the $p < 0.05$ level of probability. Readers are referred to Browner, Black, Newman, and Hulley (1988) for a complete discussion of techniques for estimating adequate sample sizes for analytic studies and other clinical experiments. Furthermore, studies that are assessing multiple predictive variables should have a test phase in which the significant variables are identified and then a validation phase in which a separate study is conducted on those variables. One variable may be significant in a study with 20 predictive variables caused by just chance alone, for example.

Subject selection is also an important factor in reducing sampling bias. Audiologists need to determine if the subject sample is representative of the clinical population that the test is intended for with various degrees of severity of the conditions that are encountered in typical health-care settings (Browner, Newman, et al., 1988). For example, assessing the performance of the *Hearing Handicap for the Elderly–Screening Version* (HHIE–S) (Ventry & Weinstein, 1982) and the Welsh-Allyn Audioscope in screening the elderly for hearing loss, Lichtenstein, Bess, and Logan (1988) included elderly subjects with various degrees of hearing loss seen in typical health-care settings of physicians' offices and hearing centers. Similarly, authors documenting new tests should report their predictive values for positive and negative results based on the prevalence for a certain disease. For example, in the aforementioned study, Lichtenstein, et al. (1988) reported those values for both the audioscope and the HHIE–S. These values are an absolute necessity to account for any difference in prevalence for the condition in the general population and that of the study sample.

Another type of systematic error comes from measurement bias. In particular, observers collecting data on the outcome variable (i.e., gold standard) must be blinded as to the results of the predictive variable (i.e., screening/diagnostic test) (Browner, Newman, et al., 1988). For example, experimenters may be less likely to accept certain head-turn responses during visual reinforcement audiometry (VRA) if they know that the infants being tested had previously failed otoacoustic emissions (OAE) screening. In addition, the study should also state procedures for technologically unsatisfactory or borderline results. Experimenters may omit subjects achieving "borderline" status (i.e., neither positive nor negative outcomes) biasing the results of the study, for example. In fact, the cut-off points for a test should be based on sound rationale, and established prior to data collection.

Regarding validity, the "gold standard" (i.e., outcome variable) used to classify patients as having a condition or not having it must have content validity, criterion validity, and construct validity. Recall that these terms were defined and discussed in Chapter 4. Briefly, content validity, or face validity, requires a subjective procedure to determine how well a diagnostic test measures the condition it claims to measure (Maxwell & Satake, 1997). Criterion validity includes both concurrent validity and predictive validity (Schiavetti & Metz, 1997). Concurrent validity is the agreement between the gold standard and some validating criterion administered at the same time (Schiavetti & Metz, 1997). It seems ironic, but true, that in using a "gold standard," audiologists should be concerned about how it has been validated by another gold standard. Similarly, predictive validity of a gold standard is how well it predicts the performance on other accepted measures (Schiavetti & Metz, 1997). Even though consideration of the criterion validity of a gold standard seems a circular process, it is necessary in establishing the credibility of a test. Lastly, the construct validity of a gold standard is the degree with which a measure either empirically or rationally purports to measure some theoretical construct (Maxwell & Satake, 1997; Schiavetti & Metz, 1997).

The second step for audiologists is to recall that performances reported in the literature are of test efficacy, not necessarily test effectiveness. Recall that in Chapter 2, we defined efficacy as performance under ideal or laboratory conditions. Effectiveness, on the other hand, is performance under "real world" conditions. For example, audiologists cannot expect all tests to perform as reported in the literature. Sensitivity and specificity values for a test are not static values, but vary dynamically within the clinical milieu. Everything within the clinical setting (e.g., audiologist behavior, patient behavior, equipment, and so forth) can have an impact on the actual sensitivity or specificity of a clinical test. All things being equal, an experienced clinician may obtain more valid results than an inexperienced clinician. Younger adults may give more reliable responses than older patients. New equipment may provide more accurate results than older equipment. The examples are seemingly endless, but the effects of these extraneous variables are reduced when controlled. The bottom line is that audiologists should follow test guidelines as closely as possible for achievement of positive diagnostic outcomes for patients. In some cases, intra-patient factors such as motivation during testing can have drastic effects on false positive rates on certain behavioral tests. For example, Silman, Silverman, and Emmer (2000) presented three case studies of children referred for a second opinion after an initial positive diagnosis, but could be coaxed with marshmallows into performing at normal levels on commonly used CAPD tests. Jerger (2000) stated that our profession can no longer tolerate false positive results such as these and that more valid tests need to be developed for diagnosing CAPD.

The third step for audiologists is to remember that, for some patients, diagnostic audiology is as much an art as it is a science. In a recent classroom discussion regarding these very issues, an inquisitive graduate student asked why audiologists spend valuable time using behavioral techniques with young children. After all, with recent advances in OAE and ABR technology, why bother? Not only do these objective measures have high sensitivity and specificity, but they also eliminate guesswork and the need for VRA assistants in the test booth, for example. The student's question has several answers, some of which go beyond the purpose of this chapter, but all are directly related to the issue at hand. First, the cross-check principle states that the results of a single test are never considered to be conclusive proof of the presence of or site of lesion of an auditory disorder (Diefendorf, 1998; Jerger & Hayes, 1976). Second, objective measurements of auditory function are only part of the picture that is not complete without assessment of children's behavioral responses to stimuli. Third, audiologists and students-in-training must realize that nothing replaces the skills, intuition, and experience of a stellar diagnostician. Some audiologists possess better skills than others, relying on an innate ability to assemble bits and pieces of information into a meaningful diagnostic patient profile. Indeed, recall the scenario presented in Chapter 1 of the audiologist who believed that establishing a universal newborn hearing screening program using automatic OAE screeners would "run itself" and found out the hard way that technology is only an audiologist's tool, not a panacea.

The fourth step for audiologists is to understand that the best tests for use in the "real world" might not be those that best perform in the laboratory. Audiologists must often practice under many limitations (e.g., financial) in providing quality patient care under the many constraints of the hearing health-care arena. In selecting diagnostic tests, audiologists consider not only the validity of an instrument, but its feasibility for use in the clinic through cost-benefit analysis. *Cost-benefit analysis* is a process by which the costs versus the benefits of various tests are weighed with the preferred procedure having the greatest benefits and the lowest costs (Turner, et al., 1999). Cost-benefit analyses can be either subjective (i.e., using subjective intuitive strategies) or objective (i.e., employing formal/logical strategies) when determining the best diagnostic procedures (Turner, et al., 1999). Objective analyses are preferred and involve assigning costs to errors (e.g., false alarms and misses), benefits to correct decisions (e.g., hits and correct rejections), and rely on difficult-to-obtain data (Turner, et al., 1999). Although audiologists consider the same variables in these analyses, each has different prioritizations and limitations unique to each clinical setting. Detailed information on cost-benefit analyses can be found in Turner, et al., (1999) and in the recommended readings section of this chapter.

The fifth step for audiologists is to acknowledge new outcomes for diagnostic testing that reflect the current emphasis on managed care and current foci of the profession. One of the advantages of managed care for patients is a continuum of coordinated care resulting in an efficient use of resources, communication among practitioners, and a case management approach for situations that require complex solutions (Johnson & Danhauer, 1999). In a similar vein, the focus on early hearing detection and intervention (EHDI) programs has established benchmarks for confirmation of hearing loss that have more to do with the timeliness and cross-disciplinary nature of diagnosis than the reliability and validity of measurements. For example, for timeliness of diagnosis, recall that in Chapter 6, one of the benchmarks for confirmation of hearing loss posited in the JCIH's Position Statement 2000 stated that infants referred from UNHS programs begin audiologic and medical evaluations before 3 months of age or 3 months after discharge for neonatal intensive care unit (NICU) infants (JCIH, 2000). Similarly, another benchmark includes that comprehensive interdisciplinary services for infants and families who are referred following screening are coordinated between the infants' medical home, family, and related professionals with expertise in hearing loss and the state and local agencies responsible for provision of services (JCIH, 2000). Clearly, these new outcomes show the importance of a seamless transition for patients through all phases of audiologic service delivery (i.e., screening, diagnosis, and rehabilitation) requiring coordinated approaches between and among related professionals, and state, and local agencies.

The sixth step for audiologists is to realize that the value placed on outcomes is

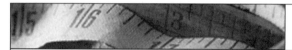

VIGNETTE 7-2

CYNTHIA AND MARGARET'S STORY

PART 2

Clearing the dishes from the dinner table, Cynthia hurried her children off to do their homework so she could have some privacy in calling her mother's physician, Dr. Dorothy "Dot" Allen. "Dr. Dot," a long-time family friend, was the kind of physician who still gave her patients her home phone number. Punching the doctor's number into her cordless phone, Cynthia was hoping that Dr. Dot was home.

"Hello?" said Dr Dot, answering the phone.

"Dr. Dot, this is Cindy Smith. I'm worried about Mother."

"What seems to be the matter?" questioned Dr. Dot.

Cynthia explained all her mother's symptoms: not answering the telephone, misunderstandings in conversation, loss of weight, clutter in a previously spotless home, and so forth.

"I'm afraid she has Alzheimer's disease," Cynthia blurted out tearfully.

"I think you might be jumping to conclusions. I saw your mother the other day at Safeway and we had a nice chat."

"Well, I see her every day and she seems to be losing it."

"Cindy, relax. Your mother is coming in for her annual physical examination in two weeks. I appreciate your input, but leave the diagnosing to me."

"Dr. Dot, is it true that there are no definitive tests for Alzheimer's disease?"

"Yes, I'm afraid so, but let's cross that bridge when we get to it. Well, goodbye Cindy," said Dr. Dot as she hung up the telephone. Dr. Dot was more worried about Cynthia than she was about her mother. Nevertheless, she was glad to have been forewarned about possible problems with one of her patients.

Early one morning two weeks later, Cynthia drove her mother to Dr. Dot's office for her yearly physical examination and picked her up at about noon to go to lunch. At the restaurant, Cynthia asked, "What did Dr. Dot have to say?" After a few moments of silence, she repeated, "Mom, what did ...?"

"Dear, I'm tired from taking so many tests and talking to so many doctors. Can we just eat?" pleaded Margaret.

"OK Mom," recoiled Cynthia.

Three days later, Cynthia answered her telephone and was surprised to find it was Dr. Dot.

"Cindy, I've already called your mother and I'd like you both in my office Monday morning at 9:00 AM."

"Dr. Dot ... Did you find ..."

CONTINUES

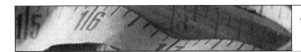

VIGNETTE 7-2

PART 2 (CONTINUED FROM PAGE 158)

"Relax, Cindy. Not to worry. See you Monday and have a good weekend. Good night."

"Good night," said Cynthia as she hung up the phone.

Nevertheless, it was a long weekend and Cynthia did not bring the subject up during their family Sunday supper, which had become a much smaller gathering during this past year with Cynthia's divorce and her father's passing.

Monday morning, Cynthia found herself sitting with her mother in Dr. Dot's waiting room. She was too nervous to read a magazine.

"Cindy and Margaret, good morning. Come in. Let's go to my office and have a seat. I usually talk with my patients confidentially regarding their results, but I've been worried about both of you. I only have good news. Margaret, you have a clean bill of health, but we need to monitor your blood pressure over the next few months, as it was a little high. However, I need to talk with both of you regarding some other results found by our audiologist, Dr Desi Bell, who told me that you have quite a hearing loss which is common for persons your age. Dr. Bell will contact you to explain the details of the evaluation, information about hearing aids, and other forms of assistance."

"So that explains why Mom is not answering the telephone and misunderstanding me. So maybe she doesn't have Alzheimer's disease." Cynthia reasoned.

"Alzheimer's disease?" exclaimed Margaret, rolling her eyes.

"Mom, I've been so worried about you," explained Cynthia. "You rarely answer your phone, you either ignore or misunderstand me, and you've been losing weight."

"Dear, I've lost weight because I'm no longer cooking as much as I used to when your father was alive. Also, your father always answered the telephone and was the outgoing one," explained Margaret with a tear in her eye. "I could understand you better if you didn't mumble!"

As Cynthia reflected, her father was the one who always answered the telephone and actually spoke for both of them covering up for her mother's apparent hearing loss until he died.

"Now, now. Margaret, Cynthia was just concerned about you. Dr. Bell can help both of you. After all, from appearances, you just didn't seem like your old self. Hearing loss is often mistaken for Alzheimer's disease and other forms of dementia. Cynthia, you will be happy to know that Dr. Bell used a test battery consisting of several objective and subjective measures. You both should understand that these tests collectively were positive for a moderate hearing loss. You should understand that a recent study by the National Council on Aging (NCOA) on over 4,000 persons with hearing impairment and their families conclusively showed that hearing loss is indeed a major health problem that is commonly misunderstood as Alzheimer's disease, dementia, and other problems associated with the elderly. Furthermore, the new high-technology hearing aids can substantially reduce the negative impact of hearing loss both for the patient and family members. Dr. Bell will discuss these options with you. It's only a hearing loss, not the end of the world. You both have been through a lot in the past year, but you have each other. Communicate with each other."

"I was just worried that I was losing you too, Mom," Cindy said, touching her mother's hand as she felt a deep sense of relief.

relative to the various stakeholders in the diagnostic process. Administrators are concerned about keeping financial costs down; audiologists want test accuracy; and patients want a quick, painless, and clear determination of the cause of their hearing difficulties. As a profession, we rarely assess patients' perceptions of the diagnostic process as it represents the middle of the service-delivery process. We began the chapter with Cynthia and Margaret's story and, in some ways, Cynthia's questions about the diagnostic process have been addressed in this chapter. However, let's return to their story in Vignette 7-2.

Confirmation of hearing loss was the missing puzzle piece that enabled Margaret's doctor to explain Margaret's behavior, ruling out other more serious causes. Positive diagnostic audiology outcomes can make all the difference as it did for the Smith family. Hearing function should be assessed for all patients, but especially for the elderly as part of a standard physical examination with their primary care physician (Bess, et al., 1999).

SUMMARY

This chapter has shown the importance of outcomes measurement for diagnostic audiology, presented methods of assessing test and protocol validity, and explained the steps that audiologists should take to have the proper perspective when considering the use of screening or diagnostic tests. Audiologists should feel confident in their understanding of basic issues involved in evaluating the validity and reliability of diagnostic tests and protocols. Furthermore, as discussed in Chapter 10, reliability and validity lie not only in the intrinsic psychometric properties of the clinical procedure, but also in its application to patients in specific clinical situations. Effective diagnostic audiology involves selecting the best procedures for unique situations, requiring a delicate balance among theoretical and practical constraints and between costs and benefits facing audiologists in the real world. Furthermore, positive diagnostic outcomes must be viewed in relation to the continuum of patient care from identification through rehabilitation.

LEARNING ACTIVITIES

- Find some investigations of commonly used diagnostic tests and complete an evaluation of them using Appendix VII-A.

- Interview three audiologists regarding their test approaches for diagnosing central auditory processing disorders (CAPD). Is it possible to classify each audiologist's approach as having parallel or series protocols and as using strict or lax criteria?

- Design a study to investigate if using reinforcers to motivate children affects the validity of CAPD testing.

RECOMMENDED READINGS

Turner, R.G., Frazer, G.J., & Shepard, N.T. (1984). Clinical performance of audiological and related diagnostic tests. *Ear and Hearing, 15,* 187-194.

Turner, R.G., Robinette, M.S., & Bauch, C.D. (1999). Clinical decisions. In F.E. Musiek & W.F. Rintelmann (Eds.), *Contemporary perspectives in hearing assessment* (pp. 437- 463). Needham Heights, MA: Allyn & Bacon.

REVIEW EXERCISES

Fill-in-the-Blank

Instructions: Please fill-in-the-blanks with the correct terms from the word bank below.

1. _____ _____ are accurate test results that identify individuals with a condition who actually have the condition.

2. _____ _____ are accurate test results that dismiss "normal" individuals as being condition-free.

3. _____ _____ are inaccurate test results that identify "normal" individuals as having a condition.

4. _____ _____ are inaccurate test results that dismiss individuals as not having a condition when they actually do have the condition.

5. A _____ _____ for an outcome variable is a recognized, highly valid test for a condition.

6. _____ is the percentage of patients who test positive on the predictor variable and actually do have the condition.

7. _____ is the percentage of patients who test negative on the predictor variable and actually do not have the condition.

8. _____ - _____ _____ or criteria of performance separate positive from negative test results.

9. _____ - _____ _____ _____ are graphs of how sensitivity and specificity of a test vary based on the use of various cut-off points.

10. _____ _____ is the prevalence of a disease for a particular individual based on the demographic and clinical characteristics estimated before performing a test.

11. _____ _____ of a _____ _____ is the likelihood that a patient with a positive test result actually has the disease.

12. _____ _____ of a _____ _____ is the likelihood that a patient with a negative test result is actually free of the disease.

13. _____ is the extent to which two tests agree on identifying patients with a condition.

14. _____ is the extent to which two tests agree on dismissing those patients without a condition.

15. A _____ is a testing process that consists of conducting two or more tests.

16. _____ protocols consist of two or more tests that are performed one right after another.

17. _____ protocols consist of tests that are performed at the same time.

18. A _____ _____ defines how many tests must be positive for a protocol to be positive.

19. _____ - _____ _____ consist of two tests conducted in sequence, requiring both tests to be positive for the protocol to be positive.

20. _____ - _____ _____ consist of two tests, one performed right after the other, pending negative results on the first test. Positive results on the first test lead to referral for treatment. Negative results on the first and second tests lead to dismissal.

21. _____ _____ _____ are those in which positive results must be obtained on two tests performed at the same time in order for a protocol to be positive leading to referral for treatment.

22. _____ _____ _____ are those that require a positive result only on one of two tests conducted at the same time for a positive protocol leading to referral for treatment.

23. _____ - _____ _____ is a process by which the costs versus

the benefits of various tests are weighed with the preferred procedure having the greatest benefits and the lowest costs.

Word Bank:
Co-negativity
Co-positivity
Cost-benefit analysis
Cut-off points
False negatives
False positives
Gold standard
Lax parallel protocols
Parallel
Predictive value of a negative test
Predictive value of a positive test
Prior probability
Protocol
Protocol criterion
Receiver-operating characteristic curves
Sensitivity
Series
Series-negative protocols
Series-positive protocols
Specificity
Strict parallel protocol
True negatives
True positives

Problems

Instructions: Complete the decision-matrix below by labeling and filling in the numbers in the appropriate boxes, then fill-in-the-blank with the correct answers below.

A new self-assessment scale for hearing loss has been developed for use with the elderly and compared against pure-tone results with the following outcomes:

- Hits =   93
- Misses =   7
- Correct Rejections = 89
- False Positives =   11

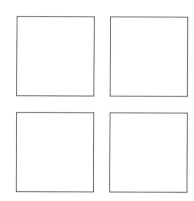

1. What is the sensitivity of the test?
_____

2. What is the specificity of the test?
_____

3. What is the predictive value of a positive test considering the prevalence of hearing loss in the elderly is 30%?
_____

4. What is the predictive value of a negative test considering the prevalence of hearing loss in the elderly is 30%?
_____

ANSWERS

Fill-in-the-Blank:
1. True positives
2. True negatives
3. False positives
4. False negatives
5. Gold standard
6. Sensitivity
7. Specificity
8. Cut-off points
9. Receiver-operating characteristic curves
10. Prior probability
11. Predictive value of a positive test
12. Predictive value of a negative test
13. Co-positivity
14. Co-negativity
15. Protocol
16. Series
17. Parallel
18. Protocol criterion
19. Series-positive protocols
20. Series-negative protocols
21. Strict parallel protocols
22. Lax parallel protocols
23. Cost-benefit analysis

Problems:

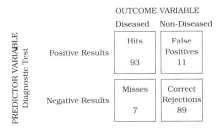

1. 93%
2. 89%
3. 78%
4. 97%

REFERENCES

Bess, F.H., Hedley-Williams, A., & Lichtenstein, M.J. (1999). Audiologic assessment of the elderly. In F.E. Musiek & W.F. Rintelmann (Eds.), *Contemporary perspectives in hearing assessment* (pp. 437–463). Needham Heights, MA: Allyn & Bacon.

Browner, W.S., Black, D., Newman, T.B., & Hulley, S.B. (1988). Estimating sample size and power. In S.B. Hulley & S.R. Cummings (Eds.), *Designing clinical research* (pp. 139–150). Baltimore, MD: Williams & Wilkins.

Browner, W.S., Newman, T.B., & Cummings, S.R. (1988). Designing a new study: III. Diagnostic tests. In S.B. Hulley & S.R. Cummings (Eds.), *Designing clinical research* (pp. 87–97). Baltimore, MD: Williams & Wilkins Co.

Cadman, D., Chambers, L., Feldman, W., & Scakett, D. (1984). Assessing the effectiveness of community screening programs. *Journal of the American Medical Association, 252,* 1580–1585.

Diefendorf, A.O. (1998). The test battery approach in pediatric audiology. In F. Bess (Ed.), *Children with hearing impairment: Contemporary trends* (pp. 71–81). Nashville, TN: Vanderbilt Bill Wilkerson Center Press.

Frattali, C.M. (1996). Outcomes data: Laying the groundwork for efficacy research and outcomes research. In *A practical guide to applying treatment outcomes and efficacy resources* (pp. 9–16). Rockville, MD: American Speech-Language-Hearing Association.

Hall, J.W. (2000). *Handbook of otoacoustic emissions.* Clifton Park, NY: Delmar Thomson Learning.

Jerger, J. (2000). Editorial: Testing with marshmallows. *Journal of the American Academy of Audiology, 11,* 56.

Jerger, J. & Hayes, D. (1976). The cross-check principle in pediatric audiometry. *Archives of Otolaryngology, 102,* 614–620.

Johnson, C.E., & Danhauer, J.L. (1999). *Guidebook for support programs in aural rehabilitation.* Clifton Park, NY: Delmar Thomson Learning.

Johnson, C.E., & Danhauer, J.L. (2001). *A survey of audiologists on outcomes measurement.* Paper presented at the 13th Annual Convention and Exposition of the American Academy of Audiology, San Diego, CA.

Joint Committee on Infant Hearing (1982). Joint Committee on Infant Hearing 1982 position statement. *ASHA, 24,* 1017–1018.

Joint Committee on Infant Hearing. (1994). Joint Committee on Infant Hearing year 1994 position statement. *ASHA, 36*(12), 38–41.

Joint Committee on Infant Hearing. (2000). Joint Committee on Infant Hearing year 2000 position statement: Principles and guidelines for early hearing detection and intervention programs. *American Journal of Audiology: A Journal of Clinical Practice, 9*(1), 9–29.

Lichtenstein, M.J., Bess, F.H., & Logan, S.L. (1988). Validation of screening tools for identifying hearing-impaired in primary care. *Journal of the American Medical Association, 259,* 2875–2878.

Martin, F.N., & Champlin, C.A. (2000). Reconsidering the limits of normal hearing.

Journal of the American Academy of Audiology, 11, 64–66.

Maxwell, D.L., & Satake, E. (1997). *Research and statistical methods in communication disorders.* Baltimore, MD: Williams & Wilkins.

Roeser, R.J. (1995). Screening for hearing loss and middle ear disorders in the schools. In R.J. Roeser & M.P. Downs (Eds.) *Auditory disorders in school children: The law, identification, remediation* (pp. 76–100). New York, NY: Thieme Medical Publishers, Inc.

Schiavetti, N., & Metz, D.E. (1997). *Evaluating research in communicative disorder* (3rd ed.) Needham Heights, MA: Allyn & Bacon.

Silman, S., Silverman, C.A., & Emmer, M.B. (2000). Central auditory processing disorders and reduced motivation: Three case studies. *Journal of the American Academy of Audiology, 11,* 57–63.

Turner, R.G., Frazer, G.J., & Shepard, N.T. (1984). Clinical performance of audiological and related diagnostic tests. *Ear and Hearing, 15,* 187–194.

Turner, R.G., Robinette, M.S., & Bauch, C.D. (1999). Clinical decisions. In F.E. Musiek & W.F. Rintelmann (Eds.), *Contemporary perspectives in hearing assessment* (pp. 437–463). Needham Heights, MA: Allyn & Bacon.

Ventry, I.M., & Weinstein, B. (1982). The Hearing Handicap Inventory for the Elderly: A new tool. *Ear and Hearing, 3,* 128–134.

Yoshinaga-Itano, C. (1997). Rationale for and outcomes from the establishment and implementation of UNHS: The Marion Downs Program. In T. Finitzo, C. Yoshinaga-Itano, Y. Sininger, & E. Cherow (Eds.), *From advocacy to intervention: Steps for successful establishment of universal newborn hearing screening (UNHS) programs* (pp. 1–34). Rockville, MD: American Speech-Language-Hearing Association.

APPENDIX VII-A

Checklist for Evaluating Investigations of Diagnostic Tests

(Adapted from Bess, Hedley-Williams, & Lichtenstein, 1999; Browner, Newman, & Cummings, 1988; Cadman, Chambers, Feldman & Scakett, 1984)

The above-referenced Appendix can be found on the companion CD-ROM.

CHAPTER 8

Outcomes Measurement in Hearing Conservation

LEARNING OBJECTIVES

This chapter will enable readers to:

- Understand comprehensive record keeping in industrial HCPs
- Acknowledge how service-delivery models can affect outcomes measurement
- Implement strategic plans for outcomes measurement in HCPs

INTRODUCTION

In 1983, the Occupational Safety and Health Administration (OSHA) estimated that 5 to 10 million workers were at risk for the hazardous effects of noise (OSHA, 1983). Today, those estimates range from 5 to 30 million noise-exposed workers (Metz, 2000). In June 2000, Ear Professional International Corporation (EPIC) sponsored a conference on Noise-Induced Hearing Loss at Lake Geneva, WI; their expert participants came to a consensus that the current paradigms for implementing hearing conservation programs (HCPs) according to the OSHA regulations have failed, particularly in (Metz, 2000):

- Measuring potential noise-induced hearing loss (NIHL)
- Assessing hearing damage after NIHL
- Placing "asset value" on NIHL
- Protecting the noise-exposed worker in industrial settings

For example, compared to traditional air- and bone-conduction thresholds, more sensitive means, such as the use of otoacoustic emissions (OAEs), have great potential to distinguish small changes in cochlear function from measurement uncertainty and to monitor cochlear function in ears exposed to noise or other hazards (Hall & Lutman, 1999). However, to state that current paradigms for implementing HCPs have failed is a pretty powerful statement. If it is true, what should be done? Metz (2000) provided some innovative directions in HCP, but should we throw the baby out with the bath water? Where are the data? What methods of program evaluation have been applied to HCPs to result in this pessimistic conclusion? What do the outcome data from current industrial HCPs show? Have national benchmarks for HCPs been established? What are the best quality indicators to measure those benchmarks? Most readers might be questioning, "Outcome data from HCPs?" Yes, outcomes measurement can and should be applied to industrial HCPs. The purpose of this chapter is to discuss current methods of HCP evaluation, record keeping, how various service-delivery models affect outcomes measurement, and strategic planning for outcomes measurement in HCPs.

INDUSTRIAL HEARING CONSERVATION PROGRAMS (HCP)

Two Approaches to Program Evaluation

There are two approaches to HCP evaluation: (1) the *prescriptive approach*, and (2) the *outcome-based approach*. The prescriptive approach is to check for the presence of key components of industrial HCPs as stipulated by the Occupational Safety and Health Administration OSHA regulations (OSHA, 1983). Complete programs meet compliance in the following areas (Stewart, 1994):

- Noise monitoring
- Employee notification of time-weighted average (TWA) exposure
- Audiometric testing program
- Qualified audiometric technician support

- Professional supervision
- Calibrated test equipment
- Audiometric test specifications
- Audiogram review and follow-up procedures
- Employee notification of standard threshold shift (STS)
- Personal hearing protective devices (HPDs)
- Fitting, training, enforcement, and replacement of HPDs
- Measurement of HPD attenuation
- Employee training
- Record keeping
- Access to records
- Transfer of records

The prescriptive approach has some advantages and disadvantages. One advantage is that evaluation is simplified through use of a checklist, such as that appearing in Appendix VIII-A, "Important Prescriptive Outcomes for Comprehensive Hearing Conservation Programs (HCPs)," on the companion CD-ROM. (Readers are advised to print out this Appendix for easy reference when reading this section.) It lists critical program components for minimal compliance with OSHA regulations in several areas, including: (1) general aspects, (2) noise monitoring, (3) noise control, (4) audiometric testing programs, (5) HPDs, (6) employee training programs, (7) ASHA accessibility, and (8) record keeping. In addition, most components list sections out of the OSHA regulations for readers who seek further information. Starred components (i.e., "*") indicate that there are some "best practices" in which minimal standards can be upgraded according to the latest recommendations by the National Institute of Industrial Occupational Safety and Health (NIOSH, 1998; Simpson, 1999).

Regarding general aspects, HCP participation should be offered to all employees at or exceeding exposure of 85 dB-A over an 8-hour period (i.e., time-weighted average) or at the 50% noise level, which is known as the

Action Level (OSHA, 1983; Stewart, 1994). Best practices, however, include offering participation in the HCP to all employees (NIOSH, 1998; Simpson, 1999).

Noise monitoring should occur for individuals who work in areas where their exposures are at or exceed the 85 dB-A TWA or 50% noise dose. In addition, HCPs should use the Permissible Exposure Level (PEL) of 90 dB-A over an 8-hour period that is considered a 100% noise dose (OSHA, 1983; Stewart, 1994). PELs are based on a 5 dB exchange rate. That is, the sound level decreases or increases 5 dB depending on the exposure time in order to maintain a 100% noise dose. For example, employees can be exposed to 95 dB-A for 4 hours, or, conversely, 85 dB-A for 16 hours, yet maintain a 100% noise dose. Noise monitoring may require the use of noise dosimetry for highly mobile workers (OSHA, 1983; Stewart, 1994). All types of sounds (i.e., continuous, intermittent, or impulse noise) ranging from 80 to 130 dB-A should be included in the measurements for determining noise dose (OSHA, 1983; Stewart, 1994). Measurements should be repeated any time a change in production has resulted in a possible increase in noise exposure (OSHA, 1983; Stewart, 1994). The maximum exposure level is 115 dB-A for 15 minutes (OSHA, 1993; Stewart, 1984). Noise measurements should be made when the level goes up. All workers at or above the Action Level should be notified and allowed to observe noise monitoring (OSHA, 1983; Stewart, 1994). Best practices include reducing the PEL from 90 dB-A to 85 dB-A over an 8-hour period (i.e., changing current 50% noise dose to 100% noise dose); using an exchange rate of 3 dB instead of 5 dB; and reducing the maximum exposure level from 115 dB-A to 110 dB-A (NIOSH, 1998; Simpson, 1999).

Regarding noise control, OSHA requires that employers use administrative (e.g., rotating worker shift) and engineering (e.g., direct reduction of noise exposure from sources) solutions so that exposures are brought below TWAs of 90 dB-A or 100% noise dose (OSHA, 1983; Simpson, 1999; Stewart, 1994). Many employers use HPDs to accomplish this requirement, but OSHA considers this a temporary solution (OSHA, 1983; Simpson, 1999). Best practices include:

- Enacting noise control procedures at 85 dB-A TWA
- Buying "quiet" equipment
- Maintaining equipment

Audiometric testing (i.e., air-conduction thresholds at 500, 1000, 2000, 3000, 4000, and 6000 Hz for each ear) using a standard audiogram should be provided for all employees at or above the Action Level. It sould be performed by a professional or a supervised technician using a calibrated audiometer (i.e., daily biologic, annual acoustic, and exhaustive biannually) in an environment meeting permissible ambient noise levels (i.e., no greater than 40 dB through 500-Hz and 1000-Hz octave bands, 47 dB through a 2000-Hz octave band, 57 dB through a 4000-Hz octave band, and 62 dB through an 8000-Hz octave band) with results recorded on a standardized form (OSHA, 1983; Stewart, 1994). Baseline audiograms must be obtained within 6 months of employment; employees who exceed the 6 months should wear HPDs until the baseline audiogram is obtained (OSHA, 1983; Stewart, 1994). Employees should have a 14-hour period of no workplace noise and an avoidance of non-occupational noise exposure prior to audiometric testing for their baseline audiograms (OSHA, 1983; Stewart, 1994). All employees at or above the Action Level should have annual audiograms (OSHA, 1983; Stewart, 1994). Each audiogram should be compared to the baseline to determine the existence of a standard threshold shift (STS) which is an average increase of 10 dB taken at 2000, 3000, and

4000 Hz in either ear in comparison to the baseline audiogram (OSHA, 1983; Stewart, 1994). Employees with STSs are retested in 30 days and notified in writing within 21 days if an STS is confirmed; that audiogram becomes the new baseline that is reviewed by audiologists, otolaryngologists, or physicians who determine the need for further evaluation (OSHA, 1983; Stewart, `1994). For work-related STSs, employees should be fit (or -refit for those currently using), trained (or retrained for those currently using), and required to wear HPDs. For nonwork related STSs, employees should be referred for an otologic evaluation. Best practices include offering audiometric testing to all employees, testing every 6 months when exposures exceed 100 dB-A, and using lower permissible ambient noise levels for testing (NIOSH, 1998; Simpson, 1999). Because OSHA does not define referral criteria, Simpson (1999) recommended the otologic referral criteria developed by the Subcommittee on Medical Aspects of Noise of the American Academy of Otolaryngology-Head and Neck Surgery (AAO-HNS, 1983) based on case history items, otoscopic findings, and audiometric results. Case history items for referral include: a history of ear pain; drainage; dizziness; sudden, fluctuating or rapidly progressing hearing loss; feelings of aural fullness or discomfort within one or both ears during the past year (AAO-HNS, 1983; Simpson, 1999). Otoscopic findings for referral include presence of excessive cerumen or foreign bodies (AAO-HNS, 1983; Simpson, 1999). Similarly, audiometric findings for referral include (AAO-HNS, 1983; Simpson, 1999):

- Average hearing loss at 500, 1000, or 2000 Hz of greater than 25 dB HL
- Difference in average hearing level between better ear and poorer ear of greater than 15 dB at 500, 1000, and 2000 Hz (low-frequency asymmetry) or

more than 30 dB at 3000, 4000, and 6000 Hz (high-frequency asymmetry)
- Shifts from baseline in average hearing levels of greater than 15 dB HL at 500, 1000, and 2000 Hz (low-frequency shift) or greater than 30 dB at 3000, 4000, and 6000 Hz (high-frequency shift).

Moreover, some have suggested that a 15 dB shift in threshold at any frequency should be used as a "red flag" for early identification of hearing loss (Royster, 1992; Simpson, 1999). Moreover, AAO-HNS (1983) suggested that baseline audiograms be defined only as the first chronologically valid test for all future comparisons with no adjustment for age.

OSHA (1983) stated that HPDs should be available to all employees and replaced when necessary (Berger, 1994). Furthermore, they are required and should be enforced to be worn by employees who:

- exceed the PEL with greater than a 100% noise dose (i.e., TWA > 90 dB-A);
- are at or above the Action Level or 50% noise dose (i.e., TWA > 85 dB-A), but who have either exceeded the 6-month time period allowed for new employees to obtain baseline audiograms or have sustained a STS.

All affected employees should have a variety of HPDs to choose from (e.g., at least two of either earmuffs, semi-permanent, or disposable HPDs) and be trained in their care and use (OSHA, 1983; Stewart, 1994). HPDs should be assessed for attenuating sound levels to 90 dB-A for employees over 100% noise dose and to 85 dB-A for those who have sustained STSs (OSHA, 1983; Stewart, 1994). Best practices include requiring HPD use for those employees at the current Action Level or at a 50% noise dose (i.e., TWA of 85 dB-A) (NIOSH, 1998; Simpson, 1999). Furthermore, the current manufacturers' estimations of noise reduction ratings (NRRs) should be multiplied by 25%, 50%, or 70%

when estimating "real world" HPD attenuation (NIOSH, 1998; Simpson, 1999).

Training programs should be required on an annual basis for employees at or above the Action Level or 50% noise dose (i.e., > or = 85 dB-A TWA) and include topics such as (Berger, 1994; OSHA, 1983; Stewart, 1994):

- Effects of noise on hearing
- Purposes, advantages, disadvantages, and attenuation of various types of HPDs and instruction on their selection, fitting, use, and care
- Purposes and procedures of audiometric testing

Best practices include (Simpson, 1999):

- Developing innovative training and instructional programs
- Using active rather than passive participation
- Advocating for one-on-one training during annual audiometric examinations
- Including employees with hearing loss to convince their colleagues about the importance of hearing conservation
- Customizing training materials for specific groups
- Using objective measures of training outcomes (e.g., employees' pre- and post-training knowledge)

Part of training can also include ensuring that workers and their representatives know that the following are available:

- OSHA (1983) standards
- Information provided by OSHA
- OSHA training materials

Regarding record keeping, OSHA requires employers to keep noise exposure measurement records for two years, and employees' audiometric data for the duration of their employment (OSHA, 1983; Simpson, 1999). Furthermore, current/former employ-

ees and OSHA should have access to these records (OSHA, 1983; Stewart, 1994). These records should include: name and job classification, audiogram date, examiner's name, date of last audiometer calibration, and the most recent noise exposure measurement (Simpson, 1999). Best practices include keeping records indefinitely or for the duration of the employee's life plus 50 years (Simpson, 1999). In addition, these data should be:

- collected, analyzed, and utilized as outcome measures;
- archived in computer-based data management systems; and
- used to track HCP performance (e.g., incidence of STSs)

Another advantage of the prescriptive approach is that it is an excellent first step in outcomes measurement in HCPs. For example, the checklist in Appendix VIII-A can be used to ensure that all program components are in place prior to measuring program performance in preventing noise-induced permanent threshold shift (NIPTS) resulting from occupational noise exposure. The disadvantage to the prescriptive approach is that a complete HCP may not be an effective one. A complete HCP may have a greater chance of being effective than an incomplete one, but measures of HCP effectiveness are necessary, requiring an outcome-based approach of HCP evaluation.

An *outcome-based approach* is to measure an HCP's effectiveness in the prevention of NIPTS according to certain quality indicators in the achievement of benchmarks. The terms "quality indicators" and "benchmarks" were defined in Chapter 6. Briefly, benchmarks are quantifiable goals or targets for monitoring and evaluation. Quality indicators reflect a measurable result in relation to stated benchmarks that are monitored using well-established practices of statistical process control to assess program consistency and stability (JCIH, 2000; Wheeler & Chambers, 1986).

In an attempt to establish national benchmarks for HCPs, the American National Standards Institute (1991) released S12.13 as the "*Draft American National Standard: Evaluating the Effectiveness of Hearing Conservation Programs*" for widespread peer review in the 1990s. The proposed standard assesses year-to-year variability and then compares the program's performance on that quality indicator to national benchmarks. For example, ANSI S12.13 (1991) uses a program's performance on three quality indicators (i.e., protocols) to determine year-to-year variability of audiometric thresholds:

■ Percent worse sequential (%Ws): The percentage of workers demonstrating a 15 dB HL or greater change toward higher (i.e., worse) thresholds at any test frequency (500–6000 Hz) in either ear between two sequential audiograms,

■ Percent better or worse sequential (%BWs): The percentage of workers demonstrating a 15 dB or greater change toward higher (i.e., worse) or lower (i.e., better) thresholds at any test frequency (500–6000 Hz) in either ear between two sequential audiograms, or

■ Standard deviation of differences (SDD) in HTLs: The standard deviation of differences in binaurally averaged HTLs between two sequential audiograms, calculated for thresholds at all test frequencies (500–6000 Hz) and at multiple frequency averages of 500 to 3000 Hz, 2000 to 4000 Hz, and 3000 to 6000 Hz (ANSI S12.13, 1991).

Through research, the Working Group established benchmarks (i.e., criterion measures) for acceptable, marginal, and unacceptable audiometric variability in HCPs (ANSI, 1991; Amos & Simpson, 1995). HCPs with little audiometric variability were believed to have a lower rate of STSs and exemplary audiometric testing programs (e.g., trained technicians, calibrated equipment, optimal testing environment, and no effects from temporary threshold shift). For example, stellar programs have trained technicians yielding valid thresholds, calibrated audiometers offering stable performance, testing environments meeting ambient noise levels, and personnel procedures requiring 14 hours of no significant exposure to workplace noise prior to testing for the baseline audiogram.

Unfortunately, recent investigations found some major problems with ANSI's S12.13 protocols. For example, Amos and Simpson (1995) found that pre-existing hearing loss and gender are confounding variables in interpreting ANSI S12.13 outcomes. Ears with poorer thresholds tend to have more test variability than ears with better thresholds. Therefore, all things being equal, HCPs that have employees with greater hearing loss may produce more audiometric variability and may be considered less effective than programs with workers having lower (better) average HTLs. Similarly, Adera, Gullickson, Helfer, Wang, and Gardner (1995) applied the ANSI S12.13 outcomes to the audiometric data collected from 82,195 Army civilian employees from 1968 to 1992 to assess the practicality, generalizability, and reliability of using the proposed standard in evaluating HCPs. Regarding practicality, the standard has some fairly stringent requirements for inclusion of data, such as annual audiometry with intervals between tests not to exceed 18 months, first audiograms within a given year with a minimum of four consecutive annual tests, and so forth (Adera, et al., 1995; ANSI, 1991). Adera, et al. (1995) found that only a mere 7% of the database was eligible for inclusion for analysis, which seriously threatened the practicality of this approach for small-to-medium HCPs that may be unable to attain adequate sample sizes. In addition, Adera, et al. (1995) stated that the results obtained on only 7% of the database could not be generalized to the study population because of systematic selection bias possibly leading to erroneous assessment of HCPs. Regarding reliability, Adera, et al. (1995) found that the ANSI S12.13 procedure yielded inconsistent results, which ran the gamut from "unacceptable" to "acceptable" (i.e., scale = unacceptable, marginal, and acceptable) from year to year and from quality indicator to quality indicator. Therefore, ANSI S12.13-1991 was seriously questioned for use as national benchmarking in evaluating the effectiveness of HCPs, except for setting general data quality guidelines (Adera, et al., 1995). Other analytic protocols that utilize audiometric data can be reviewed by readers and include Simpson (1999); Byrne and Monk (1993); Franks, Davis, and Kriegs (1989); Melnick (1984); Pell (1972); Royster (1992); and Simpson, Steward, and Kaltenbach (1994).

Generally, universal benchmarks for HCPs are difficult to devise for several reasons. First of all, workers in different industries are exposed to different types of noise, have different hearing conservation needs, and have a wide variety of demographic characteristics and noise histories. For example, noise exposure of miners (Clark & Bohl, 1999) is different from that of individuals serving in the military (Gasaway, 1994). Second, because NIPTS develops over a long period of time, assessment of HCPs' long-term effectiveness must consider data over long periods of time that are not always available for benchmarking. For example, in evaluating the effectiveness of HCPs in the Quebec mining industry, Bertrand and Zeidan (1999) employed a statistical trend analysis of the evolution of hearing threshold levels (HTLs) of 16,977 workers exposed to noise levels varying from 80 to 118 dB-A over a 15-year period as compared to the trend of HTLs based on presbycusis. Third, although the current OSHA regulations (1983) have

served as guidelines for nearly 20 years, different industries and states vary widely in the degree of adherence to those guidelines precluding the development of universal benchmarks. For example, in October 2000, the federal Mine Safety and Health Administration, an agency of the U.S. Department of Labor, issued new regulations that are expected to prevent approximately two-thirds of the possible new cases of NIPTS (Ilecki, 2000). Two important modifications of OSHA (1983) regulations include mandatory enrollment of workers at 50% noise dose (i.e., TWA of 85 dB-A) into the HCP and notification of all workers of the results of audiogram review within 10 days (Ilecki, 2000). Fourth, much is still unknown requiring research in the following areas prior to the development of universal benchmarks (Simpson, 1999):

- ways of reducing noise exposure in situations in which HPDs must be worn,
- hazardous effects of impulse noise,
- non-auditory effects of noise,
- development of high-technology noise monitoring techniques,
- improvement in laboratory methods to estimate HPD attenuation in the "real world," and
- origin and effects of ototoxic chemical exposures and possible interactions with noise.

For example, research is needed to investigate the synergistic effects of known ototoxic (i.e., affecting hearing and/or the vestibular system) industrial solvents such as toluene, styrene, and trichlorethylene and noise exposure on the human auditory system (Henderson, 1996; Mencher, Novotny, Mencher, & Gulliver, 1995). Therefore, at this point in time, some believe that the only defensible universal benchmarks for HCPs should be similar to procedures used in the field of epidemiology that are free from the problems associated with the ANSI S12.13

(1991) method. Basically, these epidemiologic methods focus on the effectiveness of HCPs preventing NIPTS such that the evolution of HTLs of employees should not be significantly different from those of non-noise exposed controls (Adera, Donahue, Malit, & Gaydos, 1993; Bertrand & Zeidan, 1999).

What about quality indicators for this benchmark? Unfortunately, the OSHA amendment (1983) did not specifically tell how to measure HCP outcomes, but it implied that lack of STSs (with the effects of age factored in) was indicative of an effective HCP (Stewart, 1994). NIOSH (1998), on the other hand, suggested monitoring the incidence of STS from year-to-year as a chronologic benchmark of effectiveness of preventive care. Recall that incidence is the number of new cases of a disease or pathologic condition that develops over a specified period of time per the number of individuals at risk (Newman, Browner, Cummings, & Hulley, 1988). Therefore, audiologists simply must determine individuals at risk, specify the time period (i.e., start and end date), measure the number of new STSs, and then make some type of comparison. The question is, however, what type of comparison? As stated, universal benchmarks for comparison are not possible at this time. Therefore, comparisons can be made to a program's previous performance. At first glance, the basic pretest and post-test paradigm seems most logical, but it may not be the most valid depending on the age and history of the HCP. New HCP programs start at ground zero with no track record for comparison. In these cases, a prescriptive approach to assessing HCP effectiveness may be the most suitable. In addition, HCP programs that change from one industrial hearing conservation company to another or from one audiologist to another, depending on service-delivery model, are in a state of flux rendering pre- and post-tests meaningless for quite sometime. For example, audiologists assuming management of HCPs may find a significantly higher number of STSs for years to come, especially if previous programming was inadequate. For example, an increase in the number of identified STSs may be indicative of stellar comprehensive audiometric monitoring implemented by a company assuming control of an HCP that had previously all but neglected workers' hearing health-care needs.

This seems fairly straightforward. But regardless of the quality indicators and benchmarks used, measuring HCP effectiveness requires the use of computer-based data management systems. These systems were discussed along with CORTI©, an example of a computer-based audiometric data management and analysis system in Chapter 5. Recall that the Bertrand-Johnson Acoustics Incorporated Company has developed CORTI© software—an effective tool for hearing conservation program (HCP) management. CORTI© helps companies to identify efficiently workers subject to noise-induced hearing loss (NIHL), controls costs, and provides full compliance with government regulations. The main features of CORTI© are data accumulation, data analysis, and individual and group reports. Regarding data accumulation, CORTI© allows for:

- unlimited aggregation of all HCP-related data (e.g., audiometric tests), job histories, noise measurements (e.g., dosimetry and sonometry), and hearing protective device information;
- use of all major audiometric microprocessors;
- import or transfer of data collected by other software packages; and
- interface with human resource information systems.

CORTI© also analyzes accumulated data to comply with OSHA regulations for:

- identification of workers exposed to or transferred to areas having levels at or above the action level or a time-weighted average of 85 dB-A,

- hearing loss classification in three main categories (e.g., normal hearing, loss caused by medical pathology, and high-frequency hearing loss),
- standard threshold shift (STS) calculation with allowance made for the aging effects according to OSHA,
- baseline adjustment upon confirmation of hearing loss,
- hearing impairment calculation according to the formula selected by the user (e.g., AAO-HNS, 1983), and
- calculation of worker time-weighted average (TWA) occupational noise exposure.

In addition to automatic data analysis, CORTI© also prepares and generates a variety of individual and group reports such as:

- Company hearing profiles
- Individual employee reports
- Industrial hygiene reports
- Medical administrative reports
- Retrospective evaluation of estimated noise exposure reports
- Standard threshold shift reports

The reports are based on user-defined parameters (e.g., age group, sex, workstations, TWA, hearing protection device (HPD), years of exposure) used permitting customization for specific information requirements and for company internal coding. Thus, CORTI© can be customized to analyze data for quality indicators such as incidence of STS in addition to those recommended by AAO-HNS (1993) for best practices.

Computer-based audiometric data analysis and management systems can assist with record keeping, which is often considered the "weak link" and all but ignored by management and technicians in the establishment of HCPs (Stewart, 1994). These systems can create an archive or permanent "paper trail"

that can protect both the worker and the company (Stewart, 1994). Successful outcomes measurement by audiologists requires an appreciation of the extent of record keeping in effective HCPs presented in Table 8-1 involving several of the following areas (Stewart, 1994):

- Records required by OSHA
- Other in-plant records
- Records maintained by audiologist
- Information needed by employers after audiogram review

Comprehensive record keeping is important for several reasons. First, record keeping is a major component of HCPs according to OSHA regulations. Second, record keeping in these areas can be used for outcome measures in specific areas of the HCPs. The reduction of incidences that employees are observed failing to wear HPDs can provide data on the effectiveness of company HPD enforcement programs, for example. Third, effective record keeping can prove invaluable in providing data for settling claims for occupational hearing loss compensation. For example, employees' and in-plant records may be used in defense of conscientious companies with aggressive hearing conservation policies against unfounded claims. Fourth, comprehensive record keeping procedures can assist in determining trends of performance revealing HCP needs. For example, failing to test all employees on an annual basis may necessitate hiring additional audiometric technicians and equipment to comply with OSHA standards.

Computer-based data analysis and management systems can use audiometric and administrative data for outcomes measurement. Recently, Helfer, Shields, and Gates (2000) explained that in August, 1996 passage of the Administrative Simplification Clause of the Health Insurance Portability and Accountability Act (HIPAA, 1996) mandated federal

Table 8-1. Record keeping in HCPs (From Stewart, A.P. (1994). The comprehensive hearing conservation program. In D. Lipscomb (Ed.), *Hearing conservation in industry, schools, and the military* (pp. 203–230) with permission from Delmar Thomson Learning).

Records Required by (OSHA, 1983)

- Employee noise exposure measurements (retained for 2 years)
- Employee audiometric tests (including name and job classification, date of test, examiner's name, date of last acoustic or exhaustive calibration of audiometer, employee's most recent noise exposure assessment (TWA), and background sound pressure levels in test room)
- Contents of employee training program

Other Necessary In-plant Measures

- Medical history (otologic) including employee's signature and date
- Previous noise exposure history (military and employment)
- Recreational noise exposure history (type, duration, and frequency)
- Audiometer (make, model, serial number of audiometer, and calibration standard)
- Audiometer calibration (biologic, acoustic, and exhaustive) including date, values, instrument ID data, and technician's name
- Additional employee audiogram data (age, sex, social security number, time of test, recent noise exposure, use of hearing protection devices (HPDs), and employee's signature)
- Otoscopic inspection of employee's ear canals
- Medical/audiologic referral history
- HPD data (initial and subsequent fitting dates, type, size for each ear, dates of training in use and care, and record of occasions when employee was found not to be satisfactorily using HPDs)
- Technician certification evidence
- Documentation of employee training (dates and signatures)

Records Maintained by the Audiologist

- Technicians train/retrain dates (dates, locations, and test scores)
- Audiometer calibration data (plant, clinical, and/or mobile van equipment)
- Test room background sound levels (plant, clinical, and/or mobile van rooms)
- Noise exposure measurements for individual plants (date and time, equipment identification data, evidence of calibration, measures obtained, examiner's name, and recommendations to the company)
- Reports of findings and recommendations during HCP evaluation visits
- Audiogram review/interpretation/recommendation data for individual plants
- Copies of all correspondence with individual plant representatives
- Records of telephone or face-to-face conversations with individual plant representatives, other HCP consultants, and individual employees
- Diagnostic audiologic evaluation data and recommendations for individual employees
- Evaluation of individual plant and corporate audiometric databases, interpretations, and recommendations
- Legal correspondence and transcripts
- System for determining when individual employees are scheduled for annual, or more frequent, hearing tests
- Industrial audiograms (to include 3000 and 6000 Hz) performed in clinic or mobile van for individual plants

(CONTINUES)

Table 8-1. (continued from page 173)

- Otologic histories, previous noise exposure histories, and recreational noise exposure histories of employees tested in clinic or mobile vans
- Otoscopic inspection findings for above employees
- HPD data (similar to in-plant list) for above employees
- Microfilming of audiograms

Information Needed by Employers After Audiogram Review

- Audiometric data and identification data for individual employees (digital or graphic)
- Individual employee notification forms (results of recent hearing test, interpretation, and recommendations)
- Otologic history data, HPD use, and noise exposure status for individual employees
- Display of previous audiograms (at least baseline) for each employee
- Individual calculations (changes from baseline audiogram, code designation of type and degree of indicated loss to facilitate follow-up activity, indication whether a significant STS according to OSHA or other criteria has occurred after appropriate age corrections have been applied, indication of degree of average hearing loss for speech and high frequencies together with changes of these degrees from baseline, other code designations, and percent of potentially compensable hearing loss for current and baseline tests)
- Specific recommendations for follow-up activity for individual employees (retests, diagnostic evaluations, hearing aid evaluations, and medical referral)
- Technical data (examiner identification, audiometer identification, test environment sound levels, and so forth)
- Scheduled dates for subsequent tests for each employee
- Lists of employees with notable findings

standards for electronic storage and transmission of administrative health-care data requiring two data elements: (1) American Medical Association's (AMA) Common Procedural Terminology (CPT) Codes (AMA, 1999a) and (2) International Classification of Disease, 9th edition, with American Clinical Modifications (ICD-9-M) Codes (AMA, 1999b). These data elements extend beyond the traditional use of audiometric data in assessing HCP effectiveness. Helfer, et al. (2000) demonstrated a method of data modeling within an administrative database for the military health system that provided high quality outcomes cost data for input into executive information and decision-making systems that have potential applications for educational and occupational HCPs in the private sector. Regardless of the type of data used, record keeping plays a critical role in the success of outcomes measurement efforts. However, at this point, it is difficult to discuss specific aspects of record keeping without discussing the effect of service-delivery models on the clinicians' role, stake, and perspective in outcomes measurement.

EFFECT OF SERVICE-DELIVERY MODELS ON OUTCOMES MEASUREMENT IN HCPS

The type of service-delivery model determines audiologists' role in, stake in, and perspective of outcomes measurement in HCPs. There are three service-delivery models in HCPs (Stewart, 1994):

1. A totally in-house program
2. A partly in-house/consultant program
3. A totally consultant program

A totally in-house program, common in larger companies, uses internal resources and personnel for running a HCP (Stewart, 1994). Audiologists are often employees of the company and typically have the responsibility for audiogram review/referral and coordination of computer-based audiometric analysis and management systems, and are considered company "insiders" (Stewart, 1994). Other HCP responsibilities are delegated to departments such as medical safety, industrial hygiene, and engineering creating an atmosphere of a HCP team (Stewart, 1994). Audiologists have considerable influence over outcomes measurement in these types of programs. For example, they can convince management of the importance of outcomes measurement, request the latest software in their budgets, select quality indicators in achievement of program benchmarks, convene the HCP team to review performance, pinpoint specific problems, and suggest remedial action for improvement. Audiologists, serving as intermediary between management and workers, often must balance the hearing health-care needs of the latter with the former's need to reduce overhead costs. Using best practices in HCPs may result in lower STSs in workers, but may come at a cost of higher false positive rates, for example. The totally in-house service-delivery model is not very common in the United States (Stewart, 1994).

The most common service-delivery model in the United States, or the combination in-house and consultant service program, is one in which the company has both in-house personnel (e.g., nurse, personnel manager, or occupational hearing conservationist) and hired consultants participate (e.g., noise surveys, mobile audiometric testing, audiogram review, and referral) in the HCPs (Stewart, 1994). Outcomes measurement is a joint responsibility between both in-house and consultant components of such HCPs. Audiologists' roles in this service-delivery model can either be as employees of the company or as hired consultants with either an "insider" or an "outsider" status, respectively, in the outcomes measurement process. Unfortunately, audiologists hired as consultants by a company can be outsiders in the outcomes measurement process. Eager audiologists with data suggesting needs for improvement may find less than enthusiastic reactions from managers who are satisfied with providing the bare minimum for OSHA (1983) compliance, for example. In these cases, program improvement efforts must be coordinated through a "team approach" requiring cooperation from "insiders" who have the greatest impact in effecting change in HCP policies (Stewart, 1994).

The totally consultant program is often used by smaller companies that do not have the resources and must "farm-out" all aspects of the HCP to consultants who provide both on-site (e.g., noise surveys, mobile van testing, or employee training sessions) and off-site services (e.g., hearing testing, HPD fitting, employee training sessions, audiogram review, or referral in the consultant's clinic) (Stewart, 1994). The totally consultant program is rarely used because of the high cost and lack of a key individual on-site who is responsible for the HCP; thus, it is not recommended for most companies. Audiologists within this program are company "outsiders," but at least have control over the outcomes measurement process and can implement reasonable quality improvement measures in the HCP. Regardless of service-delivery model, audiologists must market the importance of hearing conservation to workers and to management for programs to work. In the long run, effective HCPs are those in which the underlying motivation is for prevention of NIPTS, not workers' or management's fear of reprimand. Audiologists' consideration of service-delivery model and the dynamics of their relationships to companies, management, and employees is one of the first steps in a strategic approach to outcomes measurement in HCPs.

A STRATEGIC PLAN FOR OUTCOMES MEASUREMENT IN HCP

So far we have discussed some generalized approaches and methods for outcomes measurement in HCPs. Now, the time has come to put it all together and provide a general strategic plan for outcomes measurement that can be used by either audiologists in private practice who decide to provide HCPs to small companies or by those employed by firms requiring hearing conservation services for thousands of workers. Strategic planning can be used for both new and well-established HCPs. Appendix VIII-B, "Strategic Planning for Outcomes Measurement in Hearing Conservation Programs (HCPs)," contains a worksheet outlining the steps in a strategic plan for outcomes measurement in HCPs. (Readers are advised to print out this Appendix from the companion CD-ROM for easy reference when reading this section.)

The first step in a strategic plan for outcomes measurement is for audiologists to make a personal commitment to program excellence regardless of the service-delivery model and relationship to the particular company. A personal commitment toward HCP excellence means influencing policy to higher and higher levels of performance in whatever way possible. For example, audiologists may be hired for audiometric testing, audiogram review, and referral only, yet they can market the importance of hearing conservation through newsletters and suggest improvements in HCP programming. Although management may or may not act on those suggestions, audiologists can at least feel that they have done all within their power to make positive changes.

The second step in the plan is to determine who does what in the HCP. Appendix VIII-B lists typical HCP team members and their usual responsibilities. All HCP's are different, however. Thus, audiologists can write the names and telephone numbers of persons responsible for certain program areas to facilitate communication so that valuable time and effort is not spent trying to figure out who needs what information, for example. The most important individual is the person within the company who is ultimately responsible for the HCP. Audiologists may find that some HCPs may not have certain job designations on the list and may delegate the responsibilities of those positions to several other individuals. It is important to not only have the contact information of key HCP team members, but also the pecking order and established lines of communication. For example, non-compliance with HPDs should be reported to the HCP directors who can contact the right supervisor to enforce appropriate reprimands, if necessary. Audiologists who are "outsiders" must be especially vigilant regarding company etiquette because team members must work together, not against each other. The most effective plans for outcomes measurement are doomed for failure without the willing cooperation of those directly within the company.

The third step is to apply a prescriptive approach to evaluating effectiveness through assessing program outcomes for comprehensive HCPs with the use of Appendix VIII-A. Audiologists should interview key HCP team members to confirm the existence of key outcomes that ensure compliance with OSHA (1983) regulations. A list of program deficiencies should be noted and then reported to the HCP director. Unfortunately, the director may or may not implement suggested remedial actions, but at least audiologists should document their concerns on record and offer their expertise for program improvement. Audiologists may choose not to continue providing services to companies whose HCP policies are incomplete and place the hearing health care of their employees at risk.

The fourth step in strategic planning for outcomes measurement is to enact a formal marketing campaign about the importance of outcomes measurement in establishing and maintaining stellar HCPs. The first charge of a marketing campaign is to sell the concept that the prevention of NIPTS is in everyone's best interest. The motivation for each stakeholder may be different, but HCP success is predicated on universal cooperation in achieving HCP goals. With a spirit of cooperation, the sky is the limit! Audiologists should assess precampaign commitment by making three lists of individuals based on their alleged attitudes toward the HCP; those who:

1. already show strong support,
2. are "on the fence," and
3. do not care or are difficult to deal with.

For (2) and (3), list possible reasons for current attitudes and strategies for change. Marketing campaigns should begin at the top with those having the power to establish policies and delegate resources to make things happen. For example, audiologists may find that a two-punch approach to marketing is most effective by first garnering strong managerial support from those who set and enforce HCP policies, and second, by convincing otherwise indifferent employees that those policies are in their long-term best interests.

The fifth step in a strategic plan is to apply an outcome-based approach to assessing HCP effectiveness, requiring the use of a computer-based audiometric data analysis and management system like CORTI©, which can either be owned by the audiologist or the company. Clearly, such systems are superior to "paper and pencil" methods and are an absolute necessity for addressing the outcomes measurement needs of medium-to-large companies. With consultation from management and team members, quality indicators must be selected as an overall measure in achieving the benchmark of preventing NIPTS. Quality indicators must be understandable and agreeable by all as an overall barometer of HCP effectiveness and can vary from strict to lax. Strict criteria for program performance are usually based on the "best practices" (e.g., AAO-HNS, 1983 audiometric referral criteria) in hearing conservation that drive performance into identifying all employees at risk for NIPTS. HCPs with strict performance criteria have the benefit of being highly sensitive, but at the cost of a high false-positive rate and over-referral. In addition, a formal HCP performance review process is needed in which quality indicators are measured and reviewed by the HCP team, weaknesses are identified, and remedial strategies are implemented on a periodic regular basis. From time-to-time, outcome measures must be devised to address minor problems. For example, workers' ratings of training sessions can be used to gauge instructional improvements enacted to reduce employee absenteeism.

The sixth step in a strategic plan for outcomes measurement in HCP is to take some steps at identifying those workers at risk for NIPTS for early intervention. These steps can be as simple as identifying workers who need to be reprimanded for noncompliance with HPD policies or as sophisticated as identifying workers who are expected to develop compensable hearing loss by age 61 years through statistical modeling, taking into account age, sex, job history, and average TWA. For example, CORTI© has special features that incorporate statistical modeling that identifies workers who are susceptible to NIPTS and who may be subject to compensation in future years. For example, Figure 8-1 shows audiograms at age 45 years and audiometric projections at age 61 years that would justify compensation according to the standards for combination according to the American Medical Association (1999). Audiol-

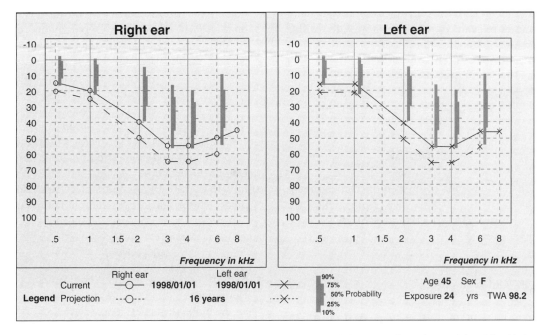

Figure 8-1. Audiograms of current and predicted thresholds for a worker at considerable risk for NIPTS (Reprinted with permission form Bertrand-Johnson Acoustics, 2001 Available Internet: www.bjainc.com/)

ogists can affect preventative measures for similar employees to circumvent the development of NIPTS. In addition, CORTI© can obtain similar summary data for a group of workers and create company hearing profiles.

In summary, a strategic plan for outcomes measurement can contribute to the improvement of HCPs regardless of service-delivery model and size of the company. Regulations will evolve and change, but a commitment to outcomes measurement and HCP program excellence should not. Audiologists can find that participation in HCPs at any level, can be not only quite lucrative, but also provide opportunities to prevent NIPTS (Florian, 2000). Prevention of hearing loss is

---

LEARNING ACTIVITIES

- Interview two audiologists involved in hearing conservation regarding their approach to outcomes measurement.

- Use Appendix VIII-A in evaluating a local HCP.

- Go to OSHA's Noise and Hearing Conservation Webpage (Available Internet: http://www.osha-slc.gov/SLTC/noisehearingconservation/index.html) and print out important documents in creation of an industrial hearing conservation notebook.

consistent with the principles of managed care and is relevant for all occupations from disc jockeys to miners (Florian, 2000). Audiologists can establish their own niches in the area of occupational audiology through meeting the increased need for HCPs and providing quality, outcome-based services (Florian, 2000).

SUMMARY

This chapter has discussed outcomes measurement in HCPs. Two approaches to evaluating the effectiveness of HCPs were discussed:

1. Prescriptive
2. Outcome-based

The prescriptive approach involves checking for the presence of key components of HCPs and is most effective for use in new HCPs. The outcome-based approach involves measuring an HCP's effectiveness in the prevention of NIPTS according to certain quality indicators in the achievement of benchmarks. Both approaches are used as part of audiologists' strategic plan for outcomes measurement regardless of service-delivery model and size of the company.

RECOMMENDED READINGS AND WEBSITES

Readings

Behar, A., Chasin, M., & Cheesman, M.E. (2000). *Noise control: A primer*. Clifton Park, NY: Delmar Thomson Learning.

Berger, E.H., Royster, L.H., Royster, J.D., Driscoll, D.P., & Layne, M. (2000). *The noise manual* (4th ed.) Fairfax, VA: American Industrial Hygiene Association (AIHA).

National Institute for Occupational Safety and Health (NIOSH). (1998). *Occupational noise exposure: Revised criteria for a recommended standard*. Department of Health and Human Services (DHHS) NIOSH Publication 98–126. Cincinnati, OH: U.S. Department of Health and Human Services, Public Health Service, Centers for Disease Control, National Institute for Occupational Safety and Health.

OSHA (2000). *OSHA CD: Noise control and hearing conservation* (1st ed.) Albany, NY: Delmar Publishers.

Villchur, E. (2000). *Acoustics for audiologists*. Clifton Park, NY: Delmar Thomson Learning.

Websites

- Military Audiology Association (MAA) Homepage:
    ⇒ Available Internet: http://www. militaryaudiology.org.html
- National Hearing Conservation Association (NHCA) Homepage:
    ⇒ Available Internet: http://www. hearingconservation.org.html
- National Institute of Occupational Safety and Health (NIOSH) Homepage:
    ⇒ Available Internet: http://www.cdc.gov/niosh/homepage. html
- Occupational Safety and Health Administration (OSHA) Noise and Hearing Conservation Page
    ⇒ Available Internet: http://www. osha-slc.gov/SLTC/noisehearing conservation/index.html

REVIEW EXERCISES

Fill-in-the-Blank

Instructions: Please fill in the blanks with the correct term from the word bank.

1. The _____ approach is to check for the presence of key components of industrial HCPs as stipulated by

OSHA regulation (OSHA, 1983).

2. An _____ - _____ approach is to measure an HCP's effectiveness in the prevention of NIPTS according to certain quality indicators in the achievement of benchmarks.

3. A totally _____ - _____ program is often used by larger companies that utilize their own resources and personnel to run a HCP.

4. A combination _____ - _____ and _____ _____ program is one in which the company has both in-house personnel and hired consultants participate in a HCP.

5. The totally _____ program is often used by smaller companies who do not have the resources and must "farm-out" all aspects of the HCP to consultants who provide both on-site and off-site services.

Word Bank:
In-house and consultant service
Consultant
In-house
Prescriptive
Outcome-based

Matching

Instructions: Please match the items below to the appropriate statements.

I. True
II. False

1. ____ All industries follow OSHA standards (1983) in exactly the same way.

2. ____ OSHA standards (1983) have considerable room for improvement in protecting workers from NIPTS.

3. ____ Universal benchmarks for HCPs should be fairly easy to establish.

4. ____ Service-delivery models in HCP can affect audiologists' role in outcomes measurement.

5. ____ The totally in-house program is the most commonly used in the United States.

Sequencing

Instructions: Please number the items below from 1 to 6 according to the order in which they take place in strategic planning for outcomes measurement.

____ Determine who does what in the HCP.

____ Apply a prescriptive approach to assessing HCP effectiveness.

____ Commit to HCP excellence.

____ Identify those workers at most risk for NIPTS.

____ Apply an outcome-based approach to assessing HCP effectiveness.

____ Enact a formal marketing campaign.

ANSWERS

Fill-in-the-Blank:
  1. Prescriptive
  2. Outcome-based
  3. In-house
  4. In-house and consultant service
  5. Consultant

Matching:
  1. II
  2. I
  3. II
  4. I
  5. II

Sequencing:
2, 3, 1, 6, 5, 4

REFERENCES

Adera,, T., Donahue, A.M., Malit, B.D., & Gaydos, J.C. (1993). An epidemiologic method for assessing the effectiveness of hearing conservation programs using audiometric data. *Military Medicine, 35,* 568–573.

Adera,, T., Gullickson, G.M., Helfer, T., Wang, L., & Gardner, J.W. (1995). Should the Audiometric Database Analysis Method

(Draft ANSI S12.13-1991) for evaluating the effectiveness of hearing conservation programs be accepted as a US national standard? *Journal of the American Academy of Audiology, 6,* 302–310.

American Academy of Otolaryngology-Head and Neck Surgery (AAO-HNS). (1983). *Otologic referral criteria for occupational hearing conservation programs.* Washington, DC: Author.

American Medical Association (1999a). *Current procedural terminology.* Chicago, IL: Author.

American Medical Association (1999b). *International classification of diseases, 9th edition (revision), clinical modification.* Salt Lake City, UT: MEDICODE.

American National Standards Institute (ANSI). (1991). *Draft American National Standard: Evaluating the effectiveness of hearing conservation programs (ANSI S12.13).* New York, NY: American National Standards Institute and the Acoustical Society of America.

Amos, N.E., & Simpson, T.H. (1995). Effects of pre-existing hearing loss and gender on proposed ANSI S12.13 outcomes for characterizing hearing conservation program effectiveness: Preliminary investigation. *Journal of the American Academy of Audiology, 6,* 407–413.

Berger, E.H. (1994). Hearing protectors—specifications, fitting, use, and performance. In D. Lipscomb (Ed.), *Hearing conservation in industry, schools, and the military* (pp. 145–191). Clifton Park, NY: Delmar Thomson Learning.

Bertrand, R.A., & Zeidan, J. (1999). A statistical approach used to evaluate the effectiveness of a hearing conservation program (HCP) in the Quebec mining industry. *Journal of Occupational Hearing Loss, 2*(2 & 3), 115–129.

Byrne, D., & Monk, W. (1993). Evaluating a hearing conservation program: A comparison of the USAEHA method and the ANSI S12.13 method [Abstract]. *Spectrum, 10*(Suppl. 1), 19.

Clark, W.H., & Bohl, C.D. (1999). Hearing levels of miners. *Journal of Occupational Hearing Loss, 2*(2 & 3), 115–129.

Florian, J. (2000). Occupational audiology: "Where audiology gets down to business." *The Hearing Journal, 53*(10), 34, 36–38.

Franks, J.F., Davis, R.R., & Krieg, E.F. (1989). Analysis of a hearing conservation program database: Factors other than workplace noise. *Ear and Hearing, 10,* 273–280.

Gasaway, D.C. (1994). Occupational hearing conservation in the military. In D. Lipscomb (Ed.), *Hearing conservation in industry, schools, and the military* (pp. 243–262). Clifton Park, NY: Delmar Thomson Learning.

Hall, A.J., & Lutman, M.E. (1999). Methods for early identification of noise-induced hearing loss. *Audiology, 38,* 277–280.

Health Insurance Portability and Accountability Act (HIPAA) of 1996. (1996). Public Law 104–191. Available Internet: www.aspe.os.dhhs.gov/admnsimp/kkimpl.html

Helfer, T.M., Shields, A.R., & Gates, K.E. (2000). Outcomes analysis for hearing conservation programs. *American Journal of Audiology: A Journal of Clinical Practice, Online: Volume 9.* Available Internet: www.asha.edoc.com/1059-0089/v9n5/helfer.html

Henderson, D. (1996). Solvents and hearing loss. *Journal of the American Academy of Audiology, 7,* 375.

Ilecki, H.J. (2000). Mine agency implements new noise standard. *The ASHA Leader, 5*(19), 1, 25.

Joint Committee on Infant Hearing. (2000). Joint Committee on Infant Hearing year 2000 position statement: Principles and guidelines for early hearing detection and intervention programs. *American Journal of Audiology: A Journal of Clinical Practice, 9*(1), 9–29.

Melnick, W. (1984). Evaluation of industrial hearing conservation programs: A review and analysis. *American Industrial Hygiene Association Journal, 45*(7), 59–67.

Mencher, G.T., Novotny, G., Mencher, L., & Gulliver, M. (1995). Ototoxicity and irriadiation: Additional etiologies of hearing loss in adults. *Journal of the American Academy of Audiology, 6*, 351–357.

Metz, M. (2000). The failed hearing conservation paradigm. *Audiology Today, 12*(5), 13–15.

National Institute for Occupational Safety and Health (NIOSH). (1998). *Occupational noise exposure: Revised criteria for a recommended standard.* Department of Health and Human Services (DHHS) NIOSH Publication 98–126. Cincinnati, OH: U.S. Department of Health and Human Services, Public Health Service, Centers for Disease Control, National Institute for Occupational Safety and Health.

Newman, T.B., Browner, W.S., Cummings, S.R., & Hulley, S.B. (1988). Designing a new study: II. Cross-sectional and case-control studies. In S.B. Hulley and S.R. Cummings (Eds.), *Designing clinical research* (pp. 75–86). Baltimore, MD: Williams & Wilkins.

Occupational Safety and Health Administration (1983, March 3). Occupational noise exposure; hearing conservation amendment; final rule. *Federal Register 46,* 9738–9785.

Pell, S. (1972). An evaluation of a hearing conservation program. *American Industrial Hygiene Association Journal, 33*(1), 60–70.

Royster, J.D. (1992). *Evaluation of different criteria for significant threshold shift in occupational hearing conservation programs.* Raleigh, NC: Environmental Noise Consultants , Inc., NTIS No. PB93-159143.

Simpson, T.H. (1999). Occupational hearing loss prevention programs. In F.E. Musiek and W.F. Rintelmann (Eds.), *Contemporary perspectives in hearing assessment* (pp. 465–484). Needham Heights, MA: Allyn & Bacon.

Simpson, T.H., Steward, M., & Kaltenbach, J.A. (1994). Early indicators of hearing conservation program performance. *Journal of the American Academy of Audiology, 5*, 300–306.

Stewart, A.P. (1994). The comprehensive hearing conservation program. In D. Lipscomb (Ed.), *Hearing conservation in industry, schools, and the military* (pp. 203–230). Clifton Park, NY: Delmar Thomson Learning.

Wheeler, D.J., & Chambers, D.S. (1986). *Understanding statistical process control.* Knoxville, TN: SPC Press, Inc.

APPENDIX VIII-A

Important Prescriptive Outcomes
for Comprehensive Hearing Conservation Programs

(Adapted from NIOSH, 1998; OSHA, 1983; Simpson, 1999; Stewart, 1994)

The above-referenced Appendix can be found on the companion CD-ROM.

APPENDIX VIII-B

Strategic Planning for Outcomes Measurement
in Hearing Conservation Programs (HCPs)

The above-referenced Appendix can be found on the companion CD-ROM.

CHAPTER 9

Outcomes Measurement in Aural Habilitation

LEARNING OBJECTIVES

This chapter will enable readers to:

- Identify reasons for the lack of reliable and valid outcomes measures for children
- Consider four questions that complicate outcomes measurement in infants and young children
- Review objective and subjective outcomes measures to be used with children
- Acknowledge alternative approaches to outcomes measurement
- Understand the complexity of outcomes measurement of intervention programs

INTRODUCTION

Positive patient outcomes in aural habilitation are very similar to critical outcomes in relay races. For example, the most successful relay teams are those that have an early start, optimum coordination in passing the baton, and cross the finish line. Successful aural habilitative outcomes require early detection of hearing loss through universal newborn hearing screening (UNHS) programs, coordination of professionals in the confirmation of hearing loss, and early intervention program development designed to meet the individualized needs of the infant and family. The relay team cannot be successful unless the final

runner crosses the finish line. No awards are given for a team that has a lightning fast reaction to the starter's pistol or runs the fastest leg, but drops the baton and does not finish. Similarly, early hearing detection and intervention (EHDI) programs that effectively identify infants with hearing loss at birth are all but useless unless those infants and their families are transferred through a seamless continuum of services with well-coordinated professionals and agencies culminating in an effective, family-centered early intervention program. But, what are effective early intervention programs? How do we measure the outcomes of pediatric hearing aid fittings? The Joint Committee on Infant Hearing Year 2000 Position Statement (JCIH, 2000) established both benchmarks and quality indicators for EHDI programs. However, state and national data have yet to be aggregated in establishing percentages for quality indicators in the confirmation of hearing loss and early intervention programs. The purpose of this chapter is to discuss outcomes measurement in aural habilitation.

OBSTACLES AFFECTING OUTCOMES MEASUREMENT IN AURAL HABILITATION

Many of the JCIH (2000) benchmarks seem straightforward and easy to assess, such as infants identified as having a hearing loss must:

- Be enrolled in a family-centered early intervention program before 6 months of age
- Begin use of amplification within one month of confirmation of hearing loss (providing no medical contraindications and as agreed upon by family)
- Receive audiologic monitoring at intervals not to exceed three months if they have amplification

These examples specifically focus on "when" or the timing of the fitting and monitoring of the amplification, but ignore the "how." If amplification is fit poorly, does the "when" matter? Yes, but audiologists should also determine the quality of their fittings through outcome measures.

Reliable and valid outcome measures for infants and young children are few and far between for several reasons (Stelmachowicz, 1999):

- Precise determination of the degree of hearing loss is often not possible

- Many physical differences exist between infants and young children versus older children and adults (e.g., ear-canal resonance, real-ear-to-coupler differences, and parent-to-child speaking proximity)
- Differences in opinions regarding the appropriate electroacoustic requirements for infants and young children (e.g., National Acoustics Laboratories versus Desired Sensation Level)
- Poor reliability (i.e., lack of cooperation) of infants and young children during audiologic testing
- Few speech perception tests geared toward the limited speech reception abilities of infants and young children
- Minimal subjective feedback provided by infants and young children

In addition, Stelmachowicz (1999) mentioned four questions that may complicate, yet must be considered, when conducting outcomes measurement with infants and young children:

- What should be used as an outcome measure?
- Over what time period should outcome measures be made?
- How can ongoing developmental changes be separated from changes specifically related to amplification?
- At what developmental age will outcome measures for adults be developed for use with children?

In spite of these obstacles, outcome measures do exist for the aural habilitation efforts of young children with hearing impairment.

OUTCOME MEASURES

Stelmachowicz (1999) stated that there are two types of outcome measures for children:

1. Objective
2. Subjective

Objective Outcome Measures

Objective outcome measures for amplification are those that assess children's speech recognition with their hearing instruments. Unfortunately, few reliable speech recognition tests exist for use with children less than 3 years of age (Stelmachowicz, 1999). However, clinicians have a wide variety of speech recognition tests for use with children 3 years of age and older. Audiologists must consider three types of variables when using speech recognition tests with children (Kirk, Diefendorf, Pisoni, & Robbins, 1997):

1. *Internal variables*
2. *External variables*
3. *Methodological variables*

Internal variables are those that have to do with the child or subject, such as vocabulary/language competency, chronologic age, and cognitive abilities (Kirk, et al., 1997). External variables are those that have to do with the speech recognition test, such as appropriate response task, utilization of reinforcement, and memory load (Kirk, et al., 1997). Methodological variables have to do with the administration of the test, such as taped versus monitored live-voice presentation, open- versus closed-set tests, and task domain in closed-set test construction (i.e., restricted or unrestricted domain) (Kirk, et al., 1997). The discussion of the effects of these variables is beyond the scope of this textbook, but readers are referred to Kirk, et al. (1997) for further reading.

Speech recognition tests for children are often classified according to whether they have an open-set or closed-set construction or response format. *Open-set* response formats are those in which patients have an infinite number of possibilities of response alternatives (Lucks Mendel & Danhauer, 1997). For example, a common open-set response paradigm for patients is simply to repeat what they hear. *Closed-set* response formats are those in which patients select a response from a group of alternatives. For example, the *Word Intelligibility by Picture Identification* (WIPI) test (Ross & Lerman, 1979) is a closed-response format test that requires children to respond by pointing to a picture out of a choice of six. Lucks Mendel and Danhauer (1997) reported that the advantages of open-set tests are:

- More flexibility because of the lack of a written answer form
- An unlimited number of response alternatives
- No guessing floor that would artificially boost scores

For example, a closed-response test with four response alternatives per item has a possible score ranging from 25 to 100% because patients can, by chance alone, receive a score of 25%. However, open-set response tests have a possible score range of 0 to 100%. The major disadvantage of open-set response tests for use with children is that their articulatory errors cannot be differentiated easily from perceptual errors invalidating test results. Lucks Mendel and Danhauer (1997) also provided the main advantages of closed-response tests:

- Manipulation of response items permits varying the difficulty and sensitivity of the test
- An equal number of response alternatives for each item
- Responses are easier to score thereby, increasing the validity and reliability of test results
- Tests can be computerized for self-recording and self-pacing of responses

Closed-response format tests also permit valid and reliable scoring of the responses of children with articulatory problems.

Closed-response test formats can further be categorized as either *unrestricted* or *restricted* regarding task domain. Kirk, et al. (1997) stated that unrestricted task domains are response tasks in which target signals are not uniquely specified for patients, but are embedded among foil items representing selected phonemic confusions, as in the WIPI (Ross & Lerman, 1979), that promote a sensory processing outcome perspective. Restricted task domains are response tasks that promote a cognitive (conceptual) processing outcome perspective with the following characteristics (Kirk, et al., 1997):

- A top-down processing approach (e.g., general knowledge and expectations based on context) is used by patients to respond correctly
- Correct responses can often be selected by a process of elimination
- Patients know what they are expected to hear

Table 9-1 shows the name, author(s), purposes, stimuli, recordings, minimum age, standardization, and additional information concerning objective speech recognition measures to be used with children (Kirk, et al., 1997).

Subjective Outcome Measures

Some subjective outcome measures used with children include teacher inventories/checklists, parent questionnaires, and use of adult subjective measures with children.

Teacher Inventories and Checklists

Other subjective outcomes measures for aural habilitation include teacher inventories and checklists. Three frequently used teacher checklists are:

1. *Fisher's Auditory Problems Checklist* (Fisher, 1985)

2. *Screening Instrument for Targeting Educational Risk* (S.I.F.T.E.R.) (Anderson, 1989) that also has a pre-school version (Anderson & Matkin, 1996)

3. *Listening Inventory for Education* (L.I.F.E.) (Anderson & Smaldino, 1996)

These checklists are brief, can be completed by teachers in a relatively short period of time, and may be quite helpful in identifying and measuring children's hearing loss and monitoring students' progress from year-to-year (Johnson, Benson, & Seaton, 1997). In addition, these checklists can be used to measure the effectiveness of intervention efforts in terms of reducing students' hearing handicap in educational environments.

The *Fisher's Auditory Problem Checklist* (Fisher, 1985) was originally developed to identify children with possible central auditory processing disorders, but it can also be used to assist in screening for hearing loss (Johnson, et al., 1997). The checklist consists of 25 items with instructions to place a check mark before each item that is considered to be a concern by the observer, who is usually a teacher, but can be a parent or teacher's aide. For example, if the child has had a long-standing history of otitis media, the observer would place a check by item 2, "Has a history of ear infection(s)." The more items checked for a child, the more concerns the observer has regarding the child's auditory processing abilities involving association, attention, attention span, auditory-visual integration, closure, comprehension, discrimination, figure-ground, identification, localization, long-term memory, motivation, performance, recognition, sensitivity, sequential memory, short-term memory, and speech-language problems. Scoring requires counting the number of items *NOT* checked and multiplying that number by 4. The checklist was normed on 280 children from kindergarten to the 6th grade (i.e., ages 5 to 12 years) and has

Table 9-1. Objective open- and closed-set speech recognition tests for use with children

OPEN-SET TESTS

NAME/ AUTHOR	PURPOSE	STIMULI	RECORDED	MINIMUM AGE	STANDARDIZATION INFORMATION
PBK-50 Word Lists (Haskins, 1949)	Not stated	3 lists of monosyllabic words (e.g., please, sled, rat, bad, bus) preceded by the carrier phrase, "Say the word"	Audio-cassette tape available from Auditec or monitored-live voice	6 years	• Low test-retest variability, lists found to be similar in difficulty • Verified on 60 children with normal hearing
Bamford-Kowal-Bench Sentences (BKB) (Bench, Kowal, & Bamford, 1979)	To assess speech recognition at a sentence level	Key words in sentences which are used to derive percent-correct score (e.g., The dog came back. She found her purse. The ball is bouncing very high.)	• Several modified recordings. • Original test contains some words that are more common in British English • Available on laser videodisc • Tyler, Preece, and Tye-Murray modified 100 sentences for use in the U.S.	6 years	Not stated
Mr. Potato Head Task (Robbins, 1994)	To assess open-set auditory comprehension in young children who are deaf	10 commands requiring object manipulation of Mr. Potato Head Toy (e.g., Give him green shoes)	Monitored-live voice	2 years for clinical use and 3 years for research purposes	Not stated
The Common Phrase Test (Robbins, Renshaw, & Osberger, 1995)	To assess open-set comprehension of familiar phrases in children with profound deafness	6 lists of 10 phrases that are 2 to 6 words in length (e.g., It is so cold outside today.)	Monitored-live voice	Not stated	Not stated

Table 9-1. (continued from page 189)

CLOSED-RESPONSE TESTS

NAME/ AUTHOR	PURPOSE	STIMULI	RECORDED	MINIMUM AGE	STANDARDIZATION INFORMATION
Monosyllabic- Trochee- Spondee Test (MTS) (Erber & Alencewicz, 1976)	To assess closed- response word identification in children with hearing impairment	12 items overall (e.g., bed, cat, button, chicken, baseball, popcorn, elephant)	Monitored-live voice	When necessary vocabulary has been acquired at approximately 4 years of age	• Reported on 67 children with hearing impairment aged 8 to 16 years • Test-retest reliability = 0.87 • Demonstrated strong relationship between test performance and pure-tone average (PTA) except for those worse than 95 dB HTL
Closed-Set Speech Perception Test for Hearing- Impaired Children- Matrix Test (Tyler & Holsted, 1978)	To evaluate the effective- ness of hear- ing aids, tactile aids, and cochlear implants in children with hearing impairment	Words in sentences 60 items and 120 items for 2 levels (e.g., Level A: small green cars, big blue bikes Level B: The teacher cuts two letters)	Monitored-live voice, but audio-cassette tapes can be used for stan- dardized pre- sentations	Level A is for chil- dren 4 to 5 years- old (chance = 50%) Level B is for chil- dren at least 6 years-old and uses more advanced vocabulary (chance = 25%)	Not stated
Word Intelligibility by Picture Identification (WIPI) (Ross & Lerman, 1979)	To compare children's abil- ity to perceive words in three conditions (i.e., speechreading with hearing aids, speech- reading with- out hearing aids, and audi- tory-only with hearing aids) in each ear	4 lists of 25 single-syllable words similar in vowels, but different in consonants (e.g., socks, box, blocks, and fox) preceded by the carrier phrase, "Show me …"	Monitored-live voice	5 to 6 years for children with mod- erate hearing loss 7 to 8 years for children with severe hearing loss	• Collected normative data on chil- dren with hearing impairments (N = 61) ranging from mild to profound; ages 4 years, 7 months to 13 years, 9 months • Reliability coefficients of 0.87 to 0.94 • High list equivalency • Scores correlate highly with degree of hearing loss • Results on 60 children with nor- mal hearing ages, 3 to 11 years, indicate greater variability among listeners and lists in the group ages 3 to 5 years

(CONTINUES)

Table 9-1. (continued from page 190)

NAME/ AUTHOR	PURPOSE	STIMULI	RECORDED	MINIMUM AGE	STANDARDIZATION INFORMATION
Northwestern University-Children's Perceptions of Speech (Elliott & Katz, 1980)	To assess speech discrimination abilities in children	Closed-set four alternative forced choice picture identification of monosyllabic words (e.g., bear, pear, hair, and chair)	Monitored-live voice or audio-cassette tapes	At least an age equivalency of 2.5 years on the Peabody Picture Vocabulary Test (PPVT)	Not stated
Auditory Numbers Test (ANT) (Erber, 1980)	To differentiate whether a child can perceive segmental features of speech or non-segmental features To be used as a screening test for initial assessment of speech perception for planning of aural rehabilitation	Numbers 1 through 5 presented sequentially or individually presented on a closed-set of five colored cards depicting groups of 1 to 5 ants with the corresponding numerals	Monitored-live voice	• 3 years-old • The ability to count to five reliably • Reliably label numbers to sets of one to five items	Test-retest results on 62 children with hearing impairment that demonstrated a maximum one point difference in scores on the five-item test with a similar bimodal distribution based on degree of hearing loss

(CONTINUES)

Table 9-1. (continued from page 191)

NAME/ AUTHOR	PURPOSE	STIMULI	RECORDED	MINIMUM AGE	STANDARDIZATION INFORMATION
GAEL-P Modified Single Word Task (Moog, Kozak, & Geers, 1983)	To assess a closed-set recognition of single word skills of children with hearing impairment	30 single words (11 multisyllabic and 19 monosyllabic) (e.g., cookie vs. table, sandwich vs. flower) presented in sets of four that change after each presentation	Monitored-live voice	2 years of age	Not stated
Minimal Pairs Test (Robbins, Renshaw, Miyamoto, Osberger, & Pope, 1988)	To assess speech perception abilities for specific segmental features in children who use cochlear implants	40 monosyllabic words (e.g., pair vs. bear) each asked twice (total of 80 items) differing in one segmental feature presented in a closed-set using a 2 alternative forced-choice picture identification	Monitored-live voice	When vocabulary is familiar to the child around 4 years of age	Not stated
Early-Speech Perception Test (ESP)- Standard Version (Moog & Geers, 1990)	To obtain accurate information about the progression of speech discrimination skills in children with profound hearing impairments	• 36 words words (e.g., show, cookie, airplane, elephant, cowboy, french fries, football, hot dog, bed, box, bite) presented in an auditory-only condition as three subsets of 12 within a closed-set picture-identification task • Words are presented twice in a random order • 1st subtest includes 12 words varying in pattern with three in each category • Child can receive pattern credit for selecting words within same category or word credit if they identify the correct word • 2nd and 3rd subtests contain 12 spondees and 12 monosyllabic words	Most clinicians use monitored-live voice, but an audio-cassette tape is available from CID	6 years of age	Test-retest reliability for digitally recorded stimuli was 0.84 to 0.93 and 0.50 to 0.62 for monitored-lived voice

(CONTINUES)

Table 9-1. (continued from page 192)

NAME/ AUTHOR	PURPOSE	STIMULI	RECORDED	MINIMUM AGE	STANDARDIZATION INFORMATION
Early Speech Perception Test (ESP) Low Verbal Version (Moog & Geers, 1990)	To assess speech perception abilities in very young children who have limited verbal abilities	Words varying in pattern in addition to spondees and monosyllabic words (e.g., aaah vs. hop hop hop, shoes vs. birthday cake, shoe vs. airplane, popcorn vs. french fries, cup vs. hat) presented in four-item closed sets of objects differing in the number of syllables or stress pattern in the first level, different spondees in the 2nd level, and different monosyllabic words in the 3rd level	Audio-cassette tape is available, but many clinicians prefer to present via monitored-live voice	2 years of age or when vocabulary has been developed	Not standardized
Screening Inventory of Perception (Osberger, Robbins, Miyamoto, Berry, Myres, Kessler, & Pope, 1991)	To assess the speech discrimination of children with profound hearing loss using single words	Four lists of single words (e.g., cowboy vs. baseball, ice cream; ball vs. fall, wall) that vary from foils by syllable number or segmental cues with two levels per level, 32 items per level (64 items total) presented in a Go/No Go Paradigm in which the child responds when the target word is heard	Monitored-live voice	3 years of age due to the Go/No Go Paradigm	Not stated
Meaningful Auditory Integration Scale (MAIS) (Robbins, Renshaw, & Berry, 1991)	To assess children's meaningful listening skills in everyday situations	10 questions scored on a scale from 0 = "never" to 4 = "always" for a total of 40 possible points examining probes for parents who must provide specific examples	Not applicable	4 years of age	Not stated

(Adapted from Kirk, Diefendorf, Pisoni, & Robbins, 1997)

mean values for each grade and for the entire sample. In addition, scores are reported for the sample for both one (i.e., 68.6%) and two (i.e., 50.4%) standard deviations below the mean. Furthermore, the cut-off score suggesting need for further evaluation is 72%.

The *Screening Instrument for Targeting Educational Risk* (S.I.F.T.E.R.) (Anderson, 1989) is a screening instrument consisting of 15 items in which teachers rate students' behavior by answering three questions in each of the following areas: academics, attention, communication, class participation, and school behavior. For example, in one question in the academics area, teachers are asked, "What is your estimate of the student's class standing in comparison to that of his/her classmates?" to which they must respond on a scale of 1 to 5 (e.g., 1 = lower, 3 = middle, and 5 = upper). Teachers are also encouraged to write pertinent comments regarding whether students have repeated a grade, had frequent absences, health problems, special support services in the classroom, and so forth in a space specifically designed for that purpose. Teachers' ratings are summed for the three questions resulting in a score for each of the five areas and are recorded on a grid and connected by lines forming a profile for each student. The scores can fall into three general areas based on the grid:

1. Pass
2. Marginal
3. Fail

The authors cautioned that the S.I.F.T.E.R. is a screening tool only and that those students failing in a particular area should be considered for further assessment (Anderson, 1989). For example, failure in the Academic area suggests educational assessment, Communication area failure suggests a speech-language evaluation, and School Behavior area failure suggests assessment by a psychologist or social worker (Anderson, 1989).

Failure in the Attention and/or Class Participation area may suggest a need for an audiologic evaluation. Anderson (1989) suggested that students in the "marginal" category should be monitored or considered for assessment depending upon their profiles.

For children 3 to 5 years of age, Anderson and Matkin (1996) stated that the purpose of the *Screening Instrument for Targeting Educational Risk in Preschool Children* (Preschool S.I.F.T.E.R.) was to identify children who were at risk for developmental or educational problems due to hearing problems warranting further observation and investigation. The instrument consists of 15 items in the same five areas as the S.I.F.T.E.R except that the academic area is the pre-academic area on the preschool version. Using a 5-point scale, teachers are asked to rate preschool students on three questions in each of the five areas. For example, in one question from the pre-academics area, teachers are asked, "How well does the child understand basic concepts when compared to classmates (e.g., colors, shapes, etc.)?" to which they must respond on a scale of 1 to 5 (e.g., 1 = below, 3 = average, and 5 = above). Similar to the S.I.F.T.E.R., teachers are also encouraged to write pertinent comments regarding whether students have had frequent absences, health problems, or other problems or handicaps in addition to hearing, in a space specifically designed for that purpose. More complicated than the S.I.F.T.E.R, the preschool version has a two-step scoring process. The first step involves summing responses for the 6 questions (i.e., items 7, 8, 9, 10, 11, and 14) for the expressive communication factor, the same for the 4 questions (i.e., items 4, 5, 6, and 13) for the socially appropriate behavior factor, recording the results, and classifying performance in these areas as either passing or at risk. The second step involves summing scores for each of the five areas (i.e., pre-academics, attention, communication, class participation, and social behavior), recording the results, and also classifying performance in these areas as either passing or at risk, Anderson and Matkin (1990) stated that the area scores might assist educators in developing a profile of the student's strengths, weaknesses, and special needs. Although the purpose of both versions of the S.I.F.T.E.R. is to identify children at educational risk, both tests can be used to assess the efficacy of intervention efforts, such as use of hearing aids, preferential seating, sound-field FM amplification systems, and so forth (Stelmachowicz, 1999). Appendix IX-A shows the addresses of where to purchase both versions of the S.I.F.T.E.R.

A relatively new pre- and post-listening questionnaire that can document the effectiveness of amplification systems for students with normal hearing and hearing impairment is the *Listening Inventory for Education: An Efficacy Tool* (L.I.F.E.) (Anderson & Smaldino, 1996). The L.I.F.E. has three inventories: (1) the Student Appraisal of Listening Difficulty, (2) Teacher Appraisal of Listening Difficulty, and (3) Teacher Opinion and Observation Checklist. The five purposes of the L.I.F.E. inventories are to provide (Anderson & Smaldino, 1999):

1. a student self-report measurement tool to identify challenging classroom listening situations for an individual student,
2. a teacher-report measurement tool to document intervention efforts to improve the listening environment of a particular student,
3. a valid and reliable pretest/post-test measurement tool to document intervention efforts to improve the classroom listening environment,
4. inservice training material for increasing the awareness of school personnel on the challenges of listening in the classroom, and

5. information for teachers and students that encourages self-advocacy for good classroom listening environments.

The Student Appraisal of Listening Difficulty was designed for use by the individual elementary school-aged student (Anderson & Smaldino, 1999). The inventory has 15 items and two main sections for classroom listening situations (i.e., 10 listening situations encountered in the classroom) and other listening situations (i.e., 5 listening situations). Accompanying the test are 10 picture cards, each depicting a classroom listening situation which can be used even with children who are deficient in reading and writing skills (Anderson & Smaldino, 1999). Students are instructed to select how often they have difficulty in the various listening situations. For example, item one has a picture of a teacher talking in front of the room to which students must indicate the proportion of time that listening difficulty is encountered using a 10-point scale in which "0" = "Always," "5" = "Sometimes," and "10" = "Never." Because this section has 10 items, each with a possible score ranging from 0 to 10 points, students can achieve scores ranging from 0 (i.e., always having listening difficulty) to 100 points (i.e., never having listening difficulty). Items from the Additional Listening Situations section are scored on the same scale except that a 20-point scale is used in which "0" still equals "Always," but "10" = "Sometimes," and "20" = "Never." Because this section has 5 items, each with a possible score ranging from 0 to 20 points, students can achieve points ranging from 0 (i.e., always having listening difficulty) to 100 points (i.e., never having listening difficulty). The student's inventory is to be used as a pre- and postintervention measure. On the back of the student inventory are suggestions for self-advocacy and rehabilitation activities keyed to each of the 15 listening situations (Anderson & Smaldino, 1999).

The Teacher Appraisal of Listening Difficulty inventory was designed to assist teachers in describing student listening and learning behaviors in the classroom (Anderson & Smaldino, 1999). The inventory consists of 16 items focusing on a student's classroom behavior and communication to be completed at the end of intervention. For example, one of the items is: "The student's focus on instruction has improved (more tuned into instruction)" to which teachers use a scale (i.e., "2" = "Agree," "0" = "Not Observed/No Change," or "−2" = "Disagree") to mark their degree of agreement with the statement. The last item on the inventory appraises the teacher's opinion of the benefit of the amplification system to the student's overall attention, listening, and learning in the classroom; it uses the same descriptors as the other items, but has scores ranging from "5" to "-5." The teacher's ratings are added together for a total appraisal score that can be categorized as: (1) "highly successful" (i.e., scores 26-35), (2) "successful" (i.e., scores 16-25), or (3) "minimally successful" (i.e., scores 5-15). The total appraisal score can be used as a measure of efficacy of classroom intervention efforts or as an indication of areas that require further intervention (Anderson & Smaldino, 1999). The back of the inventory also has suggestions for ways that teachers can take a proactive role in providing accommodations for listening and learning (Anderson & Smaldino, 1999).

The third inventory is the Teacher Opinion and Observation List consisting of 4 items in an open-ended format (Stelmachowicz, 1999). The inventory allows the teacher to comment on the effects of intervention efforts in the classroom (Anderson & Smaldino, 1999). Furthermore, the open-ended response format permits teachers to identify anticipated and unanticipated benefits or problem areas observed in the classroom (Anderson & Smaldino, 1999).

Stelmachowicz (1999) stated that the test-retest reliability of the student inventory was assessed with 19 3rd- and 4th-graders over a 1- to 3-week period indicating no significant differences between the scores of any of the test items. She also stated that these inventories are flexible and can be used to document the efficacy of amplification, classroom teaching methods, inservicing of teachers, and/or self-advocacy. For example, Kuk, Kollofski, Brown, Melum, and Rosenthal (1999) used the L.I.F.E. as a subjective rating for investigation when examining the efficacy of a digital hearing aid with a directional microphone in school-aged (i.e., 7 to 13 years old) children. Figures 9-1 and 9-2 show girls whose teachers have used checklists and inventories to document the outcome of aural habilitation efforts in the classroom.

Parent Questionnaires

With the development of EHDI programs, parents' role of participating in outcomes measurement of early intervention efforts will increase. Functional hearing aid benefit in children 3 years of age and younger should be measured on their achievement of basic auditory milestones (Osberger & Koch, 2000). One parent-report tool is the *Meaningful Auditory Integration Scale* (MAIS) (Robbins, Renshaw, & Berry, 1991) consisting of 10 questions that probe parents using a structured interview technique for the frequency of occurrence of children's meaningful listening skills used in everyday situations using a response scale (i.e., "0" = "No Skill" to "4" = "Child consistently exhibits a skill") for assessment (Kirk, et al., 1997; Stelmachowicz, 1999). The 10 questions can be broken down as follows (Yoshinaga-Itano, 2000):

■ 2 questions evaluate children's use of amplification, wearing of hearing aids, and reporting of functioning

- 5 questions assess children's ability to detect sounds; respond when their names are called in quiet and noisy situations; and be alert to environmental sounds in the home, outside the home, and in the classroom
- 3 questions appraise children's ability to discriminate suprasegmental aspects of speech, different voices, speech versus nonspeech, and the association of intonation and meaning

The MAIS is for young children with profound hearing loss because ceiling effects have been found when this instrument is used for children with greater residual hearing (Stemalchowicz, 1999). Post-cochlear implant performance on the MAIS was highly correlated (r = 0.70) with performance on the *Phonetically Balanced Kindergarten* (PBK) test (Haskins, 1949; Osberger & Koch, 2000; Robbins, Svirsky, Osberger, & Pisoni, 1998)

Zimmerman-Phillips, Osberger, and Robbins (1997) recently developed the *Infant-Toddler Meaningful Auditory Integration Scale* (IT-MAIS) which is a parent questionnaire designed to assess children's spontaneous responses to sound in everyday environments (Advanced Bionics, 2001). The questionnaire has 10 probes that parents rate on scales of "0" (lowest) to "4" (highest) (e.g., "0" = "Never" to "4" = "Always") that survey children's vocal behaviors, responses to their names in quiet and in background noise, abilities to respond to environmental sounds, to discriminate between two speakers, to distinguish speech from nonspeech stimuli, and to associate vocal-tones with specific emotions (e.g., anger, excitement, or anxiety) (Yoshinaga-Itano, 2000). For example, parents are asked, "Is the child's vocal behavior affected while wearing his/her sensory aid (hearing aid or cochlear implant)?" to which parents respond by selecting one of the following:

- 0 = Never (No difference in the child's vocalizations with or without the device)

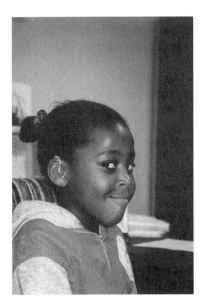
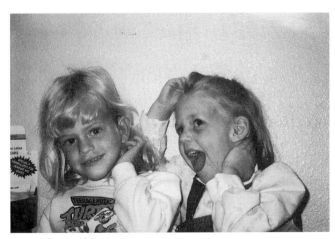

Figures 9-1 and 9-2. Girls whose teachers have used inventories and checklists to document the outcome of aural habilitation efforts in the classroom.

- 1 = Rarely (About a 25% increase in the frequency of the child's vocalizations with the device on or 25% decrease with the device off)
- 2 = Occasionally (Child vocalizes throughout the day and there is an approximately 50% increase in vocalizations with the device on or 50% decrease with the device off)
- 3 = Frequently (Child vocalizes throughout the day and there is an approximately 75% increase in vocalizations with the device on or 75% decrease with the device off)
- 4 = Always (Child's vocalizations increase 100% with the device on compared to the frequency of occurrence with the device off)

Performance is scored based on the number of points earned out of a possible 40 (i.e., 10 items × 4 point maximum = 40 points possible). Considered a parent-report scale, the IT-MAIS is administered in an interview format; any other format (e.g., parent completion) invalidates the measure. Clinicians should avoid leading parents into providing desired responses or asking questions in a way that yields yes-no answers from them (Advanced Bionics, 2001). The questions were designed to elicit a dialogue between parents and the clinician who should review the probes and all possible answers prior to administering the test (Advanced Bionics, 2001).

Both the MAIS and the IT-MAIS have been used to assess postcochlear implant performance and to determine cochlear implant candidacy in young children (Osberger, Geier, Zimmerman-Phillips, & Barker, 1997). Strict scoring criteria have been used to ensure uniformity among examiners in scoring these scales that have high inter-rater reliability (i.e., 0.90) (Osberger & Koch, 2000; Robbins, et al., 1991). Figure 9-3 serves as a reminder that parent questionnaires should be administered in the native language of the family.

Use of Adult Subjective Outcome Measures with Children

Some investigations have assessed the feasibility of using adult subjective outcome measures with children. Recently, Kopun,

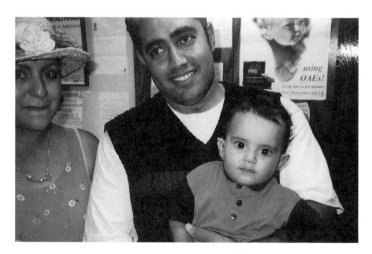

Figure 9-3. Parent questionnaires should be administered in the native language of the family.

and Stelmachowicz (in press) adapted the *Abbreviated Profile of Hearing Aid Benefit* (APHAB) (Cox & Alexander, 1995) for use by 10- to- 15 year-old children with moderate and severe sensorineural hearing losses. The APHAB is discussed in detail in Chapter 10 and appears in Appendix X-A on the companion CD-ROM. The APHAB consists of 4 subscales with 24 items in four areas: Ease of Communication (EC), Reverberation (RV), Background Noise (BN), and Aversiveness to Sounds (AV). An example of an item from the BN subscale is the phrase, "I have trouble understanding others when an air conditioner or fan is on," to which patients mark one of the following: "99%—Always," "87%—Almost Always," "75%-Generally," "50%—Half-the-Time," "25%—Occasionally," "12%—Seldom," or "1%—Never." The purposes of the APHAB are to quantify the disability associated with hearing impairment and the reduction of that disability through the use of amplification (Bentler & Kramer, 2000). The APHAB was normed on 128 (90 men, 38 women) elderly experienced, successful hearing aid users with mild-to-moderate sloping or flat sensorineural hearing loss (Cox & Alexander, 1995; Paul & Cox, 1995; Weinstein, 2000). Percentile scores have been established for a normative sample of experienced hearing aid users, but, to date, norms have not been established for new hearing aid users (Weinstein, 2000). Kopun and Stelmachowicz (in press) found a response pattern for children across the 4 subtests similar to that for aided adults (Cox & Alexander, 1995) in addition to a test-retest reliability yielding correlation coefficients ranging from 0.83 to 0.95 (Stelmachowicz, 1999). Kopun and Stelmachowicz (in press) also had the children's parents complete the APHAB in order to assess their perceptions of their children's communication problems and found low correlations between their ratings and those of their children on all four subscales (Stelmachowicz, 1999). A few explanations were

offered for these results (Kopun & Stelmachowicz, in press; Stelmachowicz, 1999):

■ Parents may have noticed communication difficulties that were not obvious to the children.
■ Parents of children 10- to-15-years-old may have had limited opportunity to observe their communication behavior in problematic situations.

Clearly, more research is needed to determine the ability of children and their parents in rating communication difficulties through observation with other tools like the *Client Oriented Scale of Improvement* (COSI) (Dillon, James, & Ginis, 1997; Moeller, 1993; Stelmachowicz, 1999). The COSI is discussed in detail in Chapter 10 and appears on the companion CD-ROM in Appendix X-E. Briefly, the COSI, was developed by Dillon, James, and Ginis (1997) and consists of up to 5 listening situations either selected from a list of 16 standardized situations or from difficult listening situations nominated by the patient that are rated two times:

■ Degree of change after wearing hearing aids by completing the following sentence, "Because of my new hearing instrument, I now hear ..." by selecting one of the following: "Worse," "No Difference," "Slightly Better," "Better," or "Much Better"
■ Final ability with the hearing instrument by completing the following sentence, "I can hearing satisfactorily ..." by selecting one of the following: "10% Hardly Ever," "25% Occasionally," "50% Half the Time," "75% Most of the Time," or "95% Almost Always."

The purpose of the COSI is to isolate up to 5 specific areas of listening difficulty and assess the degree of benefit obtained compared to that expected for the normative group (Bentler & Kramer, 2000). Stelmachowicz

(1999) stated that use of scales like the COSI may be very useful as an outcome measure for young children with hearing impairment because individual situations and goals may vary widely across children and for the same child across the various stages of auditory development.

Whitelaw, Wynne, and Williams (2001) have adapted the COSI in constructing the *Children's Outcome Worksheets* (COW) that focus on the needs of children from 4 to 12 years old. The COW identifies children's needs that are assessed according to the amount of "change" from a previous condition (e.g., unaided condition or old hearing aid) to a present condition (new hearing aid), and are rated in terms of children's final abilities. The identification and assessment of needs involves the children, and their parents and teachers as well. For example, children, parents, and teachers nominate different situations in which communication difficulty is experienced. The situations may include those on the COW specific for the three-rater groups:

1. Children (i.e., understanding others when in a car, the TV/radio at normal volume levels, conversation in distracting noises, or others in a large group [e.g., lunchroom, assembly, playground, gymnasium])
2. Parents (i.e., understanding directions in classroom and home, conversation with competing noise, or room-to-room conversation)
3. Teachers (i.e., understanding directions in the presence of competing noise, teacher and classmates in group discussions, or classmate presentations or stories)

In addition, stakeholder-specific situations can be nominated for assessment of degree of change and final ability. Children, parents, and teachers are encouraged to be as specific as possible for each situation and

to prioritize each need in order of its significance (Whitelaw, et al., 2001). After needs have been established, the COW assesses outcomes after appropriate fitting of hearing aids (i.e., "Because of the new hearing instrument, child now hears ...") and gauges children's final abilities with their hearing instruments (i.e., "Child can now hear satisfactorily ...") for each of the situations. The choices for the degree of change scale are: "Worse" (i.e., 1 point), "No Difference" (i.e., 2 points), "Slightly Better" (i.e., 3 points), "Better" (i.e., 4 points), and "Much Better" (i.e., 5 points). The choices for the final ability scale are: "Hardly Ever—10%" (i.e., 1 points), "Occasionally—25%" (i.e., 2 points), "Half-the-Time—50%" (i.e., 3 points), "Most of the Time—75%" (i.e., 4 points), and "Almost Always—95%" (i.e., 5 points). For both scales, scores for the situations are averaged and recorded on the form.

The COW presents advantages to both children and audiologists. The benefits for children are that the COW (Whitelaw, et al., 2001):

- focuses on their needs,
- forces others to focus on their strengths,
- assesses change and final ability following intervention,
- assists in the perception of their own needs and improvements, and
- quantifies success in their terms.

The benefits for audiologists are that the COW (Whitelaw, et al., 2001):

- provides structure for obtaining and using information gleaned from interactions with children, parents, and teachers;
- generates evidence that children's needs have been addressed;
- assists in the selection of appropriate hearing instruments; and
- produces outcome data to third-party payers.

In addition to individual assessment, the COW can be used for overall program evaluation by assigning individual patients' needs into standardized categories, tabulating their scores, obtaining averages, and developing norms.

ALTERNATIVE APPROACHES TO OUTCOMES MEASUREMENT IN AURAL HABILITATION

Stelmachowicz (1999) stated that there is no one approach to outcomes measurement in pediatric amplification and proposed at least three alternative approaches: (1) studies of device efficacy, (2) predictive measures for the audibility of speech, and (3) loudness measures.

Studies of Device Efficacy

With the development of new hearing aid circuitry, audiologists and parents may wonder about the use of high-technology hearing aids with young children. For example, possible advantages of digitally programmable hearing aids include (Sweetow & Tate, 1999):

- Programmability and ease of adjustment
- Multiple programs
- Advanced control of compression characteristics
- Multiple-band (multi-channel) compression

In addition to the advantages listed above, advantages of digital signal processing (DSP) hearing aids are (Sweetow & Tate, 1999):

- Fine-tuning of frequency response
- Active feedback control
- Multiple microphones
- Noise reduction strategies

Positive pediatric patient outcomes through the use of high-technology hearing aids can be facilitated through asking the following questions about children and potential hearing aids:

- How loud or disturbing are changing environmental conditions? How large are the rooms in which listening must occur? How far away are the speakers? How reverberant are these rooms? Do the children need multiple programs?
- Do the children have difficulty understanding over the telephone? How important is telephone use for the children? Do the children use an assistive listening device (ALD) requiring the use of telecoils?
- Do the children prefer hearing aids that are completely automatic versus a device with a volume-control wheel or program controls?
- What physical features do the children need on the hearing aids?
- Do the hearing aids have programming features that the children need or could use?
- Are the children in a variety of noisy listening situations and does this affect their performance?
- Is the hearing aid flexible enough to be adjusted for possible progressive, fluctuating, or unusual hearing loss?
- Are the algorithms used to program the hearing aids appropriate for the children?
- How do the hearing aids deal with potential feedback?

After considering these and other issues, audiologists should search the literature for studies of device efficacy that support the use of selected circuitry with subjects that have similar characteristics as their patients. For example, audiologists considering the use of directional or dual-microphone programmable digital hearing aids for young children would be pleased to find that Gravel, Fausel, Liskow, and Chobot (1999) demonstrated that this technology has been found to improve the signal-to-noise ratio by approximately 4.8 dB for the speech recognition of single words for two groups aged 4- to 6- and 7- to 11-years. As time goes on, the results of more and more efficacy studies will become available to audiologists for consideration in selecting high-technology hearing aids features for their pediatric patients.

Predictive Measures for the Audibility of Speech and Loudness

One of the major goals of amplification is to make soft speech audible. Evidence-based prescriptive methods, such as the DSL i/o (Cornelisse, Seewald, & Jamieson, 1995), for fitting non-linear hearing aids provide graphic displays of the audibility of average speech across the frequency range that can be used as a verification measure (Serpanos & Gravel, 2000; Stelmachowicz, 1999). The graphic displays assist audiologists in determining if targets have been met for soft, average, and loud speech so that it is audible, yet comfortable. These prescriptive methods are ideal for use with young children because they initially eliminate the need for subjective loudness judgments, but they may not be adequate for older children who may have tolerance problems (Serpanos & Gravel, 2000). Figures 9-4 and 9-5 demonstrate that real-ear probe-tube microphone measurements are important for hearing aid fittings for infants and school-aged children.

Subjective ratings of loudness are valuable outcome measures for pediatric hearing aid fittings. Unfortunately, many young children under 7 years of age cannot communicate that sounds are too loud, which may result in the rejection of amplification, and which is sometimes interpreted as stubborn-

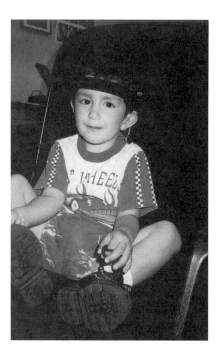 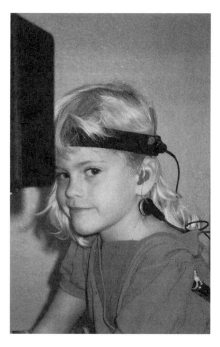

Figures 9-4 and 9-5. Real-ear probe-tube microphone measurements are important for hearing aid fittings for infants and school-aged children.

ness, anxiety, or other factors by parents and hearing health-care professionals (Bentler, 2000). The use of cross-modality matching (i.e., using the visual sense to quantify aspects of the auditory sense) shows promise as a method for young children to produce stable estimates of comfortable and uncomfortable loudness levels (Jerger, 2000). For example, Serpanos and Gravel (2000) examined the clinical feasibility, validity, and reliability of loudness growth assessment using cross-modality matching (CMM) between line length and loudness in 16 children between 4- and 12-years old with either normal hearing or moderate-to-severe bilateral sensorineural hearing loss. A group of 8 adults with normal hearing served as a comparison group. Loudness growth functions and real-ear measures were obtained for 500 Hz and 2000 Hz narrow-band noise stimuli for each subject. Results indicated no significant differences between the loudness growth functions of the adults and children with normal hearing. However, the loudness growth functions for the children with hearing loss were significantly steeper (i.e., larger) than those of the children with normal hearing. In addition, as children's hearing-threshold levels increased, so did the slope value of the loudness growth function. The authors concluded that measures of loudness growth using the CMM between line length and loudness are feasible, valid, and reliable for children as young as 6 years of age.

OUTCOMES MEASUREMENT OF INTERVENTION PROGRAMS

Some JCIH (2000) benchmarks for early intervention programs are difficult to assess. For example, one benchmark is that infants with hearing loss are enrolled in a family-centered early intervention program with professional personnel who are knowledgeable about the communication needs of infants with hearing loss. The question is, how knowledgeable is knowledgeable enough? The degree of preparedness of professionals habilitating infants with hearing loss is highly variable and often inadequate. For example, many states still permit speech therapists with bachelor's degrees to serve children with hearing impairment in the public schools. Unfortunately, those professionals have varied educational backgrounds and services. Currently, audiologists with the certificate of clinical competence in audiology (CCC-A) from the American Speech-Language-Hearing Association (ASHA), similarly certified speech-language pathologists (CCC-SLPs), and certified teachers of the deaf (CED) can all provide direct aural habilitation services to infants and young children with hearing loss. Some or all of these individuals may or may not have the necessary knowledge base or skills for providing aural habilitative services

Another issue to consider is what speech and auditory development program or aural habilitation approach to use with infants and young children. Clinicians can take two approaches for aural habilitation training: 1) *specific* and 2) *eclectic*. A specific approach is to adopt a single approach in habilitating young children and infants with hearing loss. For example, one very popular specific aural habilitation approach is the Auditory Verbal method. Other approaches include the Ling method, the Verbo-tonal method, and so forth. An eclectic approach is taking bits and pieces of various aural habilitation approaches in creation of a unique individualized technique. For example, one clinician may strictly implement the Auditory Verbal approach while another clinician may prefer to use Cued Speech with the Verbo-tonal method (i.e., eclectic).

Aural habilitation, like other areas in our field, has avoided evidence-based service provision. That is, to date, aural habilitation treatment approaches have not been required to demonstrate treatment efficacy through the use of randomized clinical trials prior to use with children. Indeed, Tharpe (1998) stated that at a time when policy makers and insurers are demanding cost containment, the field of communication sciences and disorders lacks the systematic documentation of clinical outcomes. Treatment outcome data for aural habilitation are needed for prediction of treatment duration, progress milestones, determination of likely benefit from treatment, and establishment of guidelines for the average number of visits to achieve goals (Garstecki & Erler, 2000; Task Force on Treatment Outcomes and Cost Effectiveness, 1997).

Although many audiologists do not provide direct-service therapy to children with hearing loss, they should know and advise parents of the four characteristics of fad treatments (Goldstein & Ingersoll, 1992; Tharpe, 1998). The first characteristic of a fad treatment is one that has concepts outside the mainstream, or that makes grandiose claims that lack empirical evidence (Goldstein & Ingersoll, 1992). For example, parents should be skeptical of approaches that sound too good to be true and lack sound scientific foundations with databases supporting their effectiveness. In an age of Informatics, as discussed in Chapter 5, parents should be encouraged to search the Internet (e.g., Medline searches regarding various aural habilitation approaches and other treatments for hearing loss). The second characteristic of a fad treatment is an initial popularity burst prior to demonstrated effectiveness (Goldstein & Ingersoll, 1992; Tharpe, 1998). Parents should be cautioned against being swept up in the enthusiasm for particular aural habilitation approaches. For example, as stakeholders, parents should be highly critical of wide-sweeping changes in aural habilitation programming in their public schools. The third characteristic of fad treatments is

that most of the articles written about the approaches are in non-refereed publications (Goldstein & Ingersoll, 1992; Tharpe, 1998). Parents should be taught to discriminate between refereed and non-refereed publications. For example, although most adults know not to believe everything printed in the newspapers, parents may easily be influenced by individual stories of children with deafness who defy the odds. These stories, although inspiring and often compelling, cannot infer cause and effect between the aural habilitation approach and the child's success. Moreover, parents should be taught the hierarchy of rigor for publications in the field and related professions. Articles appearing in *The Hearing Journal* are less rigorous than those appearing in the *Journal of Speech, Language, and Hearing Research*, for example. Parents should also be wary of the information obtained from the Internet, which varies widely in quality and is not subject to peer review. The fourth characteristic of fad treatments is claims of widespread effectiveness (Goldstein & Ingersoll, 1992; Tharpe, 1998). Parents should be leery of aural habilitation approaches that claim universal success and have no response for questions concerning the alternatives for children with less than positive outcomes. In summary, educating parents to be able to use the "Evaluation of Treatment Procedures, Products, and Programs" appearing in Appendix I-A can have profound repercussions regarding treatment outcomes for children with hearing loss.

One parent's efforts can make a difference for hundreds of children. Consider the efforts of one parent described in Vignette 9-1.

Indeed, Nancy showed that the power of one can make changes to improve service delivery for hundreds of students. Is this a happy ending? Yes, this is a positive outcome because service delivery was improved. However, the implementation of the approach was very costly to the school system. Thus, would the outcomes be different if another, less

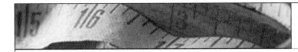

VIGNETTE 9-1

ONE PARENT CAN MAKE A DIFFERENCE

In the early 1980s, Nancy Advocatti was stunned to learn that her three-year-old son, Jamie, was diagnosed with a severe-to-profound sensorineural hearing loss, explaining his severe delay in speech and language development. Nancy was devastated, but she and her husband, Bud, faced this challenge as they had done others, head on. As soon as possible, Nancy and Bud had their son fit with binaural hearing aids.

Bud was a successful tax attorney who had provided well for his family. Nancy was into real estate that afforded her the luxury of controlling her own schedule. Since her son's diagnosis, Nancy spent most of her time researching possible treatments for her son's hearing loss, talking to various professionals, parents of children with hearing impairment, and reading everything she could get her hands on. She wanted the best for her son.

One afternoon, she heard about a promising aural habilitation program that had been used at a well-known state university and the local school system nearly 1,000 miles away. Nancy was so excited that she decided to take her son to spend the summer at that university, taking courses on the approach and enrolling her son in the summer aural habilitation program. Nancy was very motivated and pleased by the progress her son was making. He was listening better, repeating words and phrases, and enjoying his time in the program. Unfortunately, summer ended too soon and it was time for Nancy to return home as Jamie was to start preschool for children with special needs.

Even before school started, Nancy talked with the director of special education and Jamie's teachers regarding their philosophies toward aural habilitation and the types of resources available for her son. Nancy was disappointed by the lack of enthusiasm shown by the director. He seemed somewhat overwhelmed and defeated in his position. The school system was one of the largest in the country with a large immigrant, non-English speaking population. The realities were easy to understand, too many needs, too few resources.

Time passed quickly and Nancy was not pleased with Jamie's Individualized Education Plan. She was not satisfied with a total communication program and only one hour of speech therapy per week provided by a speech-language pathologist with only a bachelor's degree. Furthermore, the progress that Jamie had made during the summer seemed to have leveled off. Nancy now felt that she had to do something for her son and the other children with hearing impairment within the district. Their futures depended on it. Nancy met with other parents of children with hearing impairment within the school district to convince them that services provided to their children were not adequate and could be improved. She explained her activities during the past summer and garnered their support for change. Unfortunately, chages were too slow for her child.

As a result, Nancy and Bud decided for her to take her son, rent an apartment near the university, and enroll Jamie both in the university program and in the local school district's program for students with hearing impairment. Prior to leaving, Nancy made a videotape of Jamie's communication behaviors as evidence of his pre-intervention communication functioning. Off they went for 6 months.

CONTINUES

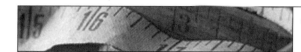

VIGNETTE 9-1

ONE PARENT CAN MAKE A DIFFERENCE   (CONTINUED FROM PAGE 205)

Nancy was thankful for the means to not have to work so she could concentrate on her son, filling her days with a ritual of driving him to school, taking him for after-school therapy, and working with the professor at the university in preparing a presentation to the school board back home. Implementation of the aural habilitation approach in the school system would require a great deal of money for special equipment, training for the speech-language pathologists, and fees for frequent consulting trips made by the professor and his training team. Both Nancy and the professor viewed their efforts as a potential "win-win" situation. The professor had a potentially lucrative opportunity to sell his special equipment and be paid for training and certifying therapists within her school system.

Again, it was time to leave for home. Jamie had blossomed from the experience and Nancy had an opportunity to videotape his communication abilities for the school board. Upon her return, Nancy scheduled a meeting for parents at her home and explained her plans to make a presentation to the school board before the summer vacation. The parents were astonished by the pre- and postintervention videotapes of Jamie; they cheered, giving Nancy the strength to move forward with her plan.

After much persistence, Nancy was placed on the school board's agenda for the last meeting of the year. That evening, over 50 parents attended the meeting to support Nancy's efforts. As her speaking time approached, Nancy could feel her heart race. She had spent months on her presentation and it was now or never. As she walked to the microphone, she was strengthened by the look of hope in the faces of the parents. She had made note cards, but found she could speak from her experience, her knowledge, and her heart. Her presentation concisely critiqued current services for children with hearing impairment and what changes should be made. The presentation concluded with the pre- and postintervention videotapes of her son and thunderous applause from those who attended the meeting. Some of the school board members had tears in their eyes. She had accomplished her goal.

In the years that followed, the school system implemented this aural habilitation at all schools with programs for children with hearing impairment. The program has served hundreds of children with good results. Today, Jamie is a college graduate, a businessman who is starting a family of his own. Nancy and Bud are enjoying an early retirement.

---

costly, approach had been used? Was the benefit worth the cost? Unfortunately, answering questions like these is practically impossible, but very important to consider for at least two reasons. First, with the reduction of state and federal funding for special education, cost-benefit ratios are important outcome measures for effective allocation of resources. Second, outcomes measurement of aural habilitation is very important in the establishment of efficacious early intervention programs.

Discerning effective from ineffective aural habilitation approaches should be fairly easy to do. The effective ones work and the ineffective ones don't. Right? After all, Yoshinaga-Itano (2000) stated that successful speech and aural habilitation approaches have:

- Skilled providers
- Hierarchical curricula
- Mass practice
- Unisensory stimulation
- Parent partnership
- Integrated activities in daily living
- Integrated auditory activities with language

Surely, if an aural habilitation approach has all these components, it should be successful, right? Not exactly. At first glance, ineffective approaches that have all these components can and do appear effective as a result of five phenomena (Tharpe, 1998). The first phenomenon causing improvement in performance with ineffective treatment is the tendency for patient performance to regress toward the mean (Tharpe, 1998). For example, patients' behavior often fluctuates. Ineffective treatment can *appear* effective if applied when performance is at its worst (i.e., far below the mean) and improves, not because of the intervention efforts, but because of the tendency for patients' behaviors to regress toward the mean. Clinicians may establish an erroneous cause-and-effect relationship between intervention efforts and improved performance. A second phenome-

non is the Hawthorne effect, described as subjects or patients behaving differently if they know that they are part of an experiment or novel treatment, thereby potentially affecting measurement of dependent variables (Schiavetti & Metz, 1997). For example, some patients and their families may be so excited about enrolling in a new treatment program that they may actually try harder and perform better as they expect intervention to have positive outcomes. The third phenomenon is the experimenter effect, that is, the bias or expectations on the part of the experimenter that may influence treatment outcomes (Tharpe, 1998). For example, proponents of particular approaches may believe so strongly in the techniques they use that they can literally influence or will their patients into performing better, thereby biasing results. Is it possible for professionals to accept the effectiveness of certain treatments without hard scientific evidence? Yes, it is very possible. Consider the use of the Verbo-tonal method in Vignette 9-2, an approach with which the authors of this text have considerable experience and confidence despite a lack of convincing scientific proof of its effectiveness.

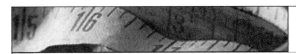

VIGNETTE 9-2

THE VERBO-TONAL METHOD—FAD OR FABULOUS?

As an undergraduate student, the first author (CEJ) was enrolled in the second author's (JLD) aural rehabilitation class at the University of California at Santa Barbara. Dr. Danhauer told his class how Petar Guberina, a phonetician-linguist, developed the Verbo-tonal method and introduced it to the United States. He told us how Petar Guberina, at the invitation of Dr. John W. Black, came to the Ohio State University in the 1960s to lecture students regarding his approach to working with young children with hearing impairment. He managed, along with Dr. Black, to obtain funding to take a study group to the SUVAG (Systems Universal Verbo-tonal Audiometry Guberina) Center in Zagreb, Yugoslavia.

CONTINUES

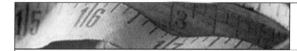

VIGNETTE 9-2

THE VERBO-TONAL METHOD(em) FAD OR FABULOUS?   (CONTINUED FROM PAGE 207)

Among those in the study group who observed the implementation of this method on a large scale were Dr. Danhauer, Dr. Patricia Kricos, Dr. Carl W. Asp, and others who went on to make a major impact on aural rehabilitation in the United States.

I remember how Dr. Danhauer showed us slides of his trip and the basic principles behind the method. I was very intrigued with this approach and wanted to learn more about it. Dr. Danhauer advised me that Dr. Carl W. Asp at the University of Tennessee knew the most about the approach and that they had a master's degree program in audiology there. I eventually completed my master's and doctoral degrees in audiology and speech and hearing sciences at the University of Tennessee. During my time at Tennessee, I had opportunities to participate in clinical experiences involving the Verbo-tonal method at the university speech and hearing clinic and in the Knox County schools system. I was so amazed at the success stories of many, many children who had undergone Verbo-tonal therapy and who were mainstreamed into regular education requiring little or no support services. In addition, in 1986, I was able to attend the International Verbo-tonal Conference and Workshop in Zagreb, Yugoslavia to learn about international developments with the method and to observe therapy at the SUVAG Center. The most striking memory I have is the love and respect that parents, children, and therapists had for Dr. Petar Guberina, affectionately known as "The Professor." He was very warm and charismatic and had an entire country believing in his method.

The Verbo-tonal method has many of the characteristics of a fad treatment mentioned by Tharpe (1998), namely, concepts outside the mainstream, non-refereed publications, claims of widespread effectiveness, and so forth. For example, my undergraduate training emphasized the importance of evidence-based treatment, so my basic belief in the effectiveness of the Verbo-tonal method clashed with the out of the mainstream ideas toward hearing impairment, the reported success rate of over 90% in Yugoslavia, and no refereed publications of results of experimental studies demonstrating the effectiveness of the method. To this day, my belief in the effectiveness of the Verbo-tonal method is not evidence-based, but I believe it works. So, even clinical researchers sometimes rely on faith more than science.

Perhaps one of the saddest outcome of the Verbo-tonal method is the fact that few, if any, investigations using formal outcomes measures have been applied to patients who have received this treatment to document the approach's successes. Although thousands of patients and their families have benefited from this method worldwide, aside from non-refereed publications and anecdotal reports, no evidence-based research exists to validate the effectiveness of the Verbo-tonal method. Although both authors have personally witnessed startling successes with deaf/hard-of-hearing children using the Verbo-tonal method and have warm feelings for its creator and trained professionals, our scientific backgrounds compel us in accepting that being evidence-based is necessary prior to widespread acceptance by the professional community. However, for many of the families who have received positive outcomes through the Verbo-tonal method, such evidence is not necessary.

For example, clinicians who provide Verbotonal training may believe in its effectiveness so much that their passion increases the likelihood of success. A fourth phenomenon is the expectation effect in which the expectations of subjects or patients can influence outcomes (Tharpe, 1998). For example, patients' expectations of expensive treatment effectiveness may result in initial positive, yet short-lived, outcomes of improved performance. After all, anything expensive should work, right? The fifth phenomenon is placebo effects, which are influences on the disease process caused by pills, potions, or procedures because of nonspecific reasons and/ or any one or combination of previously described phenomena rather than by the treatments themselves (Tharpe, 1998). Unfortunately, in spite of the scientific advances made in audiology, the placebo effect can still exert a certain amount of influence on our practices (Tharpe, 1998). Do high-cost digital hearing aids really work better than analog products with children, simply because we believe they should? Well-designed clinical trials should answer this and similar questions related to aural habilitation.

Audiologists may find it difficult to determine the exact contribution of specific approaches toward positive patient outcomes in aural habilitation. Indeed, more research is needed to determine the effectiveness of various aural habilitation approaches to be used in early intervention programs. Efficacy studies comparing various aural habilitation approaches used in early intervention programs are difficult to conduct because of the influences of possible confounding variables; they are also generally poorly controlled, have fundamental selection biases, and are not detailed enough in their description of the habilitative interventions (Bamford, 1998).

Investigators often need to examine factors beyond the type of aural habilitation program to identify critical factors for positive patient outcomes. For example, Connor,

Hieber, Arts, and Zwolan (2000) compared the effectiveness of oral versus total communication approaches in enhancing the speech, language, and education of children with cochlear implants. The study examined the speech and vocabulary performances of 147 pediatric cochlear-implant patients who had used their devices ranging from 6 months to 10 years and who were enrolled in either oral communication (OC) or total communication (TC) aural habilitation educational programs while controlling for variables such as age at implantation and type of cochlear implant (Gardner, 2000). The investigators found little difference between the speech and language performances of the children enrolled in the OC or TC programs. Even more important than the aural habilitation approach was the children's age of implantation (i.e., those children who were cochlear implant users since preschool had superior speech and language performances than children who were implanted later in childhood). Therefore, although the implications of these findings should be interpreted with caution, optimal outcomes require that children be implanted as early as possible with the latest devices having a complete active electrode array, regardless of aural habilitation programming (Conner, et al., 2000). In other words, optimal patient outcomes require a series of critical events (e.g., early identification, diagnosis, appropriate technology, and so forth) that occur as part of a seamless continuum of care for children with hearing impairment and their families.

Yoshinaga-Itano (2000) provided characteristics of complete EHDI programs:

- Parent partnerships
- Parent facilitators with specialized training and a significant number of years of experience
- Facilitators with counseling skills
- A pragmatic, socially oriented approach
- Data-driven approaches

Similarly, Bamford (1998) stated that successful EHDI programs have parents as *equal* partners, emphasize the development of communication (i.e., spoken or signed), include recursive first-class ongoing audiologic care, are multidisciplinary and seamless, provide complete information to parents prior to decision making, and involve other families. How should these attributes be measured? If an EHDI program has all these components, is it efficacious? Do we have specific outcomes measures for these programs?

Unfortunately, we do not have specific outcome measures for these purposes, but the JCIH Year 2000 Position Statement (2000) has benchmarks and quality indicators that should be indicative of EHDI program effectiveness. For example, one benchmark states that infants enrolled in early intervention achieve language development in the family's chosen communication mode that is commensurate with the infant's developmental level as documented in the Individual Family Services Plan (IFSP) and that is similar to that for hearing peers of a comparable developmental age (JCIH, 2000).

Similarly, one quality indicator is the percentage of infants who receives language evaluations at 6-month intervals (JCIH, 2000). Yoshinaga-Itano (2000) reported that Colorado EHDI programs use 6-month comprehensive evaluations to assist parents and educators to determine if the entire intervention program is achieving positive outcomes for its children. However, Bamford (1998) believed that while these short-term outcome measures are important indicators of service delivery that are predictive of long-term outcomes, hearing health-care providers must have a clearer idea of which long-term outcomes are important to the child, the family, and society. Bamford (1998) predicted that these outcomes would include development of language and communicative competence, development of age-appropriate behaviors, social and emotional development, long-term mental health, educational placement and achievement, supportive family dynamics, and social and economic opportunities, such as employment. Figure 9-6 shows a young boy who has achieved positive patient outcomes.

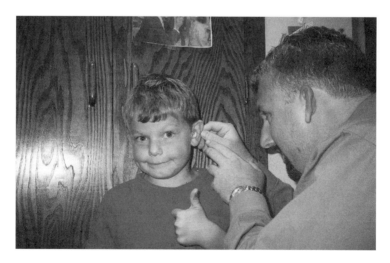

Figure 9-6. A young boy who has achieved positive patient outcomes.

SUMMARY

With the means to identify hearing loss at birth, our field must rise to the occasion and develop sensitive outcome measures to assess the effectiveness of our EHDI efforts. This chapter has reviewed the lack of outcome measures for children with hearing loss, issues that complicate outcomes measurement with young children, objective/subjective outcome measures for aural habilitation, and assessing the effectiveness of early intervention programs. Indeed, much research needs to be done, particularly in the areas of developing sensitive speech recognition tests, subjective inventories, parental inventories, modifying subjective procedures (e.g., loudness growth, quality judgments, and preferred frequency responses), and identifying objective correlates of positive aural habilitation outcomes (Stelmachowicz, 1999). We have a long way to go, but our children's futures depend on it!

LEARNING ACTIVITIES

- Provide a patient-care audit for two pediatric patients seen in your clinic; determine appropriate instances in which outcomes measurement were made or could have been made, and whether the measures that were made were appropriate; specify the other measures that should have been made.

- Make an aural habilitation outcomes measurement notebook containing measures mentioned in this chapter, score sheets, norms, and so forth.

RECOMMENDED READINGS

Bess, F. (1998). *Children with hearing impairment: Contemporary trends.* Nashville, TN: Vanderbilt Bill Wilkerson Center Press.

Lucks Mendel, L., & Danhauer, J.L. (1997). *Audiologic evaluation and management and speech perception assessment.* San Diego, CA: Singular Publishing Group.

Stelmachowicz, P.G. (1999). Hearing aid outcome measures for children. *Journal of the American Academy of Audiology, 10,* 14–25.

REVIEW EXERCISES

Fill-in-the-Blank

Instructions: Please fill in the blanks with the correct term from the word bank.

1. _____ variables are those that have to do with the child or subject, such as vocabulary/language competency, chronologic age, and cognitive abilities.

2. _____ variables are those that have to do with the speech recognition test, such as appropriate response task, utilization of reinforcement, and memory load.

3. _____ variables have to do with the administration of the test, such as taped versus monitored live-voice presentation, open- versus closed-set tests, and task domain in closed-set test construction.

4. _____ - _____ response formats are those in which patients have an infinite number of possibilities of response alternatives.

5. _____ - _____ response formats are those in which patients select a response from a group of alternatives.

6. _____ task domains are response tasks in which target signals are not uniquely specified for patients, but are embedded among foil items representing selected phonemic confusions.

7. _____ task domains are response tasks that promote a cognitive (conceptual) processing outcome perspective with the following characteristics: top-down processing approach, respondents' use of the process of elimination in responding, and expectation of the stimuli.

Word Bank:
Closed-set
Internal
External
Methodological
Open-set
Restricted
Unrestricted

Matching

Instructions: Please match the items below to the appropriate statements.

I. Adult subjective measures that may be used with children
II. Teacher checklist or inventory
III. Alternative approach
IV. Parent questionnaire

1. ___ COSI
2. ___ MAIS
3. ___ Fisher's Auditory Checklist
4. ___ APHAB
5. ___ S.I.F.T.E.R.
6. ___ Studies of device efficacy
7. ___ IT-MAIS
8. ___ Preschool S.I.F.T.E.R.
9. ___ Predictive measures
10. ___ L.I.F.E.

ANSWERS

Fill-in-the-Blank:	Matching:
1. Internal	1. I
2. External	2. IV
3. Methodological	3. II
4. Open-set	4. I
5. Closed-set	5. II
6. Unrestricted	6. III
7. Restricted	7. IV
	8. II
	9. III
	10. II

REFERENCES

Advanced Bionics Corporation. (2001). *Administration instructions: Infant-Toddler Meaningful Auditory Integration Scale.* Sylmar, CA: Advanced Bionics Corporation.

Anderson, K. (1989). *Screening Instrument for Targeting Education Risk (S.I.F.T.E.R.).* Austin, TX: Pro-Ed.

Anderson, K., & Matkin, N. (1996). *Screening Instrument for Targeting Educational Risk in preschool children (Age 3-Kindergarten) (Preschool-S.I.F.T.E.R).* Tampa, FL: Educational Audiology Association.

Anderson, K., & Smaldino, J. (1996). *The Listening Inventories for Education (L.I.F.E.): An efficacy tool .* Tampa, FL: Educational Audiology Association.

Anderson, K., & Smaldino, J. (1999). Listening inventories for education: A classroom measurement tool. *The Hearing Journal, 52*(10), 74, 76.

Bamford, J.M. (1998). Early identification ... What then? In F. Bess (Ed.), *Children with hearing impairment: Contemporary trends* (pp. 353–358). Nashville, TN: Vanderbilt Bill Wilkerson Center Press.

Bench, J., Kowal, A., & Bamford, J. (1979). The BKB (Bamford-Kowal-Bench) sentence lists for partially-hearing children. *British Journal of Audiology, 13,* 108–112.

Bentler, R.A. (2000). Amplification for the hearing-impaired child. In J.G. Alpiner and P.A. McCarthy (Eds.), *Rehabilitative* audiology: Children and adults (3rd ed., pp. 106–139).

Bentler, R.A., & Kramer, S.E. (2000). Guidelines for choosing a self-report outcome measure. *Ear and Hearing, 21*(4), 37–49.

Connor, C.M., Hieber, S., Arts, A., & Zwolan, T.A. (2000). Speech, vocabulary, and the education of children using cochlear implants: Oral or total communication. *Journal of Speech, Language, and Hearing Disorders, 43,* 1185–1204.

Cornelisse, L.E., Seewald, R.C., & Jamieson, D.G. (1995). The input/output formula: A theoretical approach to the fitting of personal amplification devices. *Journal of the Acoustical Society of America, 97,* 1854–1864.

Cox, R.M., & Alexander, G.C. (1995). The Abbreviated Profile of Hearing Aid Benefit. *Ear and Hearing, 16,* 176-183.

Dillon, H., James, A., & Ginis, J. (1997). Client Oriented Scale of Improvement (COSI) and its relationship to several measures of benefit and satisfaction provided by hearing aids. *Journal of the American Academy of Audiology, 8,* 27–43.

Elliott, L.L., & Katz, D. (1980). *Development of a new children's test of speech discrimination (Technical Manual).* St. Louis, MO: Auditec of St. Louis.

Erber, N.P. (1980). Use of the auditory numbers test to evaluate speech perception abilities of hearing-impaired children. *Journal of Speech and Hearing Disorders, 45,* 527–532.

Erber, N.J., & Alencewicz, C.M. (1976). Audiologic evaluation of deaf children. *Journal of Speech and Hearing Disorders, 41,* 256–267.

Fisher, L.I. (1985). Learning disabilities and auditory processing. In R.J. Van Hattum (Ed.), *Administration of speech language services in schools: A manual* (pp. 231–290). San Diego, CA: College-Hill Press.

Gardner, K. (2000). JSLHR in brief: How important is teaching method for children

using cochlear implants? *ASHA Leader, 5*(20), 11.

Garstecki, D.C., & Erler, S.F. (2000). Hearing care providers and individuals with hearing impairment: Continuing and new relationships in the new millennium. In J.G. Alpiner and P.A. McCarthy (Eds.), *Rehabilitative audiology: Children and adults* (3rd ed., pp. 27–59). Philadelphia, PA: Lippincott, Williams, & Wilkins.

Goldstein, S., & Ingersoll, B. (1992). Controversial treatments for children with attention deficit hyperactivity disorder. *Chadder,* Fall/ Winter.

Gravel, J., Fausel, N., Liskow, C., & Chobot, J. (1999). Children's speech recognition in noise using dual microphone hearing aid technology. *Ear and Hearing, 20,* 1–11.

Haskins, H.A. (1949). *A phonetically balanced test of speech discrimination for children.* Unpublished master's thesis, Northwestern University, Evanston, IL.

Jerger, J. (2000). Editorial: Loudness and smiling caterpillars. *Journal of the American Academy of Audiology, 11,* 180.

Johnson, C.D., Benson, P.V., & Seaton, J.B. (1997). *Educational audiology handbook.* Clifton Park, NY: Delmar Thomson Learning.

Joint Committee on Infant Hearing (2000). Year 2000 position statement: Principles and guidelines for early hearing detection and intervention programs. *American Journal of Audiology: A Journal of Clinical Practice 9*(1), 9–29.

Kirk, K.I., Diefendorf, A.O., Pisoni, D.B., & Robbins, A.M. (1997). Assessing speech perception in children. In L. Lucks Mendel & J.L. Danhauer (Eds.), *Audiologic evaluation and management and speech perception assessment* (pp. 101–132). Clifton Park, NY: Delmar Thomson Learning.

Kopun, J.G. & Stelmachowicz, P.G. (in press). The perceived communication difficulties of children with hearing loss. *Journal of the American Academy of Audiology.*

Kuk, F.K., Kollofski, C., Brown, S., Melum, A., & Rosenthal, A. (1999). Use of a digital hearing aid with directional microphones in school-aged children. *Journal of the American Academy of Audiology, 10,* 535–548.

Lucks Mendel, L., & Danhauer, J.L. (1997). Test administration and interpretation. In L. Lucks Mendel and J.L. Danhauer (Eds.), *Audiologic evaluation and management and speech perception assessment* (pp. 15–58). Clifton Park, NY: Delmar Thomson Learning.

Moeller, M.P. (1993). Auditory learning: Efficacy and evaluation. Paper presented at Developments in Pediatric Assessment and Amplification. Omaha, NE.

Moog, J.S., & Geers, A.E. (1990). *Early speech perception test for profoundly hearing-impaired children.* St. Louis, MO: Central Institute for the Deaf.

Moog, J.S., Kozak, V.J., & Geers, A.E. (1983). *Grammatical analysis of elicited language—presentence level.* St. Louis, MO: Central Institute for the Deaf.

Osberger, M.J., Geier, L., Zimmerman-Phillips, S., & Barker, M.J. (1997). Use of a parent-report scale to assess benefit in children given the Clarion cochlear implant. *American Journal of Otology, 18*(Suppl.), S79–S80.

Osberger, M.J., & Koch, D.B. (2000). Cochlear implants. In R.E. Sandlin (Ed.), *Textbook of hearing aid amplification: Technical and clinical considerations,* (2nd ed., pp. 673–703). Clifton Park, NY: Delmar Thomson Learning.

Osberger, M.J., Robbins, A.M., Miyamoto, R.T., Berry, S.W., Myres, W.A., Kessler, K.S., & Pope, M.L. (1991). Speech perception abilities of children with cochlear implants, tactile aids, or hearing aids. *American Journal of Otology, 12*(Suppl.), 105–115.

Paul, R.G., & Cox, R.M. (1995). Measuring hearing aid benefit with the APHAB: Is this as good as it gets? *American Journal of Audiology, 4*(3), 10–13.

Robbins, A.M. (1994). *Mr. Potato Head task.* Indianapolis, IN: Indiana University School of Medicine.

Robbins, A.M., Renshaw, J.J., & Berry, S.W. (1991). Evaluating meaningful auditory integration in profoundly hearing-impaired children. *American Journal of Otology, 12*(Suppl.), 144–150.

Robbins, A.M., Renshaw, J.J., Miyamoto, R.T., Osberger, M.J., & Pope, M.L. (1988). *Minimal Pairs Test.* Indianapolis, IN: Indiana University School of Medicine.

Robbins, A.M., Renshaw, J.J., & Osberger, M.J. (1995). *Common Phrases Test.* Indianapolis, IN: Indiana University School of Medicine.

Robbins, M.J., Svirsky, M., Osberger, M.J., & Pisoni, D.B. (1998). Beyond the audiogram: The role of functional assessments. In F.H. Bess (Ed.), *Children with hearing impairment: Contemporary trends* (pp. 105–124). Nashville, TN: Vanderbilt Bill Wilkerson Center Press.

Ross, M., & Lerman, J. (1979). A picture identification test for hearing impaired children. *Journal of Speech and Hearing Research, 13,* 44–53.

Schiavetti, N., & Metz, D.E. (1997). *Evaluating research in communicative disorders* (3rd ed.). Needham Heights, MA: Allyn & Bacon.

Serpanos, Y.C., & Gravel, J.S. (2000). Assessing growth of loudness in children by cross-modality matching. *Journal of the American Academy of Audiology, 11,* 190–202.

Stelmachowicz, P.G. (1999). Hearing aid outcome measures for children. *Journal of the American Academy of Audiology, 10,* 14–25.

Sweetow, R.W., & Tate, L.M. (1999). Back to school: High-tech hearing aids: Are they right for your child? *Volta Voices,* September/October, 10–14.

Task Force on Treatment Outcomes and Cost Effectiveness. (1997). Treatment outcomes data for adults in health care environments. *ASHA, 39,* 26–31.

Tharpe, A.M. (1998). Treatment fads versus evidenced-based practice. In F.H. Bess (Ed.), *Children with hearing impairment: Contemporary trends* (pp. 179–188). Nashville, TN: Vanderbilt Bill Wilkerson Center Press.

Tyler, R.S., & Holsted, B.A. (1978). *A closed-set speech perception test for hearing impaired children.* Iowa City, IA: The University of Iowa.

Weinstein, B.E. (2000). Outcome measures in rehabilitative audiology. In J.G. Alpiner and P.A. McCarthy (Eds.), *Rehabilitative audiology: Children and adults* (3rd ed., pp. 576–594). Philadelphia, PA: Lippincott, Williams, & Wilkins.

Whitelaw, G.M., Williams, C. & Wynne, M.K. (2001). Children's Outcome Worksheets (COW): Validation and efficacy. An instructional course taught at the 10th Annual Convention and Exposition of The American Academy of Audiology, San Diego, CA.

Yoshinaga-Itano, C. (2000). Assessment and intervention with preschool children who are deaf and hard-of-hearing. In J.G. Alpiner and P.A. McCarthy (Eds.), *Rehabilitative audiology: Children and adults* (3rd ed., pp. 140–177). Philadelphia, PA: Lippincott, Williams, & Wilkins.

Zimmerman-Phillips, S., Osberger, M.J., & Robbins, A.M. (1997). *Assessment of auditory skills in children two years of age or younger.* Paper presented at the 5th International Cochlear Implant Conference, New York, NY.

APPENDIX IX-A

Checklist Information for the Educational Audiology Association

Many of the teacher inventories and checklists can be purchased through the Educational Audiology Association (EAA):

ADDRESS: Educational Audiology Association
4319 Ehrlich Road
Tampa, FL 33624

PHONE: (800) 460-7EAA (7322)

FAX: (813) 968-3597

WEBSITE: www.edaud.org

CHAPTER 10

Outcomes Measurement in Aural Rehabilitation

LEARNING OBJECTIVES

This chapter will enable readers to:

- Acknowledge the conceptual frameworks for outcomes measurement in aural rehabilitation
- Recognize outcome measures in the disability and handicap domains, as well as comprehensive profiles
- Select self-report instruments
- Apply outcomes measurement in aural rehabilitative clinical practice and research
- Understand the use of outcomes measurement within the context of recommended hearing aid fitting guidelines
- Employ methods of outcomes measurement for tinnitus and vestibular/balance therapy

INTRODUCTION

When Mrs. P. came into the office, it was one of those cases where everything had gone wrong for the patient and family. It was as if the patient was a pinball that had been bumped about without rhyme or reason that somehow ended up in our waiting room. Had fate smiled upon Mrs. P? Was she finally going to be helped? Could we do it? Consider her story in Vignette 10–1.

This chapter covers outcomes measurement in aural rehabilitation. Outcomes measurement is reviewed regarding conceptual frameworks for different domains, selection of self-report instruments, and use in clinical practice and research, hearing aid fit-

tings, and tinnitus and vestibular/balance therapy. Readers might want to keep Mrs. P.'s scenario in mind while they read and think about how and when hearing health-care professionals might have used outcome measures to prevent Mrs. P.'s problems.

CONCEPTUAL FRAMEWORKS FOR OUTCOMES MEASUREMENT IN REHABILITATIVE AUDIOLOGY

A *conceptual framework* is an integrated system of ideas, terminology, variables, and

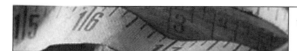

VIGNETTE 10-1

A REAL SHAME

A few months ago, a husband and wife in their 70s came into the office wanting a hearing aid consultation. The woman had been a hearing aid user for many years and had used several sets of hearing aids, which she claimed, "Never did much good." She reported that she was experiencing increased difficulty in most situations. She was very frustrated and told us her story.

"I went to a hearing aid specialist 6 months ago. He fit me with some fancy digital hearing aids that fit behind my ear for $7,000. The hearing aids did not do much good. I went to see him after 10 days and he tweaked them a bit, but he didn't seem to care about the problems I was having. They were too loud. I couldn't hear very well in restaurants or church. He told me to go home and see if things improved."

"I see. Did things improve?" I asked.

"Oh no. In fact, things got worse. They drove me crazy. I tried calling him, but his receptionist said he was away at some conference. The next week I called and he had gone fishing. Finally, two weeks later I called him and he said to come on in. He told me that he'd send them back to the manufacturer for repair. Well, they didn't get better. So he sent them back again. I wanted my money back. He told me that I had gone over the 30-day trial period. I was fit to be tied. I complained. He said that he could try something else, but the manufacturer required a $600 restocking fee. He gave me the hearing aids I have on now, which still are too loud and no damn good. Excuse me," she said as a tear rolled down her face and her husband squeezed her hand.

"Let me see your hearing aids and I'll call the manufacturer," I offered. She carefully handed them over. Upon inspection, I was horrified to find that she had spent $7,600 on basic analog programmable hearing aids, for which we would have charged about $1,700 for two. I called the manufacturer and was even more disturbed to find that no restocking fee was required if she returned the aids. I really began to have some serious doubts about her original dispenser's ethics.

"Mrs. P. you should go back to the gentleman who sold you your hearing aids and demand satisfaction or your money back. You know that as professionals, we are required to be licensed by a state board. I suggest that you complain to the licensure board if he doesn't comply with your wishes. Also, the manufacturer said that the trial period can be extended, but you must go back to the original dispenser."

"Thank you," said Mrs. P. as she left our office with her husband. I had a gut-level feeling that those hearing aids would sit in the drawer.

About 2 months later, she came back to our office and said that her husband had had a heart attack and a mild stroke, and that she was too old and frail to fight with the original dispenser. She said that it was difficult for her to get out of the house and begged for us to help her. She just wanted to start over.

We agreed to help her. "Come in and we'll hook you up to the computer," I said. Mrs. P was right. The hearing aids were set full-on with no compression. No wonder she was miserable. I reprogrammed the hearing aids to an appropriate output level with compression, as verified via real-ear probe-microphone measurement. I then re-instructed her on use and care of the hearing aids, and spent considerable time counseling Mrs. P. and her husband about the hearing aids, aural rehabilitation, and communication repair strategies. Mrs. P. thanked me and said she would try them out for a few days.

"I'd still like to try those fancy digitals if they can be set right," she offered as she left.

relationships that underlie measurement, interpretation, and prediction based on a supporting theory or a body of empirical observation (Hyde, 2000). The World Health Organization's International Classification of Impairments, Disabilities, and Handicaps (World Health Organization, 1980)—recently revised as the International Classification of Impairments, Activities, and Participation (ICIDH-2) (World Health Organization, 1999)—has provided a conceptual framework for outcomes measurement in aural rehabilitation (Hyde, 2000). These terms are precisely defined and represent abnormalities at different levels within a hierarchy ranging from basic organ structure and function (i.e., impairment) through integrated whole-body functions (i.e., disability) to high-level social role fulfillment (i.e., handicap) (Hyde, 2000; Hyde & Riko, 1994; Stephens & Hetu, 1991). Classifications for impairment can provide an objective record of hearing sensitivity for pure tones and speech that can serve as a basis for making technical decisions about electroacoustic parameters of hearing aids (Hyde & Riko, 1994; Weinstein, 1997). An example of impairment includes decreased auditory sensitivity or middle-ear disease that can be treated with selection of appropriate amplification or medical intervention, respectively (Hosford-Dunn & Huch, 2000). *Disability* has been labeled as "activity limitation," and *handicap* is defined as, "participation restriction" (Hyde, 2000). A major improvement in the ICIDH-2 is ascertaining that disability and handicap are *not* inherent characteristics of patients, but are transactions between patients and the environment (Hyde, 2000). An example of disability includes limitations in a patient's daily activities, such as not being able to hear a telephone ring from another room, unless the patient's limitation is remedied with the use of appropriate assistive listening devices (ALDs) (Hosford-Dunn & Huch, 2000). An example of handicap is not being able to listen to television with others,

because the required volume to understand is too loud for a patient's family members, unless remedied with the fitting of appropriate amplification and/or use of ALDs (Hosford-Dunn & Huch, 2000). Reduction of impairment, disability, and handicap through aural rehabilitation efforts can be measured through various methods found in Table 10–1 listing some of the more popular outcome measures in each of the three domains of impairment, disability, and handicap.

Reduction of hearing impairment can result from the achievement of certain hearing aid goals, such as making soft speech audible, normal speech comfortably loud, loud sounds tolerable, and minimizing the occlusion effect (Hosford-Dunn & Huch, 2000). Reduction of hearing impairment is measured through hearing aid verification procedures including real-ear probe-tube microphone measurements, functional gain, speech recognition measures, and so forth (Hosford-Dunn & Huch, 2000; Mueller, 1999; Weinstein, 2000). For example, Mueller (1999) stated that the *FIG-6* hearing aid prescription method is a good way to program hearing aids for patients because it can be verified through measurement of real-ear insertion gain (REIG) for three different input levels. Therefore, hearing aid *verification* involves procedures that audiologists perform to ensure that hearing aid goals have been met. Methods of hearing aid verification are beyond the scope of this handbook and readers are referred to Sandlin (2000) for further coverage. However, one self-assessment tool, the *Profile of Aided Loudness* (PAL: Palmer, Mueller, & Moriarty, 1999) can be considered as a verification measure. It determines if patients' loudness restoration is achieved through amplification (Huch & Hosford-Dunn, 2000). On the other hand, Mueller (1999) stated that hearing aid validation does not occur until after the patient has been fit and reports back through the use of some sort of self-assessment tool that the

Table 10-1. Tools and approaches to measuring impairment, disability, and handicap

IMPAIRMENT DOMAIN
- Real-ear Measures
- Functional Gain
- Speech Recognition Measures

DISABILITY DOMAIN
- Abbreviated Profile for Hearing Aid Benefit (APHAB)
- Hearing Performance Inventory (HPI)
- Hearing Aid Performance Inventory (HAPI)
- Shortened Hearing Aid Performance Inventory (SHAPI)
- Client Oriented Scale of Improvement (COSI)

HANDICAP DOMAIN
- Hearing Handicap Inventory for the Elderly (HHIE)
- Hearing Handicap Inventory for Adults (HHIA)
- Hearing Handicap for the Elderly—Screening Version (HHIE—S)
- Hearing Handicap for Adults—Screening Version (HHIA—S)

DISABILITY AND HANDICAP DOMAIN
- Communication Profile for the Hearing Impaired (CPHI)
- Glasgow Hearing Aid Benefit Profile (GHABP)

(Adapted from Weinstein, 2000).

hearing aids have provided benefit through the reduction of disability and/or handicap. Therefore, hearing aid *validation* is the perception of hearing aid benefit provided by patients and their significant others through the use of various outcome measures for disability and handicap. Tables 10-2, 10-3, and 10-4 show the name, authors, and date of publication; and description; and notes regarding common subjective self-assessment outcome measures used in aural rehabilitation for disability, handicap, and both disability and handicap, respectively. In addition, measures of hearing aid satisfaction are also important self-assessment instruments and are discussed in this chapter. Note that there are numerous other outcome measures for audiologists' use, but their inclusion is beyond the scope of this chapter.

Tools in the Disability Domain

The *Abbreviated Profile of Hearing Aid Benefit* (APHAB), was developed by Cox and Alexander (1995). The APHAB consists of 4 subscales with 24 items in four areas: Ease of Communication (EC), Reverberation (RV), Background Noise (BN), and Aversiveness to Sounds (AV), and appears in Appendix X–A, which can be found on the companion CD-ROM. An example of an item from the BN subscale is the phrase, "I have trouble understanding others when an air conditioner or fan is on," to which patients mark one of the following: 99% Always, 87% Almost Always, 75% Generally, 50% Half-the-Time, 25% Occasionally, 12% Seldom, or 1% Never. The purposes of the APHAB are to quantify the disability associated with hearing impairment

Table 10–2. The name, authors, date of publication, purpose, norms, description, and notes regarding common subjective self-assessment outcomes measures in the disability domain

NAME, AUTHORS, AND DATE OF PUBLICATION	PURPOSE	NORMS	DESCRIPTION	NOTES
Abbreviated Profile of Hearing Aid Benefit (APHAB) Cox and Alexander (1995)	To assess the perceived effects of hearing loss on social and emotional adjustment of non-institutional-ized elderly	*Normed on 128 elderly adults (90 men, 38 women) with mild-to-moderate sloping or flat loss who were successful hearing aid users *Reported percentile scores apply to these hearing aid users *Norms for new hearing aid users have not been established	4 subscales with 24 items: *Ease of Communication (EC) *Reverberation (RV) *Background Noise (BN) *Aversiveness to Sounds (AV) Example: Patient reads the phrase," have trouble understanding others when an air conditioner or fan is on" and then marks on one of the following: 99% Always, 87% Almost Always, 75% Generally, 50% Half-the-time, 25% Occasionally, 12% Seldom, 1% Never	*Can be administered one-time only (unaided versus aided) or pre- and post-measures before and after hearing aid fit-ting *Suggest a 3- to 4-week period between pre- and post-fitting measures
Hearing Performance Inventory (HPI) Giolas, Owens, Lamb, and Schubert (1979) Hearing Performance Inventory—Revised (HPI—R) (Lamb, Owens, & Schubert, 1983)	To evaluate performance in problem areas experi-enced in everyday liv-ing to deter-mine areas of communica-tion break-down	Normed on 190 adults	158 items focusing in problem areas such as: *under-standing speech *intensity of speech *response to audi-tory failure *social communication difficulties *personal communication difficulties *occupational difficulties Example: Patient reads a statement such as, "You are at a restaurant with a friend or family member and the room is fairly quiet. Can you understand the person when his/her voice is loud enough for you and you can see his/her face? And then marks on one of the following: ~100% Practically Always ~75% Frequently ~50% About Half of the Time ~25% Occasionally ~ 0% Almost Never. Later revised to 90 items through the elimination of redundant items Scoring *Scored on a 5–1 point scale (i.e., 1 for "Practically Always to 5 for "Almost Never") *Some questions in the Personal and Auditory Failure sections must be flagged and switched around prior to scoring because they are stated in the positive *Numbers are added for the individual items, the sum is then divided by the total number of items answered, and that result is then multiplied by 20 *Scores range from 20% (i.e., least amount of difficulty) to 100% (i.e., most difficulty) *The global inventory score is difficult to interpret *Individual section scores on Understanding Speech and Intensity may be more useful than the global inventory score	*Has been used in studies to measure hearing aid benefit in favorable listening conditions *Has been used to measure patients' denial of hearing loss by comparing their scores to those of significant others Advantages *Rigorous develop-ment with large num-bers of subjects with good reliability and validity *Can be used with patients with pro-found hearing loss Disadvantages *May be too long for practi-cal clinical use *Interview format can take as long as 30 to 40 minutes

(CONTINUES)

Table 10–2. (continued from page 221)

NAME, AUTHORS, AND DATE OF PUBLICATION	PURPOSE	NORMS	DESCRIPTION	NOTES
Hearing Aid Performance Inventory (HAPI) Walden, Demorest, and Helper (1984)	To evaluate the effective-ness of amplification in a variety of listening situations	Normed on 128 hearing aid users (119 men, 9 women) who wore their hearing aids an average of 10.8 hours per day and had sloping sensorineural hearing losses	64 items that quantify hearing aid benefit based on four listening situations: *Noisy listening situations *Quiet listening situations with the speaker close by *Reduced signal information *Situations with nonspeech stimuli Example: Patient reads a statement such as, "You are involved in an intimate conversation with your spouse," and then marks one of the following depending on how the hearing aid helps them in that situation: Very Helpful, Helpful, Very Little Help, No Help, Hinders Performance Scoring *Uses a 5-point scale (i.e., 1 for "Very Helpful" to 5 for "Hinders Performance"). *Numbers are added for the individual items, the sum is then divided by the total number of items answered *The closer the score is to "1," the greater the hearing aid benefit	Advantages *One of few self-assessment scales that directly asks about hearing aid benefit *Good reliabil-ity of measurement Disadvantages *Longer than SHAPI *May not be very applicable for elderly patients who are exposed to limited listening environments
Shortened Hearing Aid Performance Inventory (SHAPI) Schum (1992)	To evaluate the effective-ness of amplification in a variety of listening sit-uations using a shortened version of the HAPI	16 standardized listening situations	38 items that quantify hearing aid benefit based on four listening situations: *Noisy listening situations *Quiet listening situations with the speaker close by *Reduced signal information *Situations with nonspeech stimuli Example: Patient reads a statement such as "You are involved in an intimate conversation with your spouse," and then marks one of the following depending on how the hearing aid helps them in that situation: Very Helpful, Helpful, Very Little Help, No Help, Hinders Performance Scoring *Uses a 5-point scale (i.e., 1 for "Very Helpful" to 5 for "Hinders Performance"). *Numbers are added for the individual items, the sum is then divided by the total number of items answered *The closer the score is to "1," the greater the hearing aid benefit	Advantages *One of few self-assessment scales that directly asks about hearing aid benefit *Good reliabil-ity of measurement *Shorter than the HAPI Disadvantages *May not be very applicable for elderly patients who are exposed to limited listening environments

(CONTINUES)

Table 10–2. (continued from page 222)

NAME, AUTHORS, AND DATE OF PUBLICATION	PURPOSE	NORMS	DESCRIPTION	NOTES
Client Oriented Scale of Improvement (COSI) Dillon, James, and Ginis (1997)	To isolate up to five specific areas of listening difficulty and the degree of benefit obtained, compared to that expected for the population in similar type situations	Normed on 1,770 adults with hearing loss in Australia with 56% of the sample being new hearing aid users	16 standardized situations nominated and prioritized by the patient and the audiologist for which patients can rate two times *Their Degree of Change after wearing hearing aids by reading the statement, "Because of the new hearing instrument, I now hear ..." and marking one of the following: Worse .No difference, Slightly Better, Better, Much Better; and *Their Final Ability (with hearing instrument) by reading the statement, "I can hear satisfactorily," and marking one of the following: 10% Hardly Ever 25% Occasionally 50% Half the Time 75% Most of the Time 95% Almost Always *Patients get to decide on 5 listening situations, ranked in importance, that they need help with	* It is not simply the amount of benefit, but the importance of the listening situation to the patient *Can be used to shape patient's rehabilitation program *Final rating may highlight areas of need Advantages COSI is: *Reliable (i.e., test-retest from 0.73 to 0.84) *Simple *Brief *Patient-focused Disadvantages *Patients may have difficulty selecting and prioritizing situations *Difficult to determine to what extent patients' responses are related to how much they like their audiologists

Table 10-3. The name, authors, date of publication, purpose, norms, description, and notes regarding common subjective self-assessment outcome measures in the handicap domain

NAME, AUTHORS, AND DATE OF PUBLICATION	PURPOSE	NORMS	DESCRIPTION	NOTES
Hearing Handicap Inventory for the Elderly (HHIE) Ventry and Weinstein (1982)	To assess the perceived effects of hearing loss on social and emotional adjustment of non-institutionalized elderly	Normed on 47 non-institutionalized elderly adults using two measurement techniques: *face-to-face (20) *paper and pencil (27)	25 items with two subscales: *Emotional consequences of hearing loss (e.g., patient's attitudes and emotional responses toward hearing loss) (13 items) *Social and situational consequences of hearing loss (e.g., patient's perceived effects of hearing loss in a variety of social situations) (12 items) Example: Patient reads statement, "Does a hearing problem cause you difficulty when attending a party?" and then marks one of the following: Yes (4 points) Sometimes (2 points) No (0 points)	*Scores range from 0 to 100 (the higher the score, the greater the hearing handicap) *95% confidence interval (CI or critical difference value) is 18.7 in face-to-face administration and 36 for paper-and-pencil administration Advantages *Easy for elderly to complete *Straightforward to score and interpret *Well-established reliability and validity for elderly persons with hearing loss
Hearing Handicap for Adults (HHIA) Newman, Weinstein, Jacobson, and Hug (1990)	*To quantify perceived hearing handicap for adults under age 65 years *To assess benefit by measuring the change in perceived handicap before and after fitting of hearing aids	Normed on 28 adults (29 to 59 years of age)	25 items with two subscales: *Emotional consequences of hearing loss (13 items) *Social and situational consequences of hearing loss (12 items) Example: Patient reads statement, "Does a hearing problem cause you difficulty when attending a party?" and then marks one of the following: Yes (4 points) Sometimes (2 points) No (0 points)	*Scores range from 0 to 100 (the higher the score, the greater the hearing handicap) *95% confidence interval (CI or critical difference value) for face-to-face administration is 11.9 Advantages *High internal reliability *Excellent test-retest reliability

(CONTINUES)

Table 10–3. (continued from page 224)

NAME, AUTHORS, AND DATE OF PUBLICATION	PURPOSE	NORMS	DESCRIPTION	NOTES
Hearing Handicap Inventory for the Elderly—Screening Version (HHIE—S) Ventry and Weinstein (1982)	To screen for hearing loss in non-institutionalized elderly persons with a shortened version of the HHIE with good sensitivity and specificity		10 items <u>Example</u>: Patient reads statement, "Does a hearing problem cause you difficulty when attending a party?" and then marks one of the following: Yes (4 points) Sometimes (2 points) No (0 points)	*Scores range from 0 to 40 (the higher the score, the greater the hearing handicap) <u>Advantage</u> *Can be used as a screening tool for hearing loss
Hearing Handicap for Adults—Screening Version (HHIA—S) Newman, Weinstein, Jacobson, and Hug (1990)	To screen for hearing loss in adults under 65 years of age with a shortened version of the HHIA with good sensitivity and specificity		10 items <u>Example</u>: Patient reads statement, "Does a hearing problem cause you difficulty when attending a party?" and then marks one of the following: Yes (4 points) Sometimes (2 points) No (0 points)	*Scores range from 0 to 40 (the higher the score, the greater the hearing handicap)

(Adapted from Bentler & Kramer, 2000; Huch & Hosford-Dunn, 2000; McCarthy & Alpiner, 2000; Weinstein, 2000)

Table 10-4. The name, authors, date of publication, purpose, description, and notes regarding common subjective self-assessment outcome measures in both the disability and handicap domains

NAME, AUTHORS, AND DATE OF PUBLICATION	PURPOSE	NORMS	DESCRIPTION	NOTES
Communication Profile for the Hearing Impaired (CPHI) Demorest and Erdman (1987)	To provide a systematic and comprehensive assessment of a broad range of communication problems to define patients' hearing profiles before aural rehabilitation begins	*Normed on 827 patients at Walter Reed Army Medical Center on military and older populations *Suggested for clinicians to develop local norms	145-item questionnaire providing 3 importance ratings in 4 general areas: *Communication performance *Communication environment *Communication strategies *Personal adjustment Denial Example: Patient reads statement from Area 2, "One way I get people to repeat what they said is by ignoring them," and then marking along a scale from 1 for rarely to 5 for almost always	*Low scores are indicative of difficulty or areas warranting rehabilitative efforts *High scores reflect effective communication caused by use of compensatory strategies *Available in Spanish, Swedish, Portuguese, and Russian *Spouse and significant other forms have been developed *A pass-fail screening measure has been developed for hearing disability and handicap using data from over 1,000 respondents *Computerized scoring programs can provide profiles in less than 3 minutes. <u>Advantages</u> *Gives a wide range of clinical data for planning aural rehabilitation *Provides reliable and valid methods for profiling communication abilities of patients <u>Disadvantages</u> *Requires between 30 to 45 minutes to complete *May be impractical for common clinical use *Cost of purchasing a database for scoring may discourage offices from using this tool
Glasgow Hearing Aid Benefit Profile (GHABP) Gatehouse (1999)	To assess the aspects of hearing disability/handicap and hearing aid benefit	Normed on 293 adults (Median age 69 years)	4 pre-specified/4 subject specified items across 7 dimensions (e.g., initial disability/handicap, disability, handicap, reported hearing aid usage, reported benefit, residual disability, and satisfaction) Example: Patients read pre-specified item: "Listening to television on your own," and then answers 7 items for this situation, such as: *How often does this happen? Patients mark one of the following: 0, Never 1, Less than once a week 2, One to three days each week 3, Four to six days each week 4, Every day-under 4 hours 5, Over 4 hours every day	*Administration in interview format ensures a productive rehabilitative interaction *Can be completed in a pre- or postintervention format or postintervention only <u>Advantages</u> Before and After Approach *Identifies patients needing rehabilitative counseling prior to the fitting of amplification *Patients can review problems prior to the fitting of amplification <u>Disadvantages</u> Before and After Approach *Instrument is so short patients may remember their responses from pretest on post-test Postintervention Approach *Elderly patients may not recall preintervention state

(Adapted from Bentler & Kramer, 2000; Gatehouse, 1999, 2000; Huch & Hosford-Dunn, 2000; McCarthy & Alpiner, 2000; Weinstein, 2000.)

and the reduction of that disability through the use of amplification (Bentler & Kramer, 2000). The APHAB was normed on 128 (90 men, 38 women) elderly, experienced, successful hearing aid users with mild-to-moderate sloping or flat sensorineural hearing loss (Cox & Alexander, 1995; Paul & Cox, 1995; Weinstein, 2000). Percentile scores were established from normative group of experienced hearing aid users, but, to date, no norms have been established for new hearing aid users (Weinstein, 2000). Similar to many self-assessment tools, use of the APHAB is both criterion- and norm-referenced. Briefly, *criterion-referencing* is comparing patients' ratings made at two different times, such as pre- and postintervention. *Norm-referencing* is comparing patients' ratings to those of a sample of individuals representing the normative population. For example, criterion referencing occurs when patients complete the APHAB twice: (1) pre-hearing aid fitting, and (2) post-hearing aid fitting with a minimum of 3 to 4 weeks between administrations, and the scores are compared against themselves on all four subscales (Weinstein, 2000).

Another self-assessment tool in the disability domain is the *Hearing Performance Inventory* (HPI) developed by Giolas, Owens, Lamb, and Schubert (1979). The purpose of the HPI is to evaluate patients' performance in everyday listening situations (Wienstein, 2000). 0It was normed on 190 adults and consists of 158 items focusing on the following problem areas: understanding speech, intensity of speech, response to auditory failure, social communication difficulties, personal communication difficulties, and occupational difficulties (Bentler & Kramer, 2000). Some audiologists have classified the HPI into the handicap domain (Huch & Hosford-Dunn, 2000). The HPI is found in Appendix X–B on the companion CD-ROM. An example from the HPI is the item, "You are at a restaurant with a friend or family member and the room is fairly quiet. Can you under-

stand the person when his/her voice is loud enough for you and you can see his/her face?" Patients respond by marking one of the following: 100% Practically Always, 75% Frequently, 50% About half of the time, 25% Occasionally, or 0% Almost Never. Later, the HPI was revised (i.e., *Hearing Performance Inventory—Revised*: HPI—R) and reduced to 90 items in the same six areas (Lamb, Owens, & Schubert, 1983). The HPI is administered in an interview format that takes approximately 30 to 40 minutes. The revised version can be shortened to only 20 minutes by omitting the occupational items if the patient is unemployed (Huch & Hosford-Dunn, 2000). Possible uses of the HPI and HPI—R include (Huch & Hosford-Dunn, 2000):

- Comparison of patients' responses to those of significant others can detect denial of hearing loss such that the greater discrepancy of scores, the greater the lack of patients' acknowledgement of their problems.
- Measure of patient benefit when the HPI or HPI—R is re-administered after intervention.

Scoring involves using a 5-point scale, adding the numbers for the individual items, dividing the sum by the number of items answered, and then multiplying that result by 20 (Huch & Hosford-Dunn, 2000). Huch and Hosford-Dunn (2000) stated that scores:

- range from 20% (i.e., least amount of difficulty) to 100% (i.e., most difficulty),
- from the individual areas are more useful and easy to interpret than the global score which has low correlations with patients' audiometric results and their personal adjustment to hearing loss (Lamb, et al., 1983), and
- from the Understanding Speech and Intensity sections are most recommended for use (Lamb, et al., 1983).

The major advantages of the HPI/HPI—R are that they were rigorously developed from studies involving large numbers of subjects (i.e., good statistics and high reliability) and they can be used even with patients having profound hearing loss (Owens & Fujikawa, 1980); however, their disadvantage is that they may be too long for practical use.

The *Hearing Aid Performance Inventory* (HAPI: Walden, Demorest, & Hepler, 1984), found in Appendix X–C on the companion CD-ROM, is another self-assessment scale in the disability domain. The HAPI's purpose is to evaluate the post-fit effectiveness of amplification, using 64 items concerning four listening situations: noise, quiet with the speaker in close proximity, reduced signal information, and nonspeech stimuli (Bentler & Kramer, 2000; Huch & Hosford-Dunn, 2000; Weinstein, 2000). It was normed on 128 hearing aid users (i.e., 119 men, 9 women who wore their hearing aids an average of 10.8 hours per day and had sloping sensorineural hearing losses). An example from the HAPI is, "You are involved in an intimate conversation with your spouse," to which patients indicate how much their hearing aid(s) assist them by marking one of the following: Very Helpful, Helpful, Very Little Help, No Help, or Hinders Performance (Walden, et al., 1984). The HAPI is administered using the paper-and-pencil method when intervention is nearing completion (Huch & Hosford-Dunn, 2000). Scoring involves using a 5-point scale (i.e., 1 for "Very Helpful" to 5 for "Hinders Performance"), adding all of the numbers together, and dividing the sum by the number of items answered (Huch & Hosford-Dunn, 2000). The closer the score is to "1," the greater the amount of hearing aid benefit (Huch & Hosford-Dunn, 2000). The reliability of the HAPI is so high that other researchers have shortened the HAPI into the *Shortened Hearing Aid Performance Inventory* (SHAPI: Schum, 1992; Dillon, 1994) to decrease administration/scoring time while preserving good reliability (Huch & Hosford-Dunn, 2000). The SHAPI can be found in Appendix X-D on the companion CD-ROM. One advantage of the HAPI and SHAPI is that they help patients determine self-perceived hearing aid benefit, with the SHAPI taking less time than the HAPI. However, the major disadvantages of these tools are that they provide aided measures only and may not be applicable for use with elderly patients who are exposed to limited listening environments (Huch & Hosford-Dunn, 2000; Newman & Weinstein, 1988).

Still another self-assessment tool in the disability domain, found in Appendix X–E on the companion CD-ROM, is the *Client Oriented Scale of Improvement* (COSI) (Dillon, James, & Ginis, 1997). It was normed on 1,770 adults with hearing loss (i.e., 56% of the sample were new hearing aid users), isolates up to 5 specific areas of listening difficulty, and measures the degree of benefit obtained by patients as compared to that expected of a comparable population in similar type situations (Bentler & Kramer, 2000). Similar to the APHAB, the COSI is both criterion-referenced and norm-referenced because the selection and prioritization of situations is very patient specific and patients' responses can be compared against established norms. The COSI has 16 standardized situations, five of which are nominated and prioritized by patients in conference with their audiologists (Bentler & Kramer, 2000). Patients must be very specific about their situations; not, "I want to hear better ..." but "I want to hear better listening to the preacher in church" (Huch & Hosford-Dunn, 2000). Patients rate the situations two times: (1) on their degree of change after wearing hearing aids (i.e., Patients complete the following, "Because of the new hearing instrument I now hear_____" by marking either Worse, No Difference, Slightly Better, Better, or Much Better); and (2) on their final ability with the hearing aid (i.e., Patients complete the following, "I can hear satisfactorily_____" by marking either Hardly Ever, Occasionally, Half the Time, Most of the Time, or Almost Always) (Dillon, et al., 1997). The COSI can also be completed during planning of patients' individualized aural rehabilitation programs or a few months after fitting (Huch & Hosford-Dunn, 2000). Australian audiologists preferred using the COSI to other instruments because of its reliability (i.e., test-retest reliability ranging from 0.73 to 0.84), simplicity, brevity, and focus on patients' individual situations (Dillon, et al., 1997; Huch & Hosford-Dunn, 2000). One possible disadvantage is that patients may have a difficult time selecting and prioritizing listening situations. In addition, audiologists may find it difficult to determine to what extent patients' responses are related to how much they like their audiologists.

Tools in the Handicap Domain

The *Hearing Handicap Inventory for the Elderly* (HHIE), found in Appendix X–F on the companion CD-ROM, is a 25-item assessment tool that measures the social and emotional consequences of hearing loss on the lives of non-institutionalized elderly persons (Ventry & Weinstein, 1982). The Social Scale, consisting of 12 of the total 25 items, measures perceived effects of hearing loss in various social situations (Huch & Hosford-Dunn, 2000). For example, item S–1 asks, "Does a hearing problem cause you to use the phone less often than you would like?" to which patients respond by marking: Yes (4 points), Sometimes (2 points), or No (0 points). Similarly, the Emotional Scale, consisting of 13 of the total 25 items, measures attitudes and emotional reactions to hearing loss (Huch & Hosford-Dunn, 2000). For example, item E–2 asks, "Does a hearing problem cause you to feel embarrassed when meeting new people?" to which patients respond by marking one of the same response options mentioned above.

Scoring involves adding up the points and obtaining three scores:

1. Total score
2. Subtotal social score
3. Subtotal emotional score

Total scores range from 0 (i.e., no hearing handicap) to 100 (i.e., maximum hearing handicap). The HHIE prototype was originally pilot tested on 42 subjects with hearing loss, resulting in an internal consistency of 0.82 for the total scale, 0.83 for the Social Scale, and 0.93 on the Emotional Scale (Huch & Hosford-Dunn, 2000; Ventry & Weinstein, 1982). Items selected for the final instrument (on the basis of their strong correlations with their pure-tone sensitivity) were administered to 100 elderly persons with sensorineural hearing loss whose large variations in scores (i.e., standard deviations) were reflective of the sample's varying degrees of hearing loss (Huch & Hosford-Dunn, 2000; Ventry & Weinstein, 1982). In addition, test-retest reliability is high on the HHIE (Huch & Hosford-Dunn, 2000; Weinstein, Spitzer, & Ventry, 1986).

The HHIE is often used as a pre- and postintervention measure following a program of aural rehabilitation. When administering the HHIE for the first time, use of an interview format (i.e., face-to-face) reportedly reduces the number of responses left blank more than the paper-and-pencil method that is appropriate for postintervention or second assessments. The 95% confidence interval for the paper-and-pencil administration format is 36 points, indicating more variability in patients' responses than that of the interview format, which is 19 points (Huch & Hosford-Dunn, 2000; Weinstein, et al., 1986). When used as a benefit scale, both the Social and Emotional Scales have an 18-point confidence interval (Newman & Weinstein, 1988). Advantages of using the HHIE are that it is very simple for the elderly to complete and for audiologists to score and interpret (Huch & Hosford-Dunn, 2000).

The HHIE has a screening version, the HHIE—S, which contains 10 items from the original scale; it can be found in Appendix X–H on the companion CD-ROM. The HHIE—S was designed to detect emotional and social problems associated with hearing loss (Bess, Hedley-Williams, & Lichtenstein, 1999; Ventry & Weinstein, 1982). The scores on the HHIE—S can range from 0 to 40 points. Elderly patients (with a prior probability or prevalence rate of 30% for hearing impairment—see Chapter 7) who score between 0 to 8 points on the HHIE—S have only a 13% chance of having a hearing loss (Bess, et al., 1999). The 95% confidence interval for the HHIE—S is 10 points when administered in face-to-face format (Weinstein, 2000). Similarly, elderly patients who score between 26 and 40 points have an 84% chance of having a hearing loss (Bess, et al., 1999). An advantage of using the HHIE—S is that it can be used to screen for hearing impairment in service-delivery sites that are not conducive for pure-tone testing (Johnson & Danhauer, 1999). A disadvantage of the HHIE—S is in its misuse by audiologists who may use this as their only outcome measure. A companion to the HHIE—S is the HHIE—SP, a spouse's version that is nearly identical (i.e., changing "you" to "your spouse") and includes a spouse's perception of their partner's hearing handicap (Huch & Hosford-Dunn, 2000; Newnam & Weinstein, 1988).

The Hearing Handicap Inventory for Adults (HHIA), found in Appendix X-G on the companion CD-ROM, is a 25-item self-assessment scale that measures the same phenomena as the HHIE; both inventories are nearly identical, except for changes in one emotional and two social questions to make the HHIA more applicable for use with adults under 65 years of age (Newman, Weinstein, Jacobson, & Hug, 1990). The HHIA is scored in exactly the same way as the HHIE. The 95% confidence interval for the HHIE is 12 points using the face-to-face administration method (Weinstein, 2000). The advantages of using the HHIA include high internal reliability and excellent test-retest reliability (Newman, Weinstein, Jacobson, & Hug, 1991). The HHIA has a screening version, the HHIA—S, that has 10-items that are also designed to detect emotional and social problems associated with hearing loss. The HHIA—S appears in Appendix X–I on the companion CD-ROM.

Tools in Both the Disability and Handicap Domains

The *Communication Profile for the Hearing Impaired* (CPHI: Demorest & Erdman, 1987) is a self-assessment tool that samples both the disability and impairment domains. It was developed to provide a systematic and comprehensive assessment of a broad range of communication problems in the development of patient hearing profiles prior to aural rehabilitation efforts (Bentler & Kramer, 2000). The CPHI is a 145-item questionnaire providing 3 importance ratings on 5 general areas (Huch & Hosford Dunn, 2000):

- Communication Performance Scales—assess patients' ability to give and receive information or to carry on a conversation.
- Communication Environment Scales—assess external environmental factors and patients' strategies and emotional adjustments experienced in everyday life.
- Communication Strategies Scales—assess patients' verbal and nonverbal behaviors in different situations.
- Personal Adjustment Scales—assess patients' acceptance of and adjustment to hearing loss and reactions to the resultant communication problems using the following subscales:
  ⇒ Self-acceptance

⇒ Acceptance of hearing loss
⇒ Anger
⇒ Displacement of responsibility
⇒ Exaggeration of responsibility
⇒ Discouragement
⇒ Stress
⇒ Withdrawal
■ Denial Scales (Problem Awareness)—identify patients' responses that are surprisingly positive despite their losses.

The CPHI was normed at Walter Reed Medical Hospital on 827 active military service personnel as well as older patients (Bentler & Kramer, 2000; McCarthy & Alpiner, 2000). However, although normative studies using populations from around the country have been completed, it has been recommended that clinicians establish their own local norms (Bentler & Kramer, 2000; Huch & Hosford-Dunn, 2000). Two equivalent forms of the CPHI were developed: the Short Form (Form 1), and the Long Form (Form 2).

Both forms have undergone rigorous statistical analyses verifying their reliability and validity (Huch & Hosford-Dunn, 2000). Although scoring by "hand" is complicated and difficult, available computer programs can provide patient profiles in less than 3 minutes (Demorest & Erdman, 1987; McCarthy & Alpiner, 2000). Advantages of the CPHI include its availability in a number of languages (e.g., Spanish, Swedish, Portuguese, and Russian). Furthermore, it provides reliable and valid patient-communication profiling resulting in a wide range of clinical data for planning aural rehabilitation (Demorest & Erdman, 1987; McCarthy & Alpiner, 2000). A disadvantage is that it requires 30 to 45 minutes to complete, which may preclude its use in most practical clinical situations (Demorest & Erdman, 1987; McCarthy & Alpiner, 2000).

The *Glasgow Hearing Aid Benefit Profile* (GHABP), found in Appendix X–J on the companion CD-ROM, is a self-assessment outcome measure developed, optimized, and verified for use in evaluating the effectiveness and efficacy of aural rehabilitation services for adults with hearing impairment (Gatehouse, 1999). The GHABP was normed on 293 adults (Median age-69 years) and has a matrix design in which a variety of listening situations is inventoried providing a number of different dimensions or scales (Gatehouse, 2000):

■ Initial disability/handicap (i.e., patients' perceived difficulties prior to intervention)
■ Disability (i.e., an indication of the types/degrees of difficulty that patients experience)
■ Handicap (i.e., the impact of difficulties on patients' everyday lives)
■ Reported hearing aid usage (i.e., the percentage of time that patients report use of their hearing aids)
■ Reported benefit (i.e., the extent to which patients can hear better with their hearing aids than without them)
■ Residual disability (i.e., the extent to which patients have remaining problems that may require further audiologic or rehabilitative intervention)
■ Satisfaction (i.e., factors not related to hearing or listening, such as cosmetics or comfort)

Each dimension or scale is accounted for by a single question that patients answer for 4 pre-selected and 4 patient-selected situations. For example, patients are asked if a particular situation happens in their lives such as, "Listening to the television with other family or friends when the volume is adjusted to suit other people." Patients respond to the following question for the disability scale, "How much difficulty do you have in this situation?" by marking one of the following: Not Applicable, No Difficulty, Only Slight Difficulty, Moderate Difficulty, Great Difficulty, or Cannot Manage at All. Gatehouse (1999) suggested administering the GHABP in an interview format (instead of a self-report questionnaire) allowing for a productive rehabilitative interaction between audiologist and patient (Gatehouse, 2000). Furthermore, the GHABP can be administered in a pre- (i.e., completion of only the first two questions for initial disability/handicap) and post-intervention (i.e., completion of the rest of the instrument) fashion. Alternatively, the GHABP can be completed at the end of the rehabilitation process. There are at least two advantages of the "before and after" approach. The first advantage is that this approach provides an opportunity to identify patients needing rehabilitative counseling prior to the fitting of amplification (Gatehouse, 2000). The second advantage is that it provides patients with an opportunity to appreciate the problems that they encountered before the fitting of amplification (Gatehouse, 2000). One disadvantage is that although the test-retest reliability of the GHABP is high, it may be slightly inflated because the short instrument length may enable patients to remember their responses from administration to administration (Huch & Hosford-Dunn, 2000). A major disadvantage of the postintervention only completion of the GHABP is that questioning patients about their prefitting difficulties from past events (e.g., more than a few weeks) may be difficult for elderly patients (Gatehouse, 2000). Generally, audiologists can use these or other approaches in order to suit the needs of their patients.

Measures of Satisfaction

Over the past decade, Sergei Kochkin, Ph.D., of Knowles Electronics has conducted a series of MarkeTrak studies which have contributed a great deal of information regarding consumer satisfaction and market penetration of hearing aids in the United States. For example, one of the first MarkeTrak studies published in *The Hearing Journal* showed that overall consumer satisfaction with hearing aids was 58% for older hearing aids, but 66% for new hearing aids (Kochkin, 1993a; 1993b; 1993c; 1997). However, overall satisfaction decreased to 44% for older hearing aids, but increased to 71% for new hearing aids as documented by MarketTrak IV (Kochkin, 1997; 1998).

These studies have involved very large numbers of hearing aid users drawn from representative samples of the population of the United States using a three-step process. First, in December 1993, a short screening survey was sent to 80,000 persons from the National Family Opinion (NFO) panel consisting of households that are representative of the United States census information, with respect to market size, age of household, and income considering all regions of the country (excluding Hawaii and Alaska) and the nation's 25 largest metropolitan areas (Kochkin, 1997). Second, the results of the screening survey were analyzed identifying 13,000 persons with hearing impairment and their households (Kochkin, 1997). Third, as part of the MarkeTrak IV study, extensive surveys were sent to 3,000 non-institutionalized hearing aid users and 3,000 persons with hearing loss, but who did not use hearing aids (Kochkin, 1997). They had the following characteristics:

- Average age of 68 years
- 59% male/ 41% female
- Percentage of hearing aids by style:
  ⇒ Behind-the-ear 15%
  ⇒ In-the-ear 41%
  ⇒ In-the-canal 44%
- Average of 9.4 hours of hearing aid use per day
- 7% of the hearing aids were in a drawer
- 78% wore hearing aids 4 or more hours per day

- 30% were new hearing aids users
- 82% had bilateral hearing loss
- 65% were binaural users
- 59% viewed hearing as a problem most of the time
- 74% had difficulty conversing in noise
- Percentage of self-reported hearing loss:
  - ⇒ 5% mild
  - ⇒ 47% moderate
  - ⇒ 40% severe
  - ⇒ 7% profound

The survey included the *Hearing Satisfaction Survey* (HSS: Kochkin, 1997) measuring 34 areas on a 5-point Likert-scale (i.e., Very Satisfied, Satisfied, Neutral, Dissatisfied, and Very Dissatisfied). The HSS can be found in Appendix X-K on the companion CD-ROM. Kochkin (1997) analyzed the results of the surveys and developed norms for hearing aids one year old or less, or two years old or less to be used in the following ways:

- Comparing two or more different hearing aid technologies, or to the typical user
- Measuring improvement over time
- Using measures of hearing disability in developing predictive models of hearing aid success
- Documenting reduction in hearing disability
- Studying benefit in different listening environments
- Troubleshooting unsuccessful fittings

The norms contain percentage of dissatisfied/satisfied, mean, and standard deviations of respondents' satisfaction ratings in consumer behavior, product behavior, performance/value factors, listening environments, and dispenser service. Audiologists can administer the HSS to their patients one-year after purchase and then two-years after purchase to determine how their degree of satisfaction compares to the means and standard deviations of the normative group.

Therefore, audiologists can compare their patients' unaided and aided benefit to the norms provided by Kochkin (1997). Patients' ratings that fall more than a standard deviation below the mean on measures within a particular dimension (e.g., dispenser service) may indicate an area in need of improvement.

In addition to one-on-one work with individual patients, these more commercially oriented norms can be used in research studies investigating benefits of new hearing aid technology, or in comparing a particular manufacturer's products to the MarkeTrak norms. For example, Sandridge (1997) used the norms of the HSS, the APHAB, and the HHIE—S as baseline data (Kochkin, 1997) in assessing customer service with Oticon Multifocus hearing aids. These surveys were completed with 680 Multifocus users from 23 different states. The results of the study indicated that the Multifocus users were more satisfied with both the performance of the hearing aids and the service of their dispensers than those sampled in the MarkeTrak IV survey. In addition, Sandridge and Newman (1998) also used the HSS to compare patients' ratings of digital signal processing hearing aids to MarkeTrak norms for high-technology hearing aids and more conventional instruments. Similarly, Whichard (1997) used the HSS and found that patients' overall satisfaction with Resound hearing aids was greater than that of more traditional hearing aids as measured by MarkeTrak.

In summary, Kochkin (1997) believed that the MarkTrak IV norms could be used as the "gold standard" against which the performance of patients and their hearing aids can be compared. The contribution of the MarkeTrak studies has been significant in the industry's understanding of consumer satisfaction with and market penetration of hearing aids. MarkeTrak IV norms can be a valuable referent for outcomes measurement. However, audiologists should keep in mind the caveat that the norms must be updated to incorporate the development of new technology and the changing demographics of the general population.

Another tool is the *Satisfaction of Amplification in Daily Life* (SADL: Cox & Alexander, 1999), found in Appendix X-L on the companion CD-ROM. The purpose of the SAPL is to examine the overall outcome of amplification from the patient's perspective (Huch & Hosford-Dunn, 2000). It is a 15-item scale yielding a global satisfaction score and a profile of four subscales:

- Positive Effect subscale contains 6 items in the areas of improved performance and function (i.e., 2 items about acoustic benefit, one on sound quality, and three about psychological benefits of hearing aid use).
- Service and Cost subscale has 2 items regarding service and one on cost.
- Negative Features subscale contains 3 items each assessing a different unsatisfactory aspect of hearing aid use.
- Personal Image subscale has 3 items regarding self-image and hearing aid stigma.

Patients' responses are recorded on a 7-point scale ranging from "Not at all" (A) to "Tremendously" (G). The global score is the mean for all of the responses on the 15 items. Subscales are obtained by averaging the responses for items on each scale. The critical difference ($p < 0.01$) for test-retest global scores is 0.9 (Cox & Alexander, 1999). The scale has good content validity in that it was developed from interviews of hearing aid wearers who completed questionnaires about the relative importance of different variables affecting their satisfaction of hearing aids (e.g., What things are important to your satisfaction with a hearing aid?). The SADL is completed by patients (takes less than 15 minutes) after they have adjusted to their hearing aids (Huch & Hosford-Dunn, 2000).

SELECTING SELF-REPORT TOOLS

We have reviewed numerous scales in the disability, handicap, and both the disability/handicap domains, as well as satisfaction measures. However, what constitutes a good tool? Hyde (2000) stated 6 characteristics of a good instrument. First, an instrument should have a clear and detailed definition of its use so that it fits clinicians'/researchers' intended needs. Many of the measures have either no or only a vaguely stated purpose. Second, an instrument should specify a target population including all relevant demographic information (e.g., age, sex, and socioeconomic status), disease specific information (e.g., degree, configuration, and etiology of hearing loss), and method of administration (e.g., self-report, paper-and-pencil; interview; or computer-assisted) so that clinicians/researchers can apply the tool to patients/subjects in an appropriate way. Third, an instrument should have a definition of a conceptual framework (e.g., World Health Organization's International Classification of Impairments, Disabilities, and Impairment ICIDH-2, 1997) so that clinicians/researchers can, among other things, select an appropriate combination of tools to answer questions for specific clinical or research situations. Fourth, in development, an instrument should have undergone an iterative process for design, pilot testing (e.g., with smaller samples of fewer than 50 subjects), and validation/norming (i.e., with larger samples of greater than 200 subjects), which are necessary procedures in the seemingly endless process of a tool's acceptance in the scientific community. However, Hyde (2000) cautioned that authors should complete all revisions prior to validation and norming studies, because any changes of a scale may alter its psychometric properties and invalidate any published results not reported on the final form of an instrument. Fifth, evaluation of the reliability (e.g., internal consistency among scale items and test-retest reliability), validity (e.g., construct, content, face, and criterion), and responsiveness (i.e., the extent to which significant changes in the patient's/subject's "state" are reflected in observed values) of an instrument are critical to its widespread use. Sixth, instruments should have adequate norms that are readily available, whose method of accrual and presentation are understood easily.

Issues concerning reliability and validity of measures were discussed generally in Chapter 4. However, some focus on these issues is warranted, specifically in reference to self-report tools of impairment, disability, and handicap. Readers must be knowledgeable when assessing the reliability and validity of self-assessment scales, as these traits are interrelated and interdependent. Recall that reliability is the consistency of measurement, and validity is the truth in measurement. An instrument can have high reliability, but low validity. However, reliability without validity is worthless because an instrument can consistently produce erroneous results. It is not possible for an instrument to be valid without also being reliable because accurate measures must be consistent.

Reliability is both multifaceted and context dependent. Blanket statements that a particular instrument is a valid measure of hearing handicap are not useful unless the precise purposes/contexts of use are stated and the specific types of reliability are considered (Hyde, 2000). *Internal consistency* is the degree to which items of an instrument consistently measure the same aspects of a domain (e.g., such as handicap); this reduces error and is assessed by the following quantitative measures (Hyde, 2000):

- *Item-total correlation*—the correlation of individual items with the total score
- *Split-half reliability*—the correlation of scores obtained for two randomly selected halves of an instrument

- *Cronbach's alpha*—the variance of the total scale score to that of the individual items

When no items are correlated, then the alpha is zero; when they are perfectly correlated, a score of 1 or unity is achieved (Hyde, 2000). A high alpha is not necessarily good. As stated earlier, useful instruments adequately sample a domain with a diversity of items that may be more heterogeneous than homogeneous, which decreases the value of the alpha (Hyde, 2000). One simple solution is to construct a tool that adequately samples a domain with somewhat homogeneous items. However, in order to accomplish this feat, the length of the instrument may be too long to be feasible for use in day-to-day clinical practice.

Test-retest reliability is the degree to which scores obtained by a group of subjects correlate with the scores obtained during a second administration of an instrument. Each score is perceived as a "true" value unique to each subject plus random error. Correlation coefficients R (0 < R < 1) can be interpreted as the proportion of overall variance of the measurement that is caused by actual subject differences (Hyde, 2000). For completely reliable instruments, the correlation coefficient would be 1.0 or perfect, and the error variance would be zero. For completely unreliable instruments, the correlation coefficient would be 0 and any variation in scores would be caused by error. In addition, for highly reliable instruments, the greatest amount of variance is attributable to variability among subjects and, less to error (Hyde, 2000). The time interval between the first and second administrations of an instrument is critical. If the time interval is too short, then respondents may remember and replicate their previous responses, thereby artificially reducing the error variance and overestimating reliability (Hyde, 2000). Alternatively, if the interval between test administrations is too long, changes in responses are considered to be attributable to stability, rather than reliability with the former usually measured repeatedly over a long period of time (Hyde, 2000). Furthermore, the test-retest reliability coefficient should be assessed using intra-class correlation coefficients obtained with an analysis of variance data model that is able to accommodate more than two observations per patient, instead of the commonly used Pearson correlation for paired measurements that tends to overestimate reliability (Hyde, 2000).

Hyde (2000) summarized specific numeric criteria for evaluating the reliability of a self-assessment scale. Correlation coefficients of 0.85 or greater for internal consistency are considered adequate for health-related fields (McDowell & Newell, 1986), although some have stated that this criterion is too high and that values of 0.7 to 0.9 are more realistic (Boyle, 1991; Hyde, 2000; Streiner & Norman, 1995). For test-retest reliability, correlation coefficients must be in the range of 0.85 to 0.90 for a measurement scale to be considered of reasonable quality (Hyde, 2000; Streiner & Norman, 1995). Moreover, much higher levels of stringency are required for applications involving individual subjects (i.e., ≥ 0.9) than those for groups (i.e., ≥ 0.8) (Hyde, 2000; Nunnally, 1978). Readers are referred to further description of the reliability of measurement in Hyde (2000).

Hyde (2000) stated that validity was once believed to be an inherent characteristic of an instrument, but is now considered to have more to do with its use. Therefore as stated earlier, blanket statements about the validity of self-assessment questionnaires are meaningless unless they are provided within the context of the use of the instrument. In addition, although Chapter 4 discussed three types of validity: *content*, *criterion*, and *construct*, Hyde (2000) believed that construct is the only true type of validity and that the other two are simply facets of this phenomenon. Recall that construct validity (theoretical validity) is the degree with which a measure either empirically or rationally purports to measure some theoretical construct (Maxwell & Satake, 1997; Schiavetti & Metz, 1997). Validation of constructs is a gradual, never ending process; reflexive (i.e., testing the new measure and the construct); and involves exploring structural patterns of variation and co-variation among observable variables; and the relevance, appropriateness, and diversity of those relationships with the correlations found (Hyde, 2000). Content validity of a scale is the extent to which items represent and sample target domains, occurs early in test development, and is assessed less formally through subjective opinion (e.g., client panels, expert panels, and comparison to existing scales) rather than through quantitative means (Hyde, 2000). When evaluating content validity, instruments should have items that (Hyde, 2000):

- are brief, clear, and unambiguous;
- are unitary in theme, with no compound or multiple conditions;
- are free of jargon;
- never contain the word "not";
- include "positive" and "negative" questions;
- are appropriate culturally, educationally, and linguistically;
- are appropriate regarding response resolution;
- are low in noncompletion;
- are broad in response distribution; and
- have moderate item-total correlations (i.e., > 0.2).

Criterion validity is the degree to which an instrument statistically correlates (e.g., Pearson r for rating scale scores and continuous standard variables; Cohen's alpha for binary categorical situations; or Spearman's rho or Kendall's tau for multiple categories) to some recognized "gold standard" measure in the field (Hyde, 2000). Specific values for validity coefficients (e.g., Pearson r values) in health status measurements range from 0.2 to 0.6 and are rarely greater than 0.7 (Hyde, 2000; McDowell & Newell, 1986).

Responsiveness and *feasibility* are also important factors to evaluate prior to using an instrument. Responsiveness is how sensitive an instrument is at measuring changes in a patient's state (Hyde, 2000). Hyde (2000) stated that there are two methods to measuring change in patient state: the indirect method; and the direct method. The indirect method involves assessing the patient's state before and after an event of interest and subtracting the pre-measure score from the post-measure score to obtain a "change-score." The indirect method involves measurement of a patient's state before and after fitting of hearing aids or aural rehabilitation treatment program, for example. Many of the self-assessment instruments in the disability (e.g., APHAB, HPI, and COSI), handicap (e.g., HHIE, HHIE—S, HHIA, and HHIE—S), and combination handicap/disability domains (e.g., CPHI) encourage use of the indirect method of measuring change in patient state. An advantage of the indirect method is that two measures of the patient are made: pre-state (e.g., used for baseline reference and as a possible predictor of response to treatment) and post-state (e.g., used as an indicator of residual problem) (Hyde, 2000). The direct method, on the other hand, involves asking patients about their degree of impairment, disability, or handicap before and after intervention. Although more convenient, the direct method may not be the best for elderly patients who may have a difficult time recalling past events. Another characteristic of a tool to consider is its feasibility, or its ease of use (Hyde, 2000). Some self-assessment scales are easier to use with patients than others. For example, the CPHI, consisting of hundreds of questions, may

have been developed and normed on sound psychometric principles, but no audiologist is going to get patients to complete this instrument. The CPHI is not the only instrument that is too long to be feasible. Even the SHAPI is too long for most practical purposes and it consists of only 38 questions. Therefore, audiologists must balance the comprehensiveness of certain outcome measures with their "real world" feasibility.

USE OF SELF-ASSESSMENT TOOLS IN CLINICAL PRACTICE AND RESEARCH

We've discussed different instruments in the disability and handicap domains, as well as profiles that seem to span multiple areas of patient outcomes in addition to important considerations for selecting self-assessment scales. However, application of these principles is not possible without some concrete scenarios that vary according to measurement goals. Cox, et al., (2000) presented optimal qualities for instruments for 4 different outcomes measurement goals. For three of those goals, general characteristics, recommendations, a clinical scenario or two, and additional considerations for outcome measures are presented there.

Goal 1: To Assess Rehabilitative Outcomes for an Individual Patient

This goal focuses on measuring the rehabilitative outcomes for individual patients that are commonly encountered in clinical practice in particular, non-institutionalized elderly who are first-time hearing aid wearers with mild-to-severe sensorineural hearing losses (Cox, et al., 2000). The outcome measure should facilitate (Cox, et al., 2000):

1. Assessing patients' needs and preferences

2. Planning rehabilitation treatment
3. Determining patient dismissal criteria
4. Evaluating program success in terms of patient and family day-to-day quality of life

Furthermore, for planning and improving treatment, the instrument should be administered by the clinician and be based on individual self-report involving patient identification of items (e.g., listening situations) rather than generic situations standardized across large groups of subjects (Cox, et al., 2000). The instrument should tap into both disability and handicap domains and include measures of satisfaction and self-report from a significant other (Cox, et al., 2000). Outcomes measurement assisted the two sisters shown in Figure 10–1 in achieving positive patient outcomes through the use of amplification.

Consider the scenario encountered by Pam Pratt, Au.D., FAAA, in Vignette 10–2.

Pam's experiment with outcomes measurement with the Wanahears was a success. Using the COSI and including the patient's significant other took some time, but Pam was convinced that the time spent was justi-

fied in achieving positive patient outcomes. Pam believed that she could have achieved the same outcome had she used the GHABP in addition to the SADL. Ultimately, she now routinely uses the COSI, GHABP, and the SADL with her elderly patients.

Goal 2: To Assess the Effectiveness of Service Provided by a Clinical Unit

This goal focuses on assessing the effectiveness of the services provided by a particular clinical unit, such as a speech and hearing clinic, a private practice, or even a hearing support program in a particular health-care facility, involving a wide variety of interventions including the fitting of hearing aids, cochlear implants, and/or ALDs, or general rehabilitative services, such as hearing aid orientation groups (Cox, et al., 2000). The assessment should involve the effectiveness of an overall program rather than a specific audiologist or patient (Cox, et al., 2000). The collection of outcome data can be accomplished at two levels:

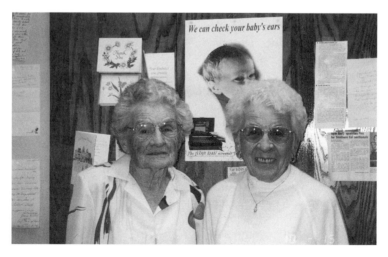

Figure 10-1 Two sisters who achieved positive patient outcomes through amplification.

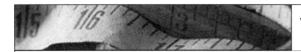

VIGNETTE 10-2

AN ADVENTURE IN OUTCOMES MEASUREMENT

Pam Pratt, Au.D., FAAA, enjoys her work as a private practice audiologist in southern California. Initially, it was a big step to resign her position as a staff audiologist at a large metropolitan hospital in Los Angeles in exchange for being her own boss in a small, but lucrative, private practice in the San Fernando Valley. In the early stages of development, Pam put in 16-hour days to build up her practice. She enjoyed her independence without having the pressure of someone always watching over her shoulder. Pam was a conscientious professional, keeping current with her continuing education hours by attending professional meetings and up-to-date with cutting-edge research findings by reading her journals over a brown-bag lunch. She had become increasingly interested in implementing outcome measures to demonstrate positive outcomes for her patients. She wanted to select measures that would be effective, but not take too much of her time and overwhelm her patients. Pam's patients primarily consisted of well-to-do senior citizens who were independent and active, and mostly had bilateral sensorineural hearing losses ranging from mild-to-severe in degree.

One day she decided to implement an outcomes measurement program with her patients, particularly those who were first-time hearing aid users. After reading the special issue of *Ear and Hearing* (2000) on outcomes measurement, she knew that for most of her patients she needed to tap into the disability and handicap domain, in addition to including a measure of overall satisfaction. Mr. Walter Wanahear was scheduled for a hearing evaluation the following week. Pam decided to study and implement outcomes measurement with him. During the next seven days, she planned her outcomes measurement strategy during her free time.

At first, Pam was overwhelmed by all the self-assessment tools available. She read a lot about reliability, validity, and so on. Her first task was to select a measure representing the disability domain. Hmmm ... there is the APHAB, the HPI, the HAPI, SHAPI, and the COSI. She immediately realized that the HPI, HAPI, and the SHAPI were far too long for her purposes. Furthermore, although the HAPI and the SHAPI asked about hearing aid benefit, they were typically completed after the fitting and acclimatization of the hearing aids. Pam wanted a measure that would assess performance pre- and post-fitting of hearing instruments. So, it was between the APHAB and the COSI. Pam called Neil Knowitall, an audiologist and friend, who had been using outcome measures in his practice.

"Hi Neil, this is Pam. How are you doing?"

"Hi Pam! I am doing fine. And you," inquired Neil.

"I am doing fine. Listen, I am starting to implement outcome measures in my practice and wanted your advice."

"Sure, go ahead," encouraged Neil.

"I am debating whether to use the COSI or APHAB with my elderly patients. What has been your experience with these tools?" asked Pam.

"Although I like the concept and the widespread use of the APHAB, it is still too long to use for most patients and many of the situations do not apply. In addition, it does not engage patients or their significant others in identifying problems or goals. Therefore, I prefer using the COSI because it is more patient-focused," explained Neil.

"Any suggestions for measures of hearing handicap?" asked Pam.

CONTINUES

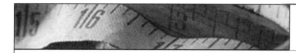

VIGNETTE 10-2

AN ADVENTURE IN OUTCOMES MEASUREMENT (CONTINUED FROM PAGE 239)

"The HHIE and HHIE—S are good tools, but even though they are short, they can take up time and are not patient-focused either. Did you see the special issue of *Ear and Hearing* focusing on outcomes measurement in rehabilitative audiology?" asked Neil.

"Yes, I did. In fact, I have read the entire issue, cover-to-cover," Pam responded.

"One of the last articles in the issue focuses on international consensus on outcomes measurement. In one clinical scenario, the authors suggested modifying the COSI to measure hearing handicap. Did you read that?" asked Neil.

"Yes, I did. I think I'll try it. The article also suggested using an overall measure of hearing aid satisfaction. I was thinking about using the SADL," Pam offered.

"The SADL is nice and short. But it still may be too long for some elderly patients," explained Neil.

"I am starting to use outcomes measurement with a 77-year-old patient next week," said Pam.

"You might consider just asking the patient at the end of the rehabilitation process if he is satisfied with the rehabilitation program," offered Neil.

"I'll keep that in mind," Pam replied.

"Recently, I've been using the GHABP by Stuart Gatehouse with my elderly patients. It is patient-focused and measures the dimensions of initial disability/handicap, hearing aid usage, reported hearing aid benefit, residual disability, and satisfaction. I can use it in a pre- and postintervention fashion or at the end of the rehabilitation process," explained Neil.

"Thanks Neil for your advice. I am excited to try these outcome measures. Good-bye," Pam concluded.

The following week, Walter Wanahear and his wife, Wilma, came in for his hearing evaluation. The case history indicated nothing out of the ordinary: family history of hearing loss, possibility of noise-induced hearing loss. Audiologic results indicated a mild sloping to severe high-frequency sensorineural hearing loss. Mr. and Mrs. Wanahear were counseled as to the styles of, circuitry for, and benefits of amplification. The Wanahears seemed very enthusiastic about amplification. Pam thought that this would be an ideal time to obtain pre-intervention "income measures." The question in Pam's mind was whether to use the COSI or the GHABP. Although enthusiastic, Mr. Wanahear had his wife fill-out all his forms for him and seemed agitated by many of the case history questions. Therefore, Pam decided to abbreviate the procedure as much as possible by using the COSI. She decided to implement the strategy suggested in the special issue of *Ear and Hearing*.

"Tell me about the problems your hearing is causing you," Pam requested.

"He can never hear me," offered Mrs. Wanahear as her husband groaned.

"Mrs. Wanahear, let's have your husband answer the question first."

"It is very difficult for me to hear in noisy places," offered Mr. Wanahear.

"Can you give me some specific situations?" asked Pam.

"Hearing my wife at crowded restaurants, hearing the preacher at church and the speaker in our lifelong learner's classes."

CONTINUES

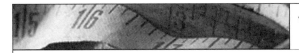

VIGNETTE 10-2

AN ADVENTURE IN OUTCOMES MEASUREMENT (CONTINUED FROM PAGE 240)

"Have these problems caused you to change the things you do or the way you do them?" asked Pam inquiring about hearing handicap.

"Yes, I don't go out to eat much, or play bingo as often, or go to many seminars anymore. If we do, it is at around 4:00 p.m. when the restaurants aren't crowded, or we sit at our own table at bingo without her chatty friends, Jim and Mary Porep" explained Mr. Wanahear.

"I thought we ate out early to take advantage of the lunch prices," chirped Mrs. Wanahear.

"No dear. It is because I wanted to listen to your sweet voice," teased Mr. Wanahear.

Pam could tell that although they had a good relationship, Mr. Wanahear's hearing loss was causing some problems for the couple.

"Mrs. Wanahear, hearing loss often causes problems for family members as well. Can you tell me about any problems that you want to solve from your point of view?" probing Mr. Wanahear's significant other about his disability and handicap.

"In addition to the problems he mentions, he can't hear very well on the telephone nor can he listen to the television at a reasonable level," offered Mrs. Wanahear.

"Has his problems with hearing caused you to change the things that you do or the way that you do them?" asked Pam.

"Yes, I resent being restricted as to when we go to restaurants. I want to sit at a bingo table with my friends. In fact, our relationship with Jim and Mary has suffered because they think we don't enjoy their company anymore. I also resent having to answer all the telephone calls. His grandchildren wonder why Grandpa doesn't like to talk with them on the phone. The television is so loud that I have to go to my room during most of the evening. I miss spending time with my husband in the evening," admitted Mrs. Wanahear with sadness in her voice.

"Dear, I had no idea," apologized Mr. Wanahear, reaching for his wife's hand.

"I appreciate your honesty. We now can focus on solving your problems. So far, these are the problems we have identified: (1) listening to conversation in a noisy restaurant, (2) listening to the preacher at church, (3) talking to your spouse at bingo, (4) listening to the speaker at lifelong learning classes/speakers during lecture, (5) talking on the telephone, and (6) watching television," checked Pam on the COSI form.

"Yes, that's about it," remarked Mr. Wanahear, looking at his wife who was nodding in agreement.

"Do you think you could rank your needs in order of their significance from most important to least important by placing a 1 for most important to 5 for least important?" Pam asked pointing out the boxes on the COSI form.

"Yes, give us a moment please," requested Mr. Wanahear."

Pam went on to counsel the Wanahears about the different options for amplification in addition to the use of assistive listening devices (ALDs). The Wanahears agreed with Pam's recommendation to try digital hearing aids with multi-microphone technology to assist with speech recognition in problem listening situations. Pam also suggested an in-line telephone amplifier to improve Mr. Wanahear's ability to talk with his grandchildren.

CONTINUES

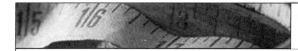

VIGNETTE 10-2

AN ADVENTURE IN OUTCOMES MEASUREMENT   (CONTINUED FROM PAGE 241)

A few weeks later, the Wanahears returned for the hearing aid fitting. Pam verified the fittings through real-ear probe-tube microphone and functional gain measures. She found the Wanahears to be enthusiastic and hopeful. Through the use of the COSI, Pam realized that Mr. Wanahear's hearing loss had put some strain on his marriage and that they required some additional counseling.

"Remember, Mr. Wanahear. You won't be able to reap the benefits of your hearing aids if you don't get out and go to dinner, sit at your friend's table at bingo, and answer the telephone," advised Pam.

"Will do doc," promised Mr. Wanahear and he walked out the door arm and arm with his wife, "See you in one week."

Pam smiled as they walked out the door. She kept her fingers crossed and hoped that Mr. Wanahear would remember all of the things that she had told them. Days passed and no calls from the Wanahears. On the day of his one-week hearing aid check, the Wanahears came in just as happy as they could be. Mr. Wanahear had a list of things that he wanted to discuss.

Pam could tell from their body language that they were communicating better without the tension or frustration that had been present during their first appointment. Mr. Wanahear went through his list of observations and questions. Pam was impressed that Mr. Wanahear had taken a proactive role in his aural rehabilitation program.

Pam addressed some minor issues by minimally reprogramming the hearing aids, after which he said, "That sounds better, but I still can't understand the preacher at church or speakers at my lifelong learners group," admitted Mr. Wanahear.

Pam thought she could try reprogramming the hearing aid further, but recalled that she had some success with other patients using a remote FM microphone and a Microlink system with the hearing aids.

"I have had patients with similar problems to yours who found success with a type of ALD known as a remote FM microphone. The microphone is placed near the speaker so that voices are picked up and sent via FM radio waves to your hearing aids. The device is moderately expensive and requires a modification of your hearing aids. Because you are on your trial period, we can exchange your current hearing aids for the same hearing aids with the special modification," explained Pam.

"But he is doing so well with the ones he has," remarked Mrs. Wanahear.

"Oh, it's the exact same hearing aids, but with this small modification. I can set his hearing aids in exactly the same way, except he will have the FM microphone option," explained Pam. "In fact, I have the same hearing aids, with modifications plus the remote FM microphone in stock. You can try this option out to see if you like it. If it doesn't work, we'll switch back to your other hearing aids."

"What do you think Sweetie?" asked Mr. Wanahear.

"Well, let's try it!"

"Great," Pam said. She quickly went to get the other hearing aids and remote FM microphone. She adjusted the new hearing aids, instructed the couple on the use of the ALD, and scheduled another appointment in one week.

CONTINUES

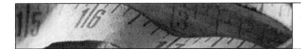

VIGNETTE 10-2

AN ADVENTURE IN OUTCOMES MEASUREMENT (CONTINUED FROM PAGE 242)

One week later, the Wanahears were all smiles as they came into the waiting room.

"You two are simply glowing!" remarked Pam, walking down the hallway to the counseling room.

"We are so pleased with the results!" offered Mr. Wanahear.

Smiling, Pam said, "These are the results audiologists hope for. Do you have any problems?"

"I am still a little confused about the switches on the microphone and the listening angle," remarked Mr. Wanahear.

Pam re-instructed and demonstrated to Mr. Wanahear the control for changing the directionality of the microphone for subtle listening angles required for various situations. The Wanahears had no doubt that they had found the solution to their communication problems and that Mr. Wanahear would keep the hearing aids complete with the remote FM microphone.

At Mr. Wanahear's 3-month hearing aid check, Pam brought out the COSI form that had served as the foundation for the rehabilitation plan.

"Do you two remember this form?" asked Pam.

"Oh yes. We do!" recalled Mr. Wanahear.

"For each of the situations, I'd like both of you to do two things. First, for each problem you identified, I'd like you to think about how much your listening experience has changed by completing the following phrase, 'Because of the new hearing instruments, I now hear ____' with one of the following: much better, better, slightly better, no difference, or worse. Second, I'd like you to complete the following phrase, 'I can hear satisfactorily ____' with one of the following: almost always (95% of the time), most of the time (75% of the time), half the time (50% of the time), occasionally (25% of the time), or hardly ever (10% of the time). Mrs. Wanahear, of course you answer the questions for your husband."

Pam found that for each of the identified needs, Mr. Wanahear and his wife indicated that he heard much better or better and that he heard satisfactorily almost always or most of the time. Although planning to have Mr. Wanahear complete the SADL, Pam noticed that Mr. Wanahear was getting a little tired, so she decided to abbreviate the hearing aid satisfaction outcome measure.

"I'd like to ask you, overall, how satisfied are you with your new hearing aids? Very satisfied, satisfied, neutral, dissatisfied, or very dissatisfied?" asked Pam.

"Very satisfied," both responded.

"Excellent," said Pam.

1. Administrative—could involve sending out an overall satisfaction questionnaire to patients and their families 3 to 6 months after initiation of aural rehabilitative programming.

2. Clinician—could involve each audiologist collecting outcome data for all or randomly selected patient(s) receiving aural rehabilitative care for aggregation, analysis, and interpretation.

Cox, et al., (2000) cautioned that successful outcome measures would have to be simple to administer, short in duration, and collected across patients. Consider the scenario involving All-in-the-Family Hearing Services, a family-owned private practice in Vignette 10-3.

The Conchas demonstrated how outcomes measurement could be implemented at both levels demonstrating positive outcomes for patients, their families, and all stakeholders in the hearing support programs. A similar outcomes measurement plan could be accomplished with a single health-care facility or nationally. Figure 10-2 shows a facility that implementated of outcomes measurement in establishing hearing support programs.

Goal 3: To Assess the Effectiveness of New Hearing Aid Technologies

Chapter 3 discussed clinical trials that fall into the Class I or experimental level of evi- dence. The future of health care will require data to support decisions for treatment and payment of health-related services (Beck, 1999). Not all audiologists have an opportunity to implement outcomes measurement within the context of a clinical trial assessing the efficacy of new treatments for hearing loss, namely, new hearing aid technologies (Cox, et al., 2000). However, hearing health-care providers will rely on the results of studies to guide clinical decision-making, patient choices, and payment for effective treatment (Beck, 1999). Chapter 3 reviewed the levels of evidence of scientific rigor required for supporting the efficacy of various therapies and devices in reducing the effects of communication disorders. Clinical trials are considered to be the "gold standard" for efficacy research at the class I level of evidence. Clinical trials are divided into four phases (ASHA, 2000; Meinert, 1995):

- Phase I trials assess a new drug or treatment on a small group of patients, between 20 to 80 individuals, for the first

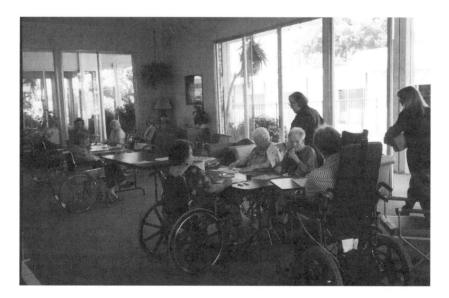

Figure 10-2 A facility in which outcomes measurement has been used in establishing hearing support programs.

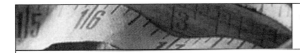

VIGNETTE 10-3

ALL-IN-THE-FAMILY

Carl Concha, Sr., Au.D., FAAA, was proud that both of his sons wanted to pursue careers in audiology. Carl Jr. and Clint were 2 years apart, but both had enrolled at the same time in the audiology graduate program at the nearby university. On graduation day, Carl Sr. knew that after a week's vacation in Mexico, both sons would start their careers as he had in the family business. Over 10 years ago, Carl Sr. had taken over Papa Concha's business, "All-in-the-Family Hearing Services" on a full-time basis. At that time, Papa Concha had advised his son that it was not necessary to obtain his master's degree in audiology, but was surprised when Carl Sr. enrolled in the University of Florida's Distance Learning Au.D. Program. Only months earlier, the family had traveled to Gainesville to watch Carl Sr. receive his Au.D.

Papa Concha first settled in Panama City Beach over 40 years ago, having been drawn to the wonderful climate and small town atmosphere of the Florida panhandle. During the first 20 years of his practice, Papa Concha had little or no competition from other hearing health-care providers, but was glad that he had now passed the business onto his son who faced increasing competition from others who had come to serve the large population of senior citizens.

In the past year, Carl Sr. had noticed the effect of increased competition on his practice. He was glad that his boys were joining him. After a trip to Mexico, the boys settled into work in the practice. After several weeks, Carl Sr. felt he needed to tell his sons that revenue was down at a time when he was investing in equipment, office space, supplies, and so forth for expanding his practice to include them.

"Boys, business is down. We're just not getting any new patients into our practice," remarked Carl Sr.

"What about those ads you ran in the Sunday paper last month?" inquired Carl Jr.

"It didn't produce the results I had hoped for," explained Carl Sr.

"If the patients aren't coming to you, why don't we go to where they are?" asked Clint.

Carl Jr. laughed at his younger brother's comment, but their father thought about the idea.

"Wait, you may have something there, son," commented Carl Sr.

"There are so many retirement communities and assistive living facilities sprouting up all over town," he observed.

Even Carl Jr. became enthusiastic and offered, "Didn't Mr. Oppenheimer say that it is too difficult for him to come downtown to our office? I bet there are many more like him who don't go to pursue hearing health-care services because they can't get to them easily."

The boys and their dad began to sketch out a plan to provide services on-site at these facilities. Clint would search the Internet for new health-care facilities and residential communities catering to the elderly. The trio had decided that they had a greater chance of providing services to newer establishments in the Panama City area. Carl Sr.

CONTINUES

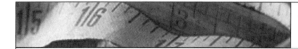

VIGNETTE 10-3

ALL-IN-THE-FAMILY   (CONTINUED FROM PAGE 244)

and Carl Jr. would work on a marketing campaign aimed at those facilities. After several drafts, the advertisements were sent to targeted facilities followed by a phone call. Surprisingly, several facilities and senior communities were interested and scheduled introductory appointments with All-in-the-Family Hearing Care. Ultimately, Heaven's Acres, Inc. showed the most interest in establishing hearing support programs in a variety of facilities including: 1 rehabilitation hospital, 6 skilled-nursing facilities, and 2 large retirement communities, all within a 60-mile radius of the main office.

The Conchas decided to establish hearing support programs for Heaven's Acres, Inc. on a trial basis. The corporation offered support for program start-up with the proviso that the hearing support programs had to document positive patient outcomes. A contract was signed providing both parties an opportunity to bow out after 6 months. In addition to designing hearing support programs to meet the needs of each type of facility, the Conchas had to implement outcomes measurement such as the COSI, APHAB, and GHABP. This was going to be difficult, considering the variety of hearing services to be provided to a heterogeneous group of elderly patients and their families.

Carl Sr. began reading up on outcomes measurement. In a special issue of *Ear and Hearing* devoted to outcomes measurement, an article by Cox, et al. (2000), gave two strategies for measuring the effectiveness of services provided in this particular context. The first strategy involved measuring the outcomes for individual patients receiving direct aural rehabilitation services through the COSI. Although the COSI is used for addressing patients' unique communication needs, those situations could be grouped into specific categories for data aggregation across patients. The second strategy involved a generic questionnaire regarding patients' and their families' evaluation of the hearing support program administered through management to ensure candid responses from stakeholders. Carl Sr. knew that the satisfaction questionnaire had to be short, but also tap into stakeholders' perceptions of the services provided through the hearing support program and their satisfaction with the program (Cox, et al., 2000). In addition, the questionnaire should provide respondents an opportunity to write down any benefits they received from the hearing support program in addition to any shortcomings (Cox, et al., 2000). Respondents' comments could be reviewed for common themes revealing areas of strength and weakness.

Carl and his sons developed the hearing support program satisfaction questionnaire and gave it to administrators for dissemination. Furthermore, they used the COSI on all their patients receiving aural rehabilitation services. Clint aggregated the results for the COSI through the use of a spreadsheet and was able to prepare an outcomes measurement report to submit to administrators after the first 3 months of the program.. Outcome data collected through the satisfaction questionnaire and the COSI demonstrated that the hearing support programs implemented by All-in-the-Family Hearing Services to Heaven's Acres, Inc. was a complete success.

time to test its safety, determine a safe dosage range, and identify side effects.

- Phase II trials examine the treatment in a larger group of patients, between 100 to 300 individuals, to assess safety and effectiveness further. Subjects often are randomly assigned to study and control groups.
- Phase III trials are used when the test treatment is given to much larger groups of subjects, between 1,000 to 3,000 individuals, to confirm its effectiveness and monitor side effects, to contrast it to commonly used treatments, to collect information that will allow the protocol to be used safely, and to validate findings of earlier clinical trials.
- Phase IV trials are conducted after the treatment has been marketed. Testing in this phase is done in order to collect data about the protocol's effect in various clinical populations, as well as any side effects associated with long-term use.

Although hearing aids are considered to be medical devices and are regulated by the Food and Drug Administration (FDA), they do not require a long series of clinical trials establishing efficacy in positive patient outcomes prior to marketing. Indeed, hearing aid manufacturers are introducing high-performance hearing aids to the hearing health-care industry on a daily basis, but often without the rigorous scientific proof of the efficacy at the Class I level of evidence. In some ways, this reality can be viewed positively in that major breakthroughs in hearing aid technology can go from the research and development laboratories of the manufacturer directly to the consumer without a lengthy approval process through the FDA. Patients with cancer and other potentially fatal diseases are often frustrated by the unavailability of new experimental treatments yet to be approved that could save their lives, for example. On the other hand,

the lack of clinical trials documenting the efficacy of hearing aids in reducing hearing handicap in persons having hearing loss may be a major factor in why hearing aids are not considered the standard of care by most health-care plans.

The Federal Trade Commission (FTC) and the Food and Drug Administration (FDA) have not, however, let the industry go unchecked. In the early 1990s, the FTC brought actions against certain hearing aid manufacturers after numerous consumer complaints regarding claims of misleading advertising about speech understanding in noise (Walden, 1997). The FDA also issued letters charging those companies with false advertising and in August, 1994 issued guidelines declaring that user-benefit claims had to be substantiated by clinical trials (Walden, 1997). The guidelines stated that standardized materials should be used for speech testing and that the experimental design is suitable for both the type of instrument and performance of its features as stated by the company (Walden, 1997). Walden (1997) felt that the guidelines fell short by not recommending a uniform protocol that would:

- permit direct comparisons among hearing devices,
- remove the temptation of manufacturers' selection of biased dependent measures,
- eliminate the need for detailed descriptions of dependent measures and test conditions with benefit claims made by manufacturers, and
- be in the best interest of the consumer and manufacturer.

Considering the results of previous research regarding the identification of dimensions of hearing aid use and benefit (Walden, Demorest, & Hepler, 1984; Cox & Gilmore, 1990), Walden (1997) concluded that clinical trials should assess benefit in four prototype listening situations (PLS):

- PLS1: Listening to Speech in Quiet (e.g., interviewing for a job in a small office or face-to-face conversation with family members at home)
- PLS2: Listening to Speech with Reduced Cues (e.g., listening in reverberation, or at a distance, or understanding dialogue at a movie or play)
- PLS3: Listening to Speech in Background Noise (e.g., conversation with others at a large noisy party or listening to the news on the car radio with family members talking)
- PLS4: Listening to Environmental Sounds (e.g., aversive sounds, but also listening to nature, music, and voice quality)

Subsequently, Walden and his colleagues at Walter Reed Army Medical Center developed a clinical trials protocol that has laboratory (i.e., objective measures of speech recognition) and field evaluations (i.e., subjective measures of benefit). The laboratory measures included presenting the *Continuous Speech Test* (CST: Cox, Alexander, & Gilmore, 1987; Cox, Alexander, Gilmore, & Pusakulich, 1988): (1) PLS1: Listening in Quiet (i.e., speech level of 50 dB-A against a 40 dB-A six-talker babble), (2) PLS2: Listening in Reverberation (i.e., speech level of 60 dB-A with 0.78 seconds of reverberation time), and (3) PLS3: Listening in Noise (i.e., speech level of 60 dB-A against a 55 dB-A six-talker babble and speech level of 70 dB-A against a 68 dB-A six-talker babble). The field evaluations included the *Profile of Hearing Aid Performance/Profile of Hearing Aid Benefit* (PHAP/PHAB: Cox & Gilmore, 1990) whose subscales correspond to patients' ratings of hearing aid benefit in each of the four prototype listening situations: (1) PLS1: Listening in Quiet (i.e., Speech Environment A [QT], Familiar Talker [FT], and Ease of Communication [EC]), (2) PLS2: Listening in Reverberation (i.e., Speech Environment B [RC], Reverberation [RV], and Reduced Cues [RC]),

(3) PLS3: Listening in Noise (i.e., Speech Environment C [BN] and Speech in Noise [BN]), and (4) PLS4: Listening to Environmental Sounds (i.e., Environmental Sounds [ES], Distortion of Sounds [DS], and Aversiveness of Sounds [AV]).

Another task for designing a clinical trial is to determine possible control test conditions and possible dimensions for defining the clinical population from which to sample. Walden (1997) stated possible control test conditions for user-benefit claims: (1) unaided (e.g., hearing device X provides significant benefit to patients having hearing impairment), (2) linear peak-clipping amplification (e.g., the compression circuitry incorporated in hearing device X provides significant benefit compared to standard amplification), (3) patient's own hearing aids (e.g., 80% of patients obtain significantly more benefit from hearing device X as compared to their own hearing aids), and (4) normal performance (e.g., performance with hearing device X is not significantly different from normal performance). Furthermore, Walden (1997) provided the following dimensions for defining clinical populations and examples from which to sample: (1) age range (e.g., pediatric, young adult, middle-aged, and geriatric), (2) severity of hearing loss (e.g., mild, moderate, and severe), (3) site of lesion (e.g., sensorineural, mixed, and conductive), (4) audiometric configuration (e.g., flat, gently sloping, precipitous), (5) speech recognition impairment (mild, moderate, and severe), and 6) hearing aid experience (e.g., inexperienced or experienced). If the subject sample involves experienced hearing aid users, then dimensions could include further subdividing into: (1) type of hearing aid (e.g., linear, compression limiter, wide dynamic range compression), (2) fitting (i.e., monaural and binaural), (3) degree of satisfaction (e.g., dissatisfied and satisfied), and (4) extent of use (e.g., infrequent, selective, and regular) (Walden, 1997).

In summary, Walden (1997) believed that there is a need to adopt a uniform core set of dependent measures and test conditions for use in manufacturer-sponsored clinical trials to substantiate hearing aid user-benefit claims. Toward this goal, Walden and his colleagues developed a model protocol for use in hearing aid clinical trials. Other researchers have stated that this approach would not result in effective and efficient trials because benefit claims vary a great deal and require the use of a variety of different measurements for different types of hearing aids (Byrne, 1998). For example, Byrne (1998) stated that the amount of benefit shown by such measures of the PHAB would vary according to subjects' degree of hearing impairment. Therefore, all trials could not use one standard measure because it might not be sensitive enough in certain studies. In addition, the most important factors in determining patient outcomes might be improved comfort or sound quality rather than improved speech recognition in everyday life (Byrne, 1998). Moreover, measures of speech recognition, alone, do not assess all possible benefits of digital signal processing (DSP) circuitry. Creative clinical trials protocols must be developed to provide Class I levels of evidence for high-technology hearing aids resulting in positive patient outcomes.

Concerned about the lack of Class I levels of evidence demonstrating the efficacy of hearing aids, the National Institute on Deafness and other Communication Disorders of the National Institutes of Health (NIDCD-NIH) and the Department of Veterans Affairs (DVA) convened in 1992 to work on several initiatives addressing the needs of persons with hearing loss. The VA/NIDCD intent was to use Class I levels of evidence, or the "gold standard" of clinical trials, in evaluating hearing aid efficacy (Beck, 1999; p. 17). Larson, et al. (2000) conducted a double-blind, 3-period, 3-treatment crossover clinical trial to compare the benefits provided to patients with

sensorineural hearing loss by 3 commonly used hearing aid circuits: linear peak-clipper (PC), compression limiter (CL), and wide dynamic range compressor (WDRC). A total of 360 patients with bilateral sensorineural hearing loss at 8 audiology laboratories at Department of Veterans Affairs medical centers were randomly assigned to 1 of 6 sequences of treatment conditions such that all subjects wore each of the 3 hearing aids (installed in identical casements) for 3 months each. The outcome measures used consisted of both verification and validation procedures. The verification measures included 2 recorded versions of the following speech recognition tests:

1. the NU-6 test presented using a single loudspeaker at a 0 degree azimuth at 62-dB-SPL, and
2. the CST also presented via a single loudspeaker at a 0 degree azimuth at 74-dB-SPL in quiet and in three background noise conditions (i.e., uncorrelated multi-talker babble at (−3 dB, 0 dB, and +3 dB S/N).

The validation measures included:

1. *Quality Ratings Test* (i.e., subjects ratings of loudness, noise interference, and overall liking in quiet and noise),
2. PHAP/PHAB, and
3. rank ordering of circuits according to preference.

The results of the study indicated that each circuit improved speech recognition for soft and loud conversational speech as compared to the unaided condition. In addition, all 3 circuits reduced the problems encountered in verbal communication. The CL and the WDRC provided better listening experiences than the PC circuits for word recognition, loudness, overall liking, aversiveness of environmental sounds, and distortion. In addition, subjects preferred the CL circuit as compared to the WDRC or PC circuits. The study group concluded that although each circuit provided significant benefit in quiet and in noisy listening conditions, the CL and WDRC circuits provided superior benefits over the PC circuit. However, the differences between the hearing aids were much less obvious than when comparing unaided to aided conditions.

Readers might be wondering if there were really only slight differences among hearing aid circuits or if the dependent measures were just not sensitive enough to show differences if they existed. For example, in a recent meta-analytic review of investigations of the effectiveness of digital signal processing (DSP) hearing aids as compared to analog hearing aids, Newman and Sandridge (2001) found that the results of laboratory measures (i.e., audibility, speech in noise, and objective sound quality), self-report measures, and satisfaction produced either equivocal or mixed results. However, they did find that for directionality and user preference, DSP were found to be superior to, although more expensive than, analog hearing aids. Newman and Sandridge's (2001) review poses some interesting questions. Do DSP hearing aids produce essentially equivocal results to analog hearing aids? Newman and Sandridge (2001) contended that no matter what outcome measures are used and whatever their results might show, patients prefer DSP to analog hearing aids. Are our verification and validation procedures not sensitive enough to measure these preferences? Readers might be wondering if outcome measures are really necessary, because, after all, the bottom-line is what patients prefer and if they are willing to pay more money for the DSP hearing aids, then so be it. Newman and Sandridge (2001) concluded that the studies reviewed on DSP hearing aids are merely a "first quarter report card" and that circuitry should continue to evolve in addition to development of appropriate outcome measures.

Cox, et al. (2000) stated that researchers must identify effective outcome measures that are relevant for clinical trials assessing the efficacy of new hearing aid technologies. To do so, audiologists must acknowledge that such clinical trials and their outcome measures have the following theoretical underpinnings (Cox, et al., 2000):

- Results of small scale studies have suggested the effectiveness of the technology
- A large number of subjects representing the population for which the treatment is indicated would be recruited
- Dependent variables would include measures of devices used in field conditions and subjective rating scales
- The null hypothesis that there is no treatment effect
- The experimental hypothesis that the new hearing technology does have a treatment effect

Cox, et al. (2000) suggested that outcome measures should be:

- Standardized (e.g., PHAP/PHAB, and SHAPI) rather than client oriented (e.g., COSI)
- Specific to conditions in which the technology is claimed to offer advantages (e.g., speech recognition in noise for DSP circuitry)
- Sensitive enough to detect minimum treatment differences
- Possessive of the following attributes (Cox, et al., 2000; Hyde, 2000):
  ⇒ Content domain relevance (e.g., if technology reduces hearing disability, then a tool measuring this domain should be used)
  ⇒ Appropriate difficulty (e.g., appropriate level of listening difficulty/realism in the test items and reading level of subjects)
  ⇒ Item applicability (e.g., subjects should perceive all or most of the test items as relevant and applicable so that non-response rate for items is low)

INCOMES MEASUREMENT

So far, this chapter has dealt with outcomes measurement or assessing patient or program outcomes at the end of intervention. However, there are considerations that audiologists should attend to at the beginning of the intervention process that can result in better patient outcomes. Are there specific things that we should do for patients with certain characteristics to increase the likelihood for success? What are critical patient characteristics that can affect patient outcomes?

Patients' personality characteristics and expectations potentially can affect responses on subjective hearing aid outcome measures. Few studies have investigated the effects of patients' personality characteristics on their responses to self-assessment items for measuring hearing aid outcome. Cox, Alexander, and Gray (1999) explored the relationship between several personality attributes and responses to the APHAB. A group of 83 elderly patients, who had worn hearing aids long enough to make a decision regarding their benefit, completed the APHAB and scales measuring anxiety (i.e., *State-Trait Anxiety Inventory* [STAI] by Speilberger, 1983), extroversion-introversion (i.e., *Myers-Briggs Type Indicator* [MBTI] form-G, revised by Myers & McCaulley, 1985), and locus of control. Results of this study indicated that although personality variables accounted for less than 10% of the variance in APHAB responses, audiologists must be aware of the findings for two personality characteristics. First, patients who were more extroverted reported greater hearing aid benefit in all speech communication situations (Cox, et al., 1999). Second, patients with a more external locus of control tended to have more negative reactions to loud sounds in the environment regardless of whether hearing aids were worn (Cox, et al., 1999). These results are in agreement with those of Kricos (2000), who completed a careful review of the litera-

ture and found that more extroverted hearing aid users reported greater hearing satisfaction than those who were introverted, while more anxious individuals yielded higher handicap self-ratings and lower ratings of hearing aid benefit, and patients with obsessive/hysteric tendencies reported less hearing aid benefit.

There are several practical implications for these findings. First, audiologists must proceed with caution when using self-assessment outcome data to measure the success of hearing aid fittings (Cox, et al., 1999). Highly introverted hearing aid users may not achieve high levels of benefit simply because they rarely socialize and/or are not involved in many activities with high communication demands. Second, clinical trials for comparing hearing aids should control for extroversion, locus of control, and anxiety (Cox, et al., 1999). For example, different groups of subjects may show more benefit on self-assessment outcome measures because of differences in personality traits of the groups rather than because of differences in hearing aid circuitry (Cox, et al., 1999).

Patients' perceived communication needs and expectations can also influence outcomes. Cox and Alexander (2000) developed a new tool assessing hearing aid users' expectations regarding amplification, called the *Expected Consequences of Hearing Aid Ownership* (ECHO) (See Appendix X–M on the companion CD-ROM) to be used as a companion to the SADL. Each item on the ECHO was reworded from an item on the SADL by converting the questions about satisfaction (i.e., "How natural is the sound from your hearing aid?") into a statement regarding expectations (i.e., "My hearing aid will have a natural sound.") (Cox & Alexander, 2000). Patients mark their degree of agreement with each of the ECHO statements using the same 7-point scale used on the SADL and responses are scored in the same way yielding (Cox & Alexander, 2000):

- A global expectation score obtained as the mean of the responses to all 15 items
- Four expectation subscale scores obtained as a mean of the responses from the items corresponding to each subscale, creating a patient profile

Additional information for scoring is that a subscale score is only valid when at least two-thirds of the items are completed and patients who do not pay for their hearing aids do not complete the item on cost (Cox & Alexander, 2000).

Cox and Alexander (2000) completed four experiments using the ECHO to:

- Determine realistic expectations for hearing aids
- Evaluate expectations of new hearing aid users
- Measure reliability of pre-fitting expectations
- Assess relationships between pre-fitting expectations and post-fitting satisfaction

For experiment 1, realistic expectations for hearing aids were obtained by securing the responses on the ECHO from 139 hearing aid users with the following characteristics (Cox & Alexander, 2000):

- A self-reported moderate or severe degree of hearing difficulty
- Hearing aids dispensed at one of three sites (i.e., a Veterans Affair Medical Center, a university-affiliated clinic, or a private practice)
- Between 60 to 89 years of age
- 25% female/75% male
- Hearing aid wearers for at least one year
- Used hearing aids at least 4 hours per day

The subjects' responses to ECHO items were scored on a scale from 1 to 7 with "tremendously" receiving a 7 on 11 of the items in which that term indicates a very positive expectation, and "not at all" receiving a 1;

whereas on 4 of the items, the number values were switched (i.e., "not at all" receiving 7, and "tremendously" receiving 1) when "tremendously" would be considered negative (Cox & Alexander, 2000). For example, "tremendously" would be scored a 7 for the item, "My hearing aids will help me understand the people I speak with most frequently," but would be scored a 1 for the item, "I will be frustrated when my hearing aids pick up sounds that keep me from hearing what I want to hear." From these data, Cox and Alexander (2000) developed norms that audiologists can apply when using the ECHO as an income measure.

For experiments 2–4, Cox and Alexander (2000) found that new hearing aid users had stable, but unrealistically high, expectations of hearing aids and that the ECHO was not very predictive of corresponding satisfaction ratings. Cox and Alexander (2000) suggested that the norms obtained in Experiment I for the ECHO can be used to:

- evaluate the pre-fitting expectations of potential hearing aid users,
- explore significant others' expectations of hearing aids, and
- counsel patients and their significant others regarding inaccurate perceptions about amplification.

Similarly, Schum (1999) used a new scale found in Appendix X–N on the companion CD-ROM, the *Hearing Aid Needed Assessment Scale* (HANA), to examine the relationship between perceived communication needs/expectations with the actual benefit eventually achieved with newly fitted hearing aids. The HANA was designed to be a companion scale to the *Hearing Aid Performance Inventory* (HAPI) (Walden, et al., 1984) and the SHAPI (Schum, 1992) and consists of 11 questions taken from the HAPI (Schum, 1999). Patients fill out the HANA for each of 11 situations prior to the hearing aid fitting process by rating how often they are in similar situations, how much difficulty they have, and how much benefit is expected from new hearing aids (Schum, 1999). A group of 42 subjects (elderly hearing aid wearers) completed both the HANA and then the SHAPI after 2 to 3 months of hearing aid use (Schum, 1999). Two important findings of the study were that (Schum, 1999):

- Hearing aid candidates expected more benefit from their hearing aids than they actually received
- Hearing aid benefit could not be predicted on the basis of patients' needs or expectations

The results of this investigation can assist audiologists in counseling hearing aid candidates by advising them that expectations often exceed achieved benefits, and that listening in noisy situations is difficult even when wearing hearing aids; it can also identify patients with unrealistically high expectations for special advisement (Schum, 1999).

Jacobson, Newman, Fabry, and Sandridge (2001) developed the *Three Clinic Hearing Aid Selection Profile* (HASP), a 40-item instrument that provides a systematic method for making some basic decisions in selecting appropriate amplification features based on patients':

- motivation to wear hearing aids,
- expectations about hearing aid performance,
- perceived importance of physical appearance,
- attitudes toward cost,
- attitudes toward technology,
- manual dexterity,
- communicative needs, and
- lifestyle and activity levels.

The HASP was developed through the following process (Jacobson, et al., 2001):

- Generation of an alpha version of the HASP, consisting of 70 items based on the collective experience of the investigators and/or information regarding consumer acceptance of hearing aids reported in the literature
- Categorization of the items into subscales, specific (i.e., motivation and expectation) and nonspecific (i.e., appearance, cost, technology, physical function, communicative needs, and lifestyle) to hearing aid use
- Administration to 130 adults at the Henry Ford Health System, the Cleveland Clinic Foundation, and the Mayo Clinic
- Analysis of data obtained from 120 of 130 subjects (i.e., 10 patients who provided incomplete HASPs were eliminated) for:
  ⇒ Cronbach's alpha (i.e., items grouped such that each subscale had an alpha of 0.70 or higher)
  ⇒ Item-total correlations (i.e., items with correlations less than or equal to 0.30 were eliminated)
- Generation of the beta (final) version of the HASP consisting of 40 items

The final version of the HASP was administered in a paper-and-pencil format to a sample of 242 patients after audiometry, but prior to any counseling at those same three clinics to assess the effects of subject characteristics on subscale scores. In addition to the HASP, subjects under 65 years of age were administered the HHIA—S, and the HHIE—S, if over 65 years of age. Data gleaned from the HASP were analyzed as a function of age, gender, hearing aid use, educational level, and severity of perceived hearing handicap. Patients under 65 years of age were more comfortable with high technology and had fewer physical limitations than those over 65 who had more communicative needs than the younger patients. Regarding gender, women had a greater motivation to wear hearing aids, had higher expectations for the devices, were more comfortable with higher technology, and believed that they had greater communicative needs than men who were more appearance conscious than women. Regarding educational level, patients with postgraduate degrees had fewer physical limitations and more active lifestyles than those with only a high school education. Previous hearing aid use had no effect on HASP subscale scores. Regarding perceived hearing handicap, patients' motivation to obtain hearing aids increased with their perceived hearing handicap. Furthermore, patients with severe hearing handicap had greater communicative needs than did those with mild-to-moderate hearing handicap.

Jacobson, et al. (2001) stated that the percentile scores generated from the study should be used to establish a referent to which the HASP results for individual patients can be compared. In addition, the HASP has the potential to provide audiologists with a number of practical benefits (Jacobson, et al., 2001):

- Counseling
- Clinician accountability
- Development of a pool of "first choice" hearing types and styles
- Teaching tool
- Documentation for multisite comparisons in quality improvement studies

In conclusion, the HASP is easily (Jacobson, et al., 2001):

- completed either at home or in the clinic setting,
- administered in a paper-and-pencil or computer format,
- used for benchmarking a given hearing aid candidate's profile against a larger sample of subjects, and
- used to assess important domains for the functioning of hearing aids.

Instruments such as the HASP encourage clinicians to go beyond the audiogram to consider other patient characteristics in the selection of hearing aid features. Johnson, Danhauer, and Krishnamurti (2000) suggested using a holistic approach in matching high-technology hearing aid features to elderly patients. Kricos and Lesner (1995) were the first to suggest a holistic approach to audiologic rehabilitation by considering elderly patients' status in at least the following domains: communication (auditory speech reception, audiovisual speech reception, conversational fluency, hearing handicap/disability, and speechreading), physical (manual dexterity/fine motor skills, general health, and visual status), psychological (attitude, depression, mental status, and motivation), and social (physical and social environments). Unfortunately, prognostic characteristics in those domains that pertain to elderly patients' use of high-techology hearing aids are scattered throughout the professional literature, and practitioners rarely have the time to gather, synthesize, and prioritize this information for clinical use. After a careful literature review, Johnson, et al. (2000) gathered and organized positive and negative prognostic indicators in four assessment domains for elderly patients' candidacy for high-technology hearing aid features into a checklist. Prognostic indicators were prioritized into flow charts for matching high-technology hearing aid features to elderly patients. Audiologists can use the checklist and accompanying flowcharts for income measures that can provide a strategy for a hearing aid selection process resulting in positive patient outcomes.

PUTTING IT ALL TOGETHER

We have discussed outcome measures that tap into different domains, are comprehensive profiles, or are satisfaction measures;

how to select and use self-assessment tools in clinical practice and research; and incomes measurement. At this point, it is important to put all this information into perspective.

Outcomes measurement concerns positive patient outcomes. Audiologists must be careful not to become so preoccupied with outcomes measurement that they forget about the patient. Positive patient outcomes begin with highly skilled clinicians who keep up with technology, preferred audiologic practices, and the scientific reports in the literature. After we presented an instructional course on outcomes measurement (Johnson & Danhauer, 2001), several participants commented that the presentation focused too much on the evaluation of research in audiology, rather than on the use of specific tools. Outcomes measurement is about research and audiologists must have adequate backgrounds in that area to be good clinicians. Unfortunately, there are no easy answers or any cookbook procedures to the use of income/outcome measures. The old adage "garbage in, garbage out" applies here.

The process should start with audiologists who decide what to offer in their product lines. The decision can be difficult when considering all the new high-technology features offered by today's manufacturers. The evaluation process should include a careful review of the literature for studies and manufacturers' advertisements demonstrating both the effectiveness and efficacy of high-technology hearing aid circuitry. Are there any studies involving specific types of circuitry? At what level of evidence are the studies? Are they case reports, single-subject design research, or quasi-experimental designs? What are the characteristics of the subject samples in studies demonstrating benefit? Are they similar to the demographic characteristics of a particular audiologist's patients? Furthermore, audiologists should consider the evidence provided in advertisements contained in manufacturers' marketing campaigns.

Have manufacturers conducted any investigations demonstrating effectiveness and/or efficacy of their products? Were the studies scientifically sound? Were the investigations conducted in-house? What other institutions, if any, participated in the studies? Only after careful scrutiny should audiologists ethically endorse products to their patients. In addition, audiologists should be wary about the language they use regarding the established efficacy of these devices. For example, audiologists should avoid phrases such as "studies have proven the superiority of DSP hearing aids with multi-microphone technology over analog hearing aids." Recall that the results are essentially equivocal in most areas (Newman & Sandridge, 2001), and at this point, audiologists should be careful about what they say regarding the effectiveness of DSP versus analog hearing aids.

Everything that good audiologists say and do should have a research base. Audiologists should strive to tailor their hearing aid fittings according to recommended guidelines. For example, ASHA's *Guidelines for Hearing Aid Fitting for Adults*" (ASHA, 1998) recommended a 6-stage process embedded in a rehabilitation plan:

1. Assessment determines the type and magnitude of the hearing loss followed by intervention planning and determining candidacy for amplification.
2. Treatment planning involves the audiologist, patient, and/or family (caregivers) reviewing the findings of the assessment stage and identifying needs.
3. Selection includes choosing the physical and electroacoustic characteristics of the hearing aids.
4. Verification consists of determining if the hearing aids meet a set of standardized measures that include basic electroacoustics, cosmetic appeal, comfortable fit, and real-ear electroacoustic performance.

5. Orientation entails counseling the patient on the use and care of the hearing aids, fostering the patient's realistic expectations of performance from the hearing aids, and exploring candidacy for ALDs and for further aural rehabilitation.

6. Validation determines the impact of the intervention on the perceived disability attributable to the hearing loss.

Figure 10-3 outlines this process which includes the recommended procedures (adapted from ASHA, 1998). The process is similar to that found in, "*Algorithm 3: Joint Audiology Committee Algorithm on Hearing Aid Selection and Fitting (Adult)*" (AAA, 2000a). Outcomes measurement should occur at strategic points during various stages of the process and is discussed according to the continuum of care suggested by ASHA (1998).

Patients enter the hearing aid fitting process during assessment. Either a patient has failed a hearing screening, been referred by a physician, or nagged by significant others to seek a hearing evaluation. Other patients may be experienced hearing aid users who feel their hearing has changed or wish to obtain the latest in hearing aid technology. Audiologists' antennae should be up and sensitive to patients' motivation and candidacy for seeking assistance or improvement in communication ability. Similarly, family members who may attend the hearing evaluation or are mentioned by the patient may be important stakeholders in the rehabilitation process and/or participants in outcomes measurement. Identification of the type and extent of hearing loss and determination of medical treatment is followed by provision of the results to the patient and family members. Use of income measures like the ECHO, HANA, and/or the HASP are appropriate at this time to obtain important information for planning intervention. For example, audiologists may use the ECHO to determine if special counseling may be

needed for patients with unrealistically high expectations for amplification. Similarly, use of the HANA may assist in determining special advisement regarding the benefits of amplification in noise.

Candidacy and rehabilitation assessment include both the determination of the effects of hearing impairment in the disability and handicap domains. Regarding disability, audiologists may consider the use of the APHAB, COSI, or HPI. Is the tool appropriate for use with this patient? Do the norms apply? Is the patient older and easily fatigued? If this is the case, then the APHAB and/or the HPI may be too long, but the COSI may be appropriate. Or one might simplify the procedure, as did Pam Pratt, Au.D. in Vignette 10-2. Regarding handicap, audiologists may consider using the HHIE if the patient is elderly, or the HHIA if the patient is under the age of 65 years. Another possibility is using the GHABP which measures multiple domains. Another consideration is whether to include the patient's significant others (e.g., spouse, adult children, or caregivers) in the outcomes measurement process. Rehabilitation assessment also includes a holistic evaluation of patients' physical, psychological, social, and communication status (Lesner & Kricos, 1995). For example, use of the HASP (Jacobson, et al., 2001) and/or checklist and flowcharts (Johnson, et al., 2000) may be helpful in matching high-technology hearing aid features to elderly patients.

Information gleaned from the candidacy and rehabilitation assessment is invaluable in the next stage of the process, treatment planning, which involves the audiologist, patient, family, and/or caregivers establishing priorities, setting goals, and acknowledging the sequence of intervention. For example, use of the COSI holds stakeholders in the intervention accountable for identified needs according to their priority. At this point, audiologists make some preliminary decisions regarding the electroacoustics of

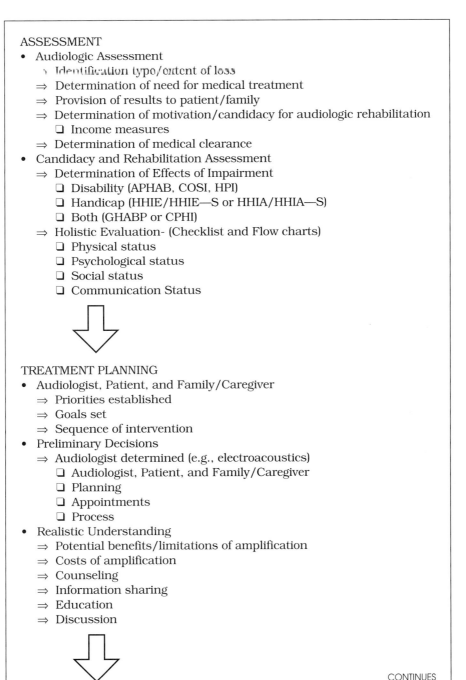

Figure 10-3. Recommended process for hearing aid fitting for adults (Adapted from ASHA, 1998).

HEARING AID SELECTION
- Electroacoustic Characteristics
    - ⇒ Frequency/gain characteristics
    - ⇒ Output sound pressure level
    - ⇒ Input-output characteristics
- Non-electroacoustic Characteristics
    - ⇒ Binaural or monaural fitting
    - ⇒ Hearing aid style
    - ⇒ Earmold/shell selection and configuration
    - ⇒ Number and size of user controls
    - ⇒ Directional/multiple microphones
    - ⇒ Volume control preferences
    - ⇒ Telecoil and telecoil sensitivity
    - ⇒ Compatibility with ALDs
    - ⇒ Programmable option
    - ⇒ Remote control
    - ⇒ Multiple memories
    - ⇒ Digital signal processing
    - ⇒ Color/shape of hearing aid
    - ⇒ Additional system features

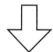

VERIFICATION
- Quality Control
    - ⇒ Electroacoustic characteristics within manufacturer's specifications
    - ⇒ Adequate visual and listening check
    - ⇒ Earmold/hearing aid feature check (e.g., color, venting, tubing, etc.)
- Physical Fit
    - ⇒ Cosmetic appeal
    - ⇒ Absence of feedback
    - ⇒ Physical comfort
    - ⇒ Ease of insertion/removal
    - ⇒ Security of fit
    - ⇒ Microphone location
    - ⇒ Ease of control operation
- Performance
    - ⇒ Real-ear probe microphone measurements
    - ⇒ Verification of audibility, comfort, and tolerance (i.e., PAL)

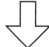

CONTINUES

Figure 10-3. (Continued)

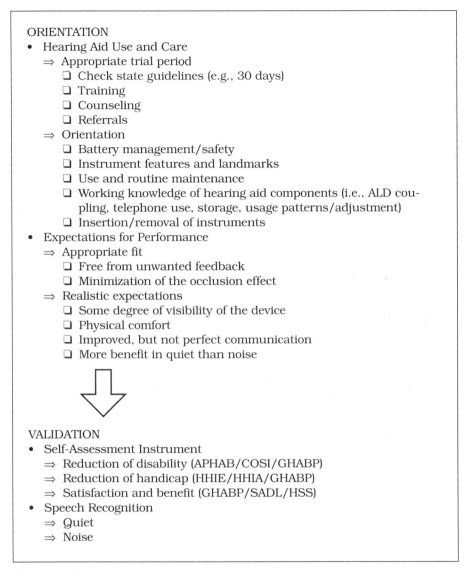

ORIENTATION
- Hearing Aid Use and Care
  - ⇒ Appropriate trial period
    - ❏ Check state guidelines (e.g., 30 days)
    - ❏ Training
    - ❏ Counseling
    - ❏ Referrals
  - ⇒ Orientation
    - ❏ Battery management/safety
    - ❏ Instrument features and landmarks
    - ❏ Use and routine maintenance
    - ❏ Working knowledge of hearing aid components (i.e., ALD coupling, telephone use, storage, usage patterns/adjustment)
    - ❏ Insertion/removal of instruments
- Expectations for Performance
  - ⇒ Appropriate fit
    - ❏ Free from unwanted feedback
    - ❏ Minimization of the occlusion effect
  - ⇒ Realistic expectations
    - ❏ Some degree of visibility of the device
    - ❏ Physical comfort
    - ❏ Improved, but not perfect communication
    - ❏ More benefit in quiet than noise

VALIDATION
- Self-Assessment Instrument
  - ⇒ Reduction of disability (APHAB/COSI/GHABP)
  - ⇒ Reduction of handicap (HHIE/HHIA/GHABP)
  - ⇒ Satisfaction and benefit (GHABP/SADL/HSS)
- Speech Recognition
  - ⇒ Quiet
  - ⇒ Noise

Figure 10-3. (Continued)

hearing aids. They also make some decisions with the patient and family, and/or caregivers (e.g., planning, appointments, and process). Incomes measurement and the rehabilitation assessment can assist audiologists in counseling patients and their families regarding potential benefits/limitations and costs of amplification. For example, low percentile rankings of HASP subscale scores may indicate the need for educating, counseling, and sharing information with patients ensuring realistic expectations about hearing aid performance, perceived importance of physical appearance, and attitudes toward cost.

:omes measurement is also valuable
le hearing aid selection process for
both electroacoustic and non-electroacoustic
features. For example, the COSI can identify
communication needs in varied listening situations (e.g., listening to live music performances and understanding speech in noisy
restaurants), and may suggest the use of DSP
circuitry with multimicrophone technology
(e.g., omnidirectional microphones for listening at the symphony and directional microphones for understanding speech in a noisy
restaurant). Moreover, the COSI may indicate
patients' needs in a variety of situations (e.g.,
listening on the telephone or in a reverberant
church) that suggest the use of multimemory
or programmable hearing aids. Similarly,
results on the HASP and the checklists and
flow charts (Johnson, et al., 2000) can be an
effective "one-two punch" when matching
high-technology hearing aid features to elderly patients. For example, strong degrees of
agreement on the appearance (e.g., "I am concerned that wearing a hearing aid will make
me look older") and physical function (e.g., "I
do not have arthritis in my fingers" and "I
have good sensation in my fingertips") subscales may assist audiologists in using
checklists and flowcharts in discerning candidacy for CIC hearing aids.

The verification stage involves measures
made by the audiologist for ensuring quality,
good physical fit, and appropriate performance. For example, real-ear probe-tube
microphone measurements verify that targets for gain and output have been met. In
addition, verification of audibility, comfort,
and tolerance are critical for patient satisfaction. The PAL can be used to ensure that
most sounds are tolerable for patients. Furthermore, items on the HAPI, SHAPI, and
SADL measure long-term aspects of comfort
and tolerance during the validation stage.

Patients' responses on previously mentioned income measures (e.g., ECHO, HANA,
and the HASP) and outcome measures like

the COSI can assist audiologists in gearing
the hearing aid orientation to the needs of
patients. For example, the ECHO can help
patients who need special counseling during
the hearing aid orientation about the realistic
expectations of amplification during trial
periods that can be problem laden requiring
numerous visits to the hearing health-care
professional for adjustments. Moreover, the
COSI can alert audiologists to the need for
specialized instructions in achieving maximum benefit in patients' problem situations
during the trial period.

The validation stage, the hallmark for
outcomes measurement, determines the
impact of the intervention on the patient and
the family or caregivers. Validation should
occur after an appropriate period of acclimatization, or about 1 to 3 months after the
initial fitting. Validation should involve re-
administration of the outcome measures used
during the rehabilitation assessment for
measuring any change in patient state that
can be attributed to the intervention. Recall
that the indirect method involves assessing
the patient's state before and after an event of
interest and subtracting the pre-measure
score from the post-measure score to obtain a
"change-score." Audiologists must remember
two things when using the indirect method.
First, they must consult the literature regarding the confidence intervals for specific tests
which may vary according to different methods of administration. For example, the 95%
confidence interval for the paper-and-pencil
administration format of the HHIE is 36
points, indicating more variability in patients'
responses than that of the interview format,
which is 19 points (Huch & Hosford-Dunn,
2000; Weinstein, et al., 1986). Second,
patients must be clear regarding what conditions are to be compared. For example, conditions for comparison using the COSI vary
depending on whether patients are first-time
(i.e., unaided versus aided conditions) or
experienced hearing aid users (i.e., old versus

new hearing aids). Validation can also occur simply by administering outcome measures at the end of the rehabilitation process. This can involve the direct method of measuring the change in patient state by asking patients to compare their communication difficulties prior to intervention and then with amplification, using the GHABP, for example. Or, some outcome measures are completed post-fitting only and can either assess patients' performance (e.g., HAPI/SHAPI) or satisfaction with hearing aids (e.g., SADL or HSS).

Many audiologists believe that the ultimate outcome is whether patients decide to keep their hearing aids at the end of the trial period. We hope readers can now see the potential benefits of using income/outcome measures for enhancing the hearing aid fitting process. Furthermore, outcome measures can assist audiologists and patients in determining communication needs that may require additional intervention such as counseling or use of an ALD. For example, spouses may disagree regarding the continued effects of hearing impairment on their relationship necessitating referral to a mental health professional. Similarly, lingering communication difficulties in selected situations may require the use of an ALD. For example, in Vignette 10-2, Mr. Wanahear's continued difficulty understanding the speaker at his lifelong learner's group necessitated the purchase of a remote FM microphone. Audiologists must remember that dispensing of ALDs should follow a specific protocol including the achievement of specific orientation and fitting outcomes through use of Appendix X–O, "ALD Selection Protocol" and Appendix X–P, "ALD Orientation and Fitting Checklist" (ASHA, 1997), both of which can be found on the companion CD-ROM.

In summary, no matter how skilled the audiologist or sophisticated the technology, some patients may never achieve positive patient outcomes. We've all had those cases that break our hearts leaving us feeling ineffective in improving patients' quality of life. For example, take J.T., a 56 year-old woman with a progressive bilateral severe-to-profound sensorineural hearing loss, who one of the authors of the text has served for nearly 20 years. J.T. relies on her hearing for her passion, music performance. It has been frustrating trying to find hearing solutions because she knows that her most important sense is failing her. We have no outcome measures that can quantify the aspects of hearing that are critical for her. One way that we can understand her frustration is through her poetry. Vignette 10-4 contains her poignant poem, "On Growing Deaf ... Music." So, why is outcomes measurement important? It is important for JT whose hearing impairment affects her soul. How can we ever begin to measure what she experiences? We hope readers are motivated to pursue vigorously the use and development of outcome measures that are applicable to all patients. Although most patients' major complaint is their inability to hear, aural rehabilitation also includes management of those that experience tinnitus and vestibular and/or balance problems. We conclude this chapter with a discussion concerning outcomes measurement for tinnitus and vestibular rehabilitation therapy.

OUTCOMES MEASUREMENT FOR TINNITUS AND VESTIBULAR REHABILITATION THERAPY

Outcomes Measurement for Tinnitus Therapy

It has been estimated that 40 to 50 million individuals in the United States have experienced tinnitus at some time or another; as many as 2.5 million report being debilitated by this condition (AAA, 2000b). Tinnitus results in (Noble, 2000):

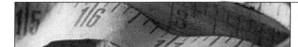

VIGNETTE 10-4

ON GROWING DEAF ... MUSIC
By Janet Thomas

I have come unprepared into the world of silence.
It is as soft as down, or the first snow of winter,
      blanketing the world with false reality.
It has subtly crept into my life day by sneaky day, year by flowing year, until
It consumes my every moment ... every thought ... every passion.

The echoes of the past appear with suddenness and fury;
The sounds that once were all around no longer give comfort to the ear.
Music that found a home in my soul as I was still growing into womanhood,
      that held harmonies and bass lines that I followed until
      my body was breathless with youthful fulfillment,
Now are but a puzzle to be solved as each measure passes.

Those heroes who boldly lit up my heart with passion that flamed
      throughout my life—Bach, Beethoven, Rachmaninoff, Tchaikovsky—
      remain the same, but I am different:
Different because my perception of their gifts has atrophied.
Whose music was once a dearest friend has become a challenge to be
      understood, and therefore like any other obstacle in life.
The solace and safety of their music has been ripped from me
      like the slow erosion of the mountain beneath one's home.

I think, "I know that sound ... It's part of who I am!"
And yet it pays respectful distance to the here and now.
Hear and Now. Hear and Know.

Know the clarity of violins soaring high upon their resin-coated strings,
Sometimes only a wisp of a sound as if on angels' wings
But also used by masters for a melody that throbs with soul-searing intensity
      determined to deliver its song atop the orchestra.

Know the cello as it sings and wends its way through the mid- to-lower range;
      "Ah yes!" I cry, "I recognize ... I think I know this tune!"
And then tones mingle into shades, a melody so strange,
Unrecognizable at first to my offended ear, then all too plain and sure,
      The one I've heard and known for years has now become a blur.

The horn and winds blow slowly into my understanding;
I hear the oboe's edge the best.
But flute and tymp are all but lost in tonal comprehension,
For highs and lows, those cowardly tones, have finally been laid to rest.

The bass that shook my floor and soul is not a factor now.
Instead, bereft of certainty, I tread on satan's power:
      Destruction of my dearest gift,
      Each week, each day, each hour.

When some lone instrument can pierce the fog in which I lie,
My spirit begs to know its song, or otherwise to die.

- disabilities (e.g., interference with and distortion of normal auditory perception),
- handicaps (e.g., emotional distress, interference with sleep, and social life), and
- non-auditory factors (e.g., chronic depression and high self-focused attention).

According to their scope of practice (ASHA, 1996), audiologists are qualified to evaluate, diagnose, develop management strategies, and provide treatment for patients with tinnitus (AAA, 2000b). Several treatments for tinnitus have been developed, such as cognitive-behavioral individual and group therapies, habituation/tinnitus retraining therapy, hypnosis, biofeedback, and relaxation techniques (Henry & Wilson, 2001). Other management procedures include: counseling, use of hearing aids/tinnitus instruments, maskers/home-masking devices, self-help and support/education groups, stress management, and alternative treatments (e.g., acupuncture, homeopathy, and herbal remedies such as ginkgo biloba) (AAA, 2000b). Unfortunately, the effectiveness, efficiency, and efficacy of many of these treatments are based more on faith than on scientific proof. For example, there is no evidence to support the effectiveness of alternative treatments for tinnitus (AAA, 2000b). The American Academy of Audiology's *Audiologic Guidelines for the Diagnosis and Management of Tinnitus Patients* stated that tinnitus treatment and management procedures should be validated using randomized clinical trials, investigations with appropriate placebo controls, and the valid and reliable use of questionnaires.

Self-report questionnaires are used to measure the cognitive, behavioral, emotional, and social effects of tinnitus for the following purposes (Henry & Wilson, 2001):

- The identification of patients who are particularly bothered (e.g., impaired or distressed) by tinnitus who may benefit from intervention

- The evaluation of specific disabilities encountered by patients
- The evaluation of the outcome of treatments for individual patients

Self-assessment tinnitus questionnaires can also be used for the following research purposes (Henry & Wilson, 2001):

- Provide a basis for understanding the psychological aspects of tinnitus.
- Enable standardization of patient-selection criteria.
- Provide a means of evaluating the short- and long-term effectiveness of treatment.

Self-assessment questionnaires can be classified by what they measure. Specifically, there are instruments that measure one or more of the following (Henry & Wilson, 2000):

- distress, impairment, and handicap;
- negative and positive thought processes; and
- coping strategies.

Other outcome measures include those evaluating depression and anxiety and some daily self-monitoring tinnitus methods.

Questionnaires for Distress, Impairment, and Handicap

Wilson, Henry, Bowen, and Haralambous (1991) developed the *Tinnitus Reduction Questionnaire* (TRQ) which measures the psychological distress caused by tinnitus using 4 symptom categories, described by Tyler and Baker (1983) (Henry & Wilson, 2001). The scale consists of 26 items with several that "load" onto more than one of the 4 factors (Noble, 2000):

1. Distress (feelings of anger and despair)
2. Interference with work and leisure
3. Severe distress (crying, loss of sleep,

and feelings of going crazy)
4. Activity avoidance

All items are negative descriptors rated on a 5-point scale (e.g., 0 to 4) with higher scores representing a greater degree of distress. The TRQ score correlated with standard measures of depression and anxiety ($r \geq 0.60$) and other measures of tinnitus, but only minimally correlated with measures of neuroticism ($r = 0.27$) (Henry & Wilson, 2001; Noble, 2000). Therefore, the construct validity of the TRQ as a measure of distress is good (Henry & Wilson, 2001).

Kuk, Tyler, Russell, and Jordan (1990) developed the *Tinnitus Handicap Questionnaire* (THQ). It consists of 28 items, all negative statements except for items 26 (i.e., "I think I have a healthy outlook on tinnitus.") and 27 (i.e., "I have support from my friends regarding my tinnitus.") that were developed to measure the handicapping effects of tinnitus on hearing, lifestyle, health, and emotional status (Henry & Wilson, 2001). Respondents are instructed to provide a rating from 0 (i.e., no agreement) to 100 (i.e., strong agreement) to reflect their degree of agreement with each statement (Henry & Wilson, 2001). Although covering a broader range of factors than the TRQ, the THQ is not that different and has some similar items in common (Noble, 2000). The THQ has a high internal consistency (Cronbach's alpha = 0.94) with item to total-score correlations ranging from 0.15 to 0.81 (Kuk, et al., 1990) and good test-retest reliability (Newman, Wharton, & Jacobson, 1995). Factor analysis determined that the scale measures three factors:

1. Social, emotional, and physical effect
2. Effects of tinnitus and hearing acuity
3. Appraisal of tinnitus

The *Tinnitus Questionnaire* (TQ) or the *Tinnitus Effects Questionnaire* (TEQ) is a 52-item instrument that measures the dimensions of patients' complaints about their tinnitus (Hallam, Jakes, & Hinchcliffe, 1988; Henry & Wilson, 2001). Respondents are instructed to indicate their degree of agreement to statements by circling one of three possible responses with their point values in parentheses (Henry & Wilson, 2001):

1. "true" (2 points)
2. "partly true" (1 point)
3. "not true" (0 points)

Affirmative responses (i.e., "true") are identified as complaints about tinnitus with the exception of items: 1, 7, 32, and 49 which are reverse scored because they are positive statements about tinnitus (e.g., "I can sometimes ignore the noises even when they are there.") (Henry & Wilson, 2001). Several studies have performed factor analysis on responses on the TEQ and have yielded a variety of factors (Noble, 2000). For example, Henry and Wilson (2001) identified 5 interpretable factors on the TEQ:

1. Coping orientation
2. Loudness, unpleasantness, and intrusiveness of the noise
3. Effects on communication and hearing acuity
4. Sleep disturbance
5. Effects on physical well-being

The TEQ has been found to have a high internal consistency (Cronbach alpha of 0.91 to 0.95) and high test-retest reliability (R of 0.91 to 0.94). Furthermore, the TEQ is highly correlated with the TRQ and THQ (Henry & Wilson, 2001).

Questionnaires for Cognitions (i.e., Thoughts) and Coping Strategies

The *Tinnitus Cognitions Questionnaire* (TCQ) (Wilson & Henry, 1998) assesses patients' thoughts in response to their tinnitus (Henry & Wilson, 2001). The TCQ consists of 26 items of which 13 are positive statements (e.g., "I can learn to live with it.") and 13 are negative statements (e.g., "The noise will drive me crazy.") (Noble, 2000). Respondents are instructed to, "indicate how often you have been aware of thinking a particular thought on occasions when you have noticed the tinnitus," by using a 5-point Likert scale (e.g., ranging from 0 = "never" to 4 = "very frequently" for negative statements and reverse scoring for positive statements) (Henry & Wilson, 2001). The higher the total score, the greater is the tendency for patients to engage in negative thought processes about their tinnitus (Noble, 2000). Factor analysis of patients' responses on the TCQ resulted in 4 factors (Henry & Wilson, 2001): positive thoughts, hopelessness, helplessness/victimization, and an active coping outlook that could be further reduced to two factors of positive and negative thoughts. Furthermore, Wilson and Henry (1998) found that the TCQ had high internal consistency (Cronbach alpha of 0.91) and test-retest validity (R of 0.88) showing a good stability of responses from patients over time (Henry & Wilson, 2001).

Outcomes Measurement for Vestibular and Balance Rehabilitation

ASHA's Scope of Practice for Audiologists (ASHA, 1996) states that the following functions are within their professional area of expertise:

- canalith repositioning procedures (e.g., techniques of moving the body to reposition the otoconia and/or other material from abnormal positions in the semi-circular canals back into the vestibule), and
- consultation to and/or serving as a member of a multidisciplinary team managing patients with balance disorders and/or dizziness

Other functions include:

- Habituation activities (e.g., focus on specific planes of motion or visual motions that elicit symptoms)
- Vestibular-ocular reflex (VOR) exercise (e.g., activities that stress the VOR)
- Balance activities (e.g., those that involve a variety of both static and dynamic gait)

ASHA (1999) has outlined specific training for these functions in its "*Guidelines on the Role of Audiologists in Vestibular and Balance Rehabilitation Programs.*"

The general goals of a vestibular and balance rehabilitation program are to (ASHA, 1999):

- Promote the central vestibular system compensation process.
- Reduce the patient's sensitivity to head, eye, or visual motion activity that produces symptoms of vertigo, disequilibrium, unsteadiness, and so forth.
- Reduce risk for falls by improvement in static and dynamic balance through the use of various gait activities.
- Improve the maintenance of the compensation process via increased lifestyle activities associated with head and eye movements.

The treatment efficacy of vestibular and balance rehabilitation seems to be population specific such that the best prognosis is for patients with uncompensated or decompensated unilateral peripheral lesions (ASHA, 1999). Table 10-5 shows the author, date of publication, questions investigated, experimental designs, results, and conclusions for some studies investigating the efficacy of vestibular and balance rehabilitation (ASHA, 1999). As shown in Table 10-5, several studies have demonstrated the efficacy of certain vestibular and balance rehabilitation programs with patients having a variety of balance disorders of different etiologies.

Table 10-5. Author, date of publication, question investigated, experimental designs, results, and conclusions of studies demonstrating effectiveness of vestibular rehabilitation (Adapted from ASHA, 1999)

AUTHOR/DATE OF PUBLICATION	QUESTION INVESTIGATED	EXPERIMENTAL DESIGNS	RESULTS	CONCLUSIONS
Norre (1987)	Do patients with benign paroxysmal positional vertigo (BPPV) benefit from habituation exercises?	Three groups of patients were compared: (1) Active habituation treatment group. (2) Sham exercise group, or (3) Non-treated control group	Active habituation treatment group (1) showed superior results compared to groups (2) and (3).	Patients in the habituation treatment group had a significant improvement of their BPPV condition compared to those in a sham exercise group or those who received no treatment at all.
Horak, Jones-Rycewicz, Black, & Shumway-Cook (1992)	Do patients with BPPV benefit from a customized program of vestibular rehabilitation?	Three groups of patients were compared: (1) Active habituation treatment group, (2) Medical therapy (i.e., meclizine or diazepam) group, or (3) Sham exercises (i.e., aerobic exercises and strength training)	All three groups reported subjective decreases in dizziness with the greatest effects shown with the vestibular rehabilitation group.	The vestibular rehabilitation group showed greater decreases in subjective dizziness than those groups undergoing medical therapy or participating in a sham exercise group.
Shepard & Telian (1995)	Is a customized vestibular and balance program more efficacious than a generic program of vestibular exercises for patients with vestibular dysfunction?	Clinical trial involving random assignment of patients to two groups: (1) Customized therapy group, or (2) Generic therapy group	Customized therapy group showed statistically significant decreases in spontaneous nystagmus, rotational chair asymmetries, and motion sensitivity than the generic therapy group. In addition, they had a greater performance on clinical measures of static and dynamic balance ability than the other group.	The customized therapy group achieved a superior level of vestibular compensation than the generic therapy group.

(CONTINUES)

Table 10–5. (continued from page 266)

AUTHOR/DATE OF PUBLICATION	QUESTION INVESTIGATED	EXPERIMENTAL DESIGNS	RESULTS	CONCLUSIONS
Lynn, Pool, Rose, Brey, & Suman (1995)	Is a single vestibular rehabilitation program (i.e., a single office visit for benign positional vertigo–particle reposition procedure) effective for patients with unilateral BPPV?	Clinical trial involving random assignment of 36 patients with unilateral BPPV to two groups to receive a: (1) Modified Epley (1992) procedure (i.e., treatment group), or a (2) Sham procedure (i.e., control group) Patients and audiologists were double-blinded to group assignments	At 1-month post-treatment, 89% of the treatment group and only 27% of the control group had negative Halpike maneuvers.	A single office visit procedure (i.e., Epley) was effective in reducing symptoms of BPPV as measured by the Hallpike maneuver.
Krebs, Gill-Body, Riley, & Parker (1993)	Does therapy for gait benefit patients with significant bilateral peripheral vestibular paresis?	Clinical trial involving random assignment of patients to two groups: (1) Gait therapy (i.e., treatment group), or a (2) Control group	Group receiving gait therapy had statistically significantly greater improvement in measures of gait compared to the control group.	Patients with bilateral peripheral vestibular system paresis can benefit from gait therapy.
Herdman, Clendaniel, Mattox, Holliday, & Niparko (1995) [a]	Is a series of activities designed to increase vestibular-ocular reflex gain effective in increasing postural control in patients following an acoustic neuroma resection?	Clinical trial involving random assignment of patients following acoustic nerve resection (i.e., 3 days post-surgery) into two groups: (1) Generic therapy designed to increase vestibulo-ocular reflex gain (e.g., head and eye movement plus a walking program), or a (2) Control group receiving eye movement exercises and walking	The group receiving a generic therapy program demonstrated a statistically significant greater improvement in postural control than the control group. Furthermore, the generic therapy group reported a significantly lesser amount of disequilibrium than the control group during days 5 and 6 post-surgery.	Patients receiving an acoustic nerve resection can benefit from a generic exercise program.

(Adapted from ASHA, 1999)

Audiologists providing vestibular and balance rehabilitation need outcome measures to demonstrate the efficacy of these treatments for patients measuring both balance function impairment and handicap. Recall that the terms impairment and handicap were defined earlier in this chapter. Several self-assessment scales have been well-documented in the literature and standardized in measuring handicap resulting from vestibular dysfunction. Balance function impairment may be considered an abnormality in any of three interdependent systems involved in maintaining stability (Newman & Jacobson, 1997): vision, proprioception (e.g., gravity-sensing apparatus located in the muscles, tendons, and joints), and the vestibular system.

Newman and Jacobson (1997) stated that balance system impairment is most often measured through vestibulometric and/or posturographic tests. Balance function handicap, on the other hand, is more difficult to quantify because it is highly individualistic and determined by a number of factors, including personality, age, occupational status, psychosocial adjustment, and general physical health (Newman & Jacobson, 1997).

There are at least four methods of assessing the effectiveness of vestibular and balance rehabilitation (Gans & Crandell, 2000; Newman & Jacobson, 1997):

1. Formula method
2. Subjective disability and symptom measure
3. Handicap inventories
4. Quality of life assessments

The Formula Method

The Committee on Hearing and Equilibrium of the American Academy of Ophthamology and Otolaryngology (AAOO) developed a formula for providing a single number to express the change in dizzy spells following intervention (Newman & Jacobson, 1997). The formula involves 3 steps:

1. obtaining the number of dizzy spells per month 6 months prior to treatment and 24 months after the initiation of treatment,
2. dividing the number of post-treatment spells by the number of pretreatment spells, and
3. multiplying the dividend by 100.

The product is then placed in one of 5 categories, depending on the score:

1. 0 = complete control of definitive spells
2. 1 to 40 = substantial control of definitive spells
3. 41 to 80 = limited control of definitive spells
4. 81 to 120 = insignificant control of definitive spells
5. over 120 = worse (poorer) control of definitive spells

For example, if a patient has 10 spells 6 months prior to the initiation of treatment and only one spell 24 months after the initiation of treatment, the patient has substantial control of definitive spells with a final score of 10 (i.e., $1 / 10 = 0.1 \times 100 = 10$). The advantage of the formula method is that the calculations are easy to perform and may provide information regarding the overall success of treatment (Newman & Jacobson, 1997). However, the definition of a definitive spell was provided by the AAOO and may not be completely clear to patients who must self-monitor their episodes, thereby casting doubt on the validity of the outcome measure (Newman & Jacobson, 1997).

Subjective Disability and Symptom Measures

Shepard, Telian, and Smith-Wheelock (1990) developed two measures involving clinician assessment of the effectiveness of their management programs which focused on reducing the motion provoked/positional sensitivity and correcting deficits of balance/gait (Newman & Jacobson, 1997):

1. *Subjective Disability Scale* (SDS)—administered pre- and post-therapy
2. *Post-therapy Symptom Scale* (PSS)

The SDS consists of 6 categories with corresponding scores and descriptors:

1. 0 = No Disability (e.g., negligible symptoms)
2. 1 = No Disability (e.g., no bothersome symptoms)
3. 2 = Mild Disability (e.g., performs usual work responsibilities, but symptoms interfere with outside activities)
4. 3 = Moderate Disability (e.g., symptoms interfere with work duties and outside activities)
5. 4 = Recent Severe Disability (e.g., on medical leave or had to change jobs because of symptoms)
6. 5 = Long-term Disability (e.g., unable to work for more than one year or permanent disability)

The PSS scoring involves using the following 5 categories with corresponding scores and descriptors:

1. 0 = No symptoms remaining at the end of therapy
2. 1 = Marked improvement in symptoms with mild symptoms remaining
3. 2 = Mild improvement in symptoms, with definite persistence of symptoms remaining
4. 3 = No change in symptoms relative to pretreatment
5. 4 = Symptoms worsened with treatment on a consistent basis relative to pretreatment

The SDS and the PSS have the following three advantages (Newman & Jacobson, 1997): they provide a 2-dimensional approach for assessing treatment outcomes, are quick, and easy to perform.

Three disadvantages of these scales are (Newman & Jacobson, 1997):

1. lack of a quantitative method for classifying "marked improvement" or "mild improvement,"
2. a focus on work and outside activity limitations, and
3. the use of clinician-assigned scores instead of patients scoring of their own disability and symptoms.

Self-Assessment and Handicap Scales

Several self-assessment scales have been developed that measure the effectiveness of vestibular and balance rehabilitation. The *Dizziness Handicap Inventory* (DHI), developed by Jacobson and Newman (1990), assesses patients' perception of the effect of vestibular dysfunction on their emotional/functional adjustment and corresponding limitations. The DHI has 25 items distributed over 3 categories:

1. Functional (9 items)
2. Emotional (9 items)
3. Physical (7 items)

Patients respond to each question (e.g., P-1 = "Does looking up increase your problem?") by marking either "yes" (i.e., assigned 4 points), "sometimes" (i.e., assigned 2 points), or "no" (i.e., assigned 0 points). Scores obtained on all questions are added together resulting in a total score ranging from 0 (i.e., no perceived handicap) to 100 (i.e., significant perceived balance handicap) points (Newman & Jacobson, 1997).

The DHI has good reliability and validity. For example, the final version of the DHI was administered to 106 patients yielding good internal consistency for the total inventory (i.e., Cronbach's alpha coefficient of 0.89), and for the functional (i.e., Cronbach's alpha coefficient of 0.85), emotional (i.e., Cronbach's alpha coefficient of 0.72), and physical categories (i.e., Cronbach's alpha coefficient of 0.70). Furthermore, the DHI has good content validity (e.g., items drawn from case histories of dizzy patients), and a criterion validity demonstrating a significant association between components of the balance function examination (e.g., ENG, rotational testing, and posturography) and DHI scores (Newman & Jacobson, 1997). The advantages of the DHI include (Newman & Jacobson, 1997):

- good reliability and validity;
- short administration time;
- ease of scoring;
- identification of specific functional, emotional, and physical problems; and
- information as a basis for making referrals to other professionals.

A limitation of the DHI is its use of a single form that may result in practice effects (Newman & Jacobson, 1997). Other self-assessment scales include: *Vestibular Disorder Activities of Daily Living Scale* (Cohen, Kimball, & Adams, 2000) *Activities of Daily Living Questionnaire* (Black, Angel, Pesznecker, & Gianna, 2000).

Quality of Life Measures

More recently, hearing health-care providers have considered using generic quality of life self-assessment instruments to measure clinical outcomes (Bess, 2000). *Clinimetrics* is a subjective measurement of patients' health status that has been found to be a highly effective indicator of treatment efficacy (Gans & Crandell, 2000). These types of instruments may be particularly sensitive to measuring the effectiveness of rehabilitation in improving the quality of life for patients debilitated by vestibular and balance problems.

For example, the *Medical Outcomes Study* (MOS—SF-36) (Ware & Sherbourne, 1992), the most popular multidimensional outcome measure for quality of life, was designed to monitor patient outcomes in medical and research settings (Bess, 2000). The SF-36 is a shortened version of the MOS consisting of a 36-item, self-report questionnaire that assesses 8 different health concepts (Bess, 2000):

1. Physical functioning
2. Role limitations because of functional health
3. Bodily pain
4. Social functioning
5. General mental health
6. Role limitation because of emotional problems
7. Vitality
8. General health perceptions

The SF-36 Health Survey Questionnaire takes only 5 to 10 minutes to complete and is well-recognized among the health-care and medical communities (Bess, 2000; Gans & Crandell, 2000).

Gans and Crandell (2000) performed a pilot study using 12 subjects (10 females, 2 males) ranging in age from 51 to 83 years diagnosed with a posterior canalithiasis form of BPPV who completed the SF-36 Health Survey Questionnaire before and 30 to 45 days after being treated with a modified Canalith Repositioning Manuever. Pre-, post-, and individual subscale SF-36 scores were submitted to paired-comparison t-tests that showed that mean post-treatment scores were significantly higher than pretreatment scores, indicating an improvement in functional and general health status (Gans & Crandell, 2000). Therefore, audiologists performing canalithic repositioning treatment can reduce vestibular impairment and also improve patients' quality of life (Gans & Crandell, 2000).

SUMMARY

This chapter opened with a vignette that represents one of the worst outcomes that patients and their families could experience. Outcomes measurement at any point might have prevented many of the patient's problems. Readers were asked to consider the scenario while reading about outcomes measurement and may be wondering, what outcome measures should have been used; when should they have been administered; and how the results should be used to achieve positive patient outcomes. The coverage of outcomes measurement in aural rehabilitation should help readers answer these questions. However, as with all clinical situations, there is no one single answer. Readers should now know that there are both appropriate and inappropriate uses of outcomes measurement in aural rehabilitation. Furthermore, outcomes measurement will continue to play a significant role in newer areas of rehabilitative audiology, such as tinnitus and vestibular/balance therapy.

LEARNING ACTIVITIES

- Divide your class into groups and have each construct a scenario for Vignette 10–1 in which outcomes measures might have been used to prevent Mrs. P.'s problems.

- Create a notebook for aural rehabilitation that includes selected outcome measures with a short write-up on each.

- Survey audiologists in your local area regarding their use of outcomes measurement in aural rehabilitation.

RECOMMENDED READINGS

Hosford-Dunn, H. & Huch, J.L. (2000). Acceptance, benefit, and satisfaction measures of hearing aid user attitudes. In R. Sandlin (Ed.), *Textbook of hearing aid amplification* (pp. 467–487). Clifton Park, NY: Delmar Thomson Learning.

Huch, J.L., & Hosford-Dunn, H. (2000). Inventories of self-assessment measurements of hearing aid outcome. In R. Sandlin (Ed.), *Textbook of hearing aid amplification* (pp. 489–521). Clifton Park, NY: Delmar Thomson Learning.

Proceedings of the 1999 Audiological Workshop at Eriksholm, Denmark. *Ear and Hearing, 21*(4).

REVIEW EXERCISES

Fill-in-the-Blank

Instructions: Please fill-in-the-blank with the correct term from the word bank below.

1. _____ _____ are integrated systems of ideas, terminology, variables, and relationships that underlie measurement, interpretation, and prediction based on a supporting theory or a body of empirical evidence.

2. _____ involves procedures that audiologists perform to ensure that hearing aid goals have been met.

3. _____ is the perception of hearing aid benefit provided by patients and their significant others through

the use of various outcome measures for disability and handicap.

4. _____ is activity limitation.

5. _____ is participation restriction.

6. _____ - _____ is comparing patients' ratings made at two different times, usually pre- and postintervention.

7. _____ - _____ is comparing patients' ratings to that of a sample of individuals representing the normative population.

8. _____ _____ is the degree to which items of an instrument consistently measure the same aspects of a domain (e.g., such as handicap) that reduces error and is assessed by quantitative measures.

9. _____ - _____
_____ is the correlation of individual items with the total score.

10. _____ - _____
_____ is the correlation of scores obtained for two randomly selected halves of an instrument.

11. _____ _____ relates the variance of the total score to that of the individual items.

12. _____ _____ (theoretical validity) is the degree with which a measure either empirically or rationally purports to measure some theoretical construct.

13. _____ _____ of a scale is the extent to which items represent and sample target domains, occurs early in test development, and is assessed less formally through subjective opinion.

14. _____ _____ is the extent to which an instrument statistically correlates to some recognized "gold standard" measure in the field.

15. _____ is how sensitive an instrument is at measuring changes in

a patient's state.

16. _____ is the ease of use of an instrument.

17. _____ is subjective measurement of patients' health status that has been found to be a highly effective indicator of treatment efficacy.

Word Bank:
Clinimetrics
Conceptual frameworks
Construct validity
Content validity
Criterion-referencing
Criterion validity
Cronbach's alpha
Disability
Feasibility
Handicap
Internal consistency
Item-total correlation
Norm-referencing
Responsiveness
Spilt-half reliability
Validation
Verification

Matching

Instructions: Please match the following items with the correct statements and terms below.

  I. Handicap domain
 II. Disability domain
III. Income measure
 IV. Both disability and handicap
  V. Satisfaction

1. ____ APHAB
2. ____ SADL
3. ____ HASP
4. ____ ECHO
5. ____ HHIE
6. ____ GHABP
7. ____ HAPI
8. ____ CPHI
9. ____ HANA

10. ____ HSS
11. ____ HHIA
12. ____ SHAPI
13. ____ COSI
14. ____ HPI
15. ____ Checklists and Flow Charts

ANSWERS

Fill-in-the-Blank:	Matching:
1. Conceptual frameworks	1. II
2. Verification	2. V
3. Validation	3. III
4. Disability	4. III
5. Handicap	5. I
6. Criterion-referencing	6. IV
7. Norm-referencing	7. II
8. Internal consistency	8. IV
9. Item-total correlation	9. III
10. Split-half reliability	10. V
11. Cronbach's alpha	11. I
12. Construct validity	12. II
13. Content validity	13. II
14. Criterion validity	14. II
15. Responsiveness	15. III
16. Feasibility	
17. Clinimetrics	

REFERENCES

American Academy of Audiology. (2000a). Statement 3. Joint audiology committee statement on hearing aid selection and fitting (adult). *Audiology Today, 12*(Special Issue), 42.

American Academy of Audiology. (2000b). *Audiologic guidelines for the diagnosis and management of tinnitus.* McLean, VA: Author.

American Speech-Language-Hearing Association. (1996). Scope of practice in audiology. *ASHA, 38*(Suppl. 16), 12–14.

American Speech-Language-Hearing Association. (1997). *Preferred practice patterns for the profession of audiology.* Rockville, MD: Author.

American Speech-Language-Hearing Association. (1998). Guidelines for hearing aid fitting for adults: Ad-Hoc Committee on Hearing Aid Selection and Fitting. *American Journal of Audiology: A Journal of Clinical Practice, 7*(1), 5–13.

American Speech-Language-Hearing Association. (1999). Role of audiologists in vestibular and balance rehabilitation: Position statement, guidelines, and technical report. *ASHA, 41*(Suppl. 19), 13–22.

American Speech-Language-Hearing Association. (2000). *Research facts: Clinical trials and communication sciences and disorders.* Rockville, MD: Author.

Beck, L.B. (1999). Audiology service delivery in the new millennium: Are you ready? *Audiology Today, Special Issue: Audiology and the New Millenium, 11*(10), 28.

Bentler, R.A., & Kramer, S.E. (2000). Guidelines for choosing a self-report outcome measure. *Ear and Hearing, 21*(Suppl. 4), 37S–49S.

Bess, F.H. (2000). The role of generic health-related quality of life measures in establishing audiological rehabilitation outcomes. *Ear and Hearing, 21*(Suppl. 4), 74S–99S.

Bess, F.H., Hedley-Williams, A., & Lichtenstein, M.J. (1999). Audiologic assessment of the elderly. In F.E. Musiek & W.F. Rintelmann (Eds.), *Contemporary perspectives in hearing assessment* (pp. 437–463). Needham Heights, MA: Allyn & Bacon.

Black, F.O., Angel, C.R., Pesznecker, S.C., & Gianna, C. (2000). Outcome analysis of individualized vestibular rehabilitation protocols. *American Journal of Otology, 21,* 543–551.

Boyle, C.M. (1991). Does item homogeneity indicate internal consistency or item redundancy in psychometric scales? *Personality and Individual Differences, 12,* 291–294.

Byrne, D. (1998). Hearing aid clinical trials: Specific benefits need specific measures. *American Journal of Audiology: A Journal of Clinical Practice, 7,* 17–19.

Cohen, H.S., Kimball, K.T., & Adams, A.S. (2000). Application of the vestibular disorders activities of daily living scale. *Laryngoscope, 110*, 1204–1209.

Cox, R.M., & Alexander, G.C. (1995). The Abbreviated Profile of Hearing Aid Benefit. *Ear and Hearing, 16*, 176–183.

Cox, R.M., & Alexander, G.C. (1999). Measuring satisfaction with amplification in daily life: The SADL Scale. *Ear and Hearing, 20*, 306–320.

Cox, R.M., & Alexander, G.C. (2000). Expectations about hearing aids and their relationship to fitting outcome. *Journal of the American Academy of Audiology, 11*, 368–382.

Cox, R.M., Alexander, G.C., & Gilmore, C. (1987). Development of the Connected Speech Test. *Ear and Hearing, 8*(Suppl. 5), 119S–126S.

Cox, R.M., Alexander, G.C., Gilmore, C., & Pusakulich, K.M. (1988). Use of the Connected Speech Test (CST) with hearing-impaired listeners. *Ear and Hearing, 9*, 198–207.

Cox, R.M., Alexander, G.C., & Gray, G. (1999). Personality and the subjective assessment of hearing aids. *Journal of the American Academy of Audiology, 10*, 1–13.

Cox, R.M., & Gilmore, C. (1990). Development of the Profile of Hearing Aid Performance. *Journal of Speech and Hearing Research, 33*, 343–357.

Cox, R., Hyde, M., Gatehouse, S., Noble, W., Dillon, H., Bentler, R., Stephens, D., Arlinger, S., Beck, L., Wilkerson, D., Kramer, S., Kricos, P., Gagne, J.P., Bess, F., & Hallberg, L. (2000). Optimal outcome measures, research priorities, and international cooperation. *Ear and Hearing, 21*(Suppl. 4), 106S–115S.

Demorest, M.E., & Erdman, S.A. (1987). Development of the communication profile for the hearing impaired. *Journal of Speech and Hearing Disorders, 52*, 129–139.

Dillon, H. (1994). Shortened Hearing Aid Profile Inventory for the Elderly. *Australian Journal of Audiology, 16*, 34–37.

Dillon, H., James, A., & Ginis, J. (1997). Client Oriented Scale of Improvement (COSI) and its relationship to several other measures of benefit and satisfaction provided by hearing aids. *Journal of the American Academy of Audiology, 8*, 27–43.

Gans, R.E., & Crandell, C.C. (2000). Overview of BPPV: Evaluating treatment outcomes with clinimetrics. *The Hearing Review 7*(11), 50, 52–54, 75.

Gatehouse, S. (1999). The Glasgow Hearing Aid Benefit Profile: Derivation and validation of a client-centered outcome measure for hearing aid services. *Journal of the American Academy of Audiology, 10*, 80–103.

Gatehouse, S. (2000). The Glasgow Hearing Aid Benefit Profile: What it measures and how to use it. *The Hearing Journal, 53*(3), 10, 12, 14, 16, 18.

Giolas, T.J., Owens, E., Lamb, S.H., & Schubert, E.D. (1979). Hearing Performance Inventory. *Journal of Speech and Hearing Disorders, 44*, 169–195.

Hallam, R.S., Jakes, S.C., & Hinchcliffe, R. (1988). Cognitive variables in tinnitus annoyance. *British Journal of Clinical Psychology, 27*, 213–222.

Henry, J.L., & Wilson, P.H. (2001). *The psychological management of chronic tinnitus: A cognitive-behavioral approach.* Boston, MA: Allyn & Bacon.

Herdman, S.J., Clendaniel, R.A., Mattox, D.E., Holliday, M.J., & Niparko, J.K. (1995). Vestibular adaptation exercises and recovery: Acute stage after acoustic neuroma resection. *Journal of the American Academy of Otolaryngology—Head and Neck Surgery, 113*, 77–87.

Horak, F., Jones-Rycewicz, C., Black, F.O., & Shumway-Cook, A. (1992). Effects of vestibular rehabilitation on dizziness, and imbalance. *Journal of the American Acad-*

emy of Otolaryngology—Head and Neck Surgery, 106, 175–180.

Hosford-Dunn, H. & Huch, J.L. (2000). Acceptance, benefit, and satisfaction measures of hearing aid user attitudes. In R. Sandlin (Ed.), *Textbook of hearing aid amplification* (2nd ed., pp. 467–487). Clifton Park, NY: Delmar Thomson Learning.

Huch, J.L., & Hosford-Dunn, H. (2000). Inventories of self-assessment measurements of hearing aid outcome. In R. Sandlin (Ed.), *Textbook of hearing aid amplification* (2nd ed., pp. 489–521). Clifton Park, NY: Delmar Thomson Learning.

Hyde, M.L. (2000). Reasonable psychometric standards for self-report outcome measures in audiological rehabilitation. *Ear and Hearing, 21*(Suppl. 4), 24S–36S.

Hyde, M.L. & Riko, K. (1994). A decision-analytic approach to audiological rehabilitation. In J.P. Gagne & N. Tye-Murray (Eds.), *Research in audiological rehabilitation: current trends and future directions monograph. Journal of the Academy of Rehabilitative Audiology, 27,* 337–374.

Jacobson, G. P., & Newman, C.W. (1990). The development of the Dizziness Handicap Inventory. *Archives of Otolaryngology— Head and Neck Surgery, 116,* 424–427.

Jacobson, G.P., Newman, C.W., Fabry, D.A., & Sandridge, S.A. (2001). Development of the Three-Clinic Hearing Aid Selection Profile (HASP). *Journal of the American Academy of Audiology, 12,* 128–141.

Johnson, C.E., & Danhauer, J.L. (1999). *Guidebook for support programs in aural rehabilitation.* Clifton Park, NY: Delmar Thomson Learning.

Johnson, C.E., & Danhauer, J.L. (2001). *Outcomes measurement: From A to Z.* An instructional course presented at the 13th Annual Convention and Exposition of the American Academy of Audiology, San Diego, CA.

Johnson, C.E., Danhauer, J.L., & Krishnamurti, S. (2000). A holistic model for matching high technology hearing aids to elderly patients. *American Journal of Audiology, 9*(2), 112–123.

Kochkin, S. (1993a). MarkeTrak III: Why 20 million in U.S. don't use hearing aids for their hearing loss I. *The Hearing Journal, 46*(1), 20–27.

Kochkin, S. (1993b). MarkeTrak III: Why 20 million in U.S. don't use hearing aids for their hearing loss II. *The Hearing Journal, 46*(2), 26–31.

Kochkin, S. (1993c). MarkeTrak III: Why 20 million in U.S. don't use hearing aids for their hearing loss III. *The Hearing Journal, 46*(4), 36–37.

Kochkin, S. (1996). MarkeTrak IV: 10–year trends in the hearing aid market: Has anything changed? *The Hearing Journal, 48*(1), 23–24.

Kochkin, S. (1997). MarkeTrak norms: Subjective measures of satisfaction & benefit: Establishing norms. *Seminars in Hearing, 18*(1), 37–48.

Kochkin, S. (1998). MarkeTrak IV: Correlates of hearing aid purchase intent. *The Hearing Journal, 51*(1), 3–41.

Krebs, D.E., Gill-Body, K.M., Riley, P.O., & Parker, S.W. (1993). Double-blind, placebo-controlled trial of rehabilitation for bilateral vestibular hypofunction: Preliminary report. *Journal of the American Academy of Otolaryngology—Head and Neck Surgery, 109,* 735–741.

Kricos, P.B. (2000). The influence of nonaudiological variables on audiological rehabilitation outcomes. *Ear and Hearing, 21*(Suppl. 4), 7S–14S.

Kricos, P.B. & Lesner, S.A. (1995). *Hearing care for the older adult: Audiologic rehabilitation.* Boston, MA: Butterworth-Heinemann.

Kuk, F.K., Tyler, R.S., Russell, D., & Jordan, H. (1990). The psychometric properties of a tinnitus handicap questionnaire. *Ear and Hearing, 11,* 434–445.

Lamb, S.H., Owens, E., & Schubert, E.D. (1983). The revised form of the Hearing

Performance Inventory. *Ear and Hearing, 4,* 152–157.

Larson, V.D., Williams, D.W., Henderson, W.G., Luethke, L.E., Beck, L.B., Noffsinger, D., Wilson, R.H., Dobie, R.A., Haskell, G.B., Bratt, G.W., Shanks, J.E., Stelmachowicz, P., Studebaker, G.A., Boysen, A.E., Donahue, A., Canalis, R., Fausti, S.A., & Rappaport, B.Z. (2000). Efficacy of 3 commonly used hearing aid circuits: A crossover trial. *Journal of the American Medical Association, 284,* 1806–1813.

Lesner, S.A., & Kricos, P.B. (1995). Audiologic rehabilitation assessment: A holistic approach. In P.B. Kricos & S.A. Lesner (Eds.), *Hearing care for the older adult: Audiologic rehabilitation* (pp. 21–58). Boston, MA: Butterworth-Heinemann.

Lynn, S., Pool, A., Rose, D., Brey, R., & Suman, V. (1995). Randomized trail of the canalith repositioning procedure. *Journal of the American Academy of Otolaryngology—Head and Neck Surgery, 113,* 712–720.

Maxwell, D.L., & Satake, E. (1997). *Research and statistical methods in communication disorders.* Baltimore, MD: Williams & Wilkins.

McCarthy, P.A., & Alpiner, J.G. (2000). *Rehabilitative audiology: Children and Adults* (3rd ed.) Baltimore, MD: Lippincott, Williams & Wilkins.

McDowell, I., & Newell, C. (1986). *Measuring health: A guide to rating scales and questionnaires.* New York, NY: Oxford University Press.

Meinert, C.L. (1995). *Clinical trials: Design, conduct, and analysis.* New York, NY: Oxford University Press.

Mueller, H.G. (1999). Just make it audible, comfortable, and loud, but okay. *The Hearing Journal, 52*(1), 10, 12,14,16.

Myers, I.B., & McCaulley, M.H. (1985*). Manual: A guide to the development and use of the Myers-Briggs Type Indicator.* Palo Alto, CA: Consulting Psychologists Press.

Newman, C.W., & Jacobson, G.P. (1997). Balance handicap assessment. In G.P. Jacobson, C.W. Newman, & J.M. Kartush (Eds.), *Handbook of balance function testing* (pp. 380–391). Clifton Park, NY: Delmar Thomson Learning.

Newman, C.W., Jacobson, G.P., Hug, G.A., Weinstein, B.E., & Malinoff, R.L. (1991). Practical methods for quantifying hearing aid benefit in older adults. *Journal of the American Academy of Audiology, 2,* 70–75.

Newman, C.W., & Sandridge, S.A. (2001). *Digital signal processing hearing aids: A report card.* Paper presented at the 13th Annual Convention and Exposition of the American Academy of Audiology, San Diego, CA.

Newman, C.W., & Weinstein, B.E. (1988). The Hearing Handicap Inventory for the Elderly as a measure of hearing aid benefit. *Ear and Hearing, 9,* 81–85.

Newman, C.W., & Weinstein, B.E. (1989). Test-retest reliability of the Hearing Handicap Inventory for the Elderly using two administration approaches. *Ear and Hearing, 10,* 190–191.

Newman, C.W., Weinstein, B.E., Jacobson, G.P., & Hug, G.A. (1990). The Hearing Handicap Inventory for Adults: Psychometric adequacy and audiometric correlates. *Ear and Hearing, 11,* 430–433.

Newman, C.W., Weinstein, B.E., Jacobson, G.P., & Hug, G.A. (1991). Test-retest reliability of the hearing handicap inventory for adults. *Ear and Hearing 12,* 355–357.

Newman, C.W., Wharton, J.A., & Jacobson, G.P. (1995). Retest stability of the Tinnitus Handicap Questionnaire. *Annals of Oto-Rhino-Laryngology, 104,* 718–723.

Newman, C.W., Wharton, J.A., & Jacobson, G.P. (1997). Self-focused and somatic attention in patients with tinnitus. *Journal of the American Acedemy of Audiology, 8,* 143–149.

Noble, W. (2000). Self-reports about tinnitus and about cochlear implants. *Ear and Hearing, 21*(Suppl. 4), 50S–59S.

Norre, M.E. (1987). Rationale of rehabilitation treatment for vertigo. *American Journal of Otolaryngology, 8,* 31–35.

Nunnally, J.C. (1978). *Psychometric theory* (2nd ed.) New York, NY: McGraw-Hill.

Owens, E.O., & Fujikawa, S. (1980). The Hearing Performance Inventory and hearing aid use in profound hearing loss. *Journal of Speech and Hearing Research, 23,* 470–479.

Palmer, C.V., Mueller, H.G., & Moriarty, M. (1999). Profile of Aided Loudness: A validation procedure. *The Hearing Journal, 52*(6), 34, 36, 40–42.

Paul, R.G., & Cox, R.M. (1995). Measuring hearing aid benefit with the APHAB: Is this as good as it gets? *American Journal of Audiology, 4*(3), 10–13.

Sandlin, R. (2000). *Textbook of hearing aid amplification* (2nd ed.) Clifton Park, NY: Delmar Thomson Learning.

Sandridge, S.A. (1997). Consumer satisfaction with Multifocus hearing aids. *Seminars in Hearing, 18*(1), 67–72.

Sandridge, S.A., & Newman, C.W. (1998). *Subjective satisfaction ratings for digital signal processing hearing aids.* Paper presented at the Annual Convention of the American Speech-Language-Hearing Association, San Antonio, TX.

Schiavetti, N., & Metz, D.E. (1997). *Evaluating research in communicative disorders* (3rd ed.) Needham Heights, MA: Allyn & Bacon.

Schum, D.J. (1992). Responses of elderly hearing aid users on the Hearing Aid Performance Inventory. *Journal of the American Academy of Audiology, 3,* 308–314.

Schum, D.J. (1999). Perceived hearing aid benefit in relation to perceived needs. *Journal of the American Academy of Audiology, 10,* 40–45.

Shepard, N.T., & Telian, S.A. (1995). Programmatic vestibular rehabilitation. *Journal of the American Academy of Otolaryngology—Head and Neck Surgery, 112,* 173–182.

Shepard, N.T., Telian, S.A., & Smith-Wheelock, M. (1990). Habituation and balance retraining therapy. *Neurology Clinic, 8,* 159–475.

Speilberger, C.D. (1983). *State-Trait Anxiety Inventory.* Palo Alto, CA: Consulting Psychologists Press.

Stephens, D., & Hetu, R. (1991). Impairment, disability, and handicap in audiology: Towards a consensus. *Audiology, 30,* 185–200.

Streiner, D.L., & Norman, G.R. (1995). *Health measurement scales: A practical guide to their development and use.* New York, NY: Oxford University Press.

Tyler, R.S., & Baker, L.J. (1983). Difficulties experienced by tinnitus sufferers. *Journal of Speech and Hearing Disorders, 48,* 150–154.

Ventry, I.M., & Weinstein, B.E. (1982). The hearing inventory for the elderly: A new tool. *Ear and Hearing, 3,* 128–134.

Walden, B.E. (1997). Toward a model clinical-trials protocol for substantiating hearing aid user-benefit claims. *American Journal of Audiology: A Journal of Clinical Practice, 6,* 13–24.

Walden, B.E., Demorest, M.E., & Hepler, E.L. (1984). Self-report approach to assessing benefit derived from amplification. *Journal of Speech and Hearing Research, 27,* 49–56.

Ware, J.E., & Sherbourne, C.D. (1992). The MOS 36-item Short-Form Health Survey (SF-36). *Medical Care, 30,* 473–483.

Weinstein, B.E. (1997). Introduction: Customer satisfaction with and benefit from hearing aids. *Seminars in Hearing, 18*(1), 3–5.

Weinstein, B.E. (2000). Outcome measures in rehabilitative audiology. In J.G. Alpiner and P.A. McCarthy (Eds.), *Rehabilitative audiology: Children and adults.* (3rd ed., pp. 575–594). Baltimore, MD: Lippincott, Williams, & Wilkins.

Weinstein, B.E., Spitzer, J.B., & Ventry, I.M. (1986). Test-retest reliability of the Hearing

Handicap Inventory for the Elderly. *Journal of Speech and Hearing Research, 27,* 49–56.

Whichard, S. (1997). Auditory benefits of resound sound processing technology. *Seminars in Hearing, 18*(1), 63–66.

Wilson, P.H., & Henry, J.L. (1998). Tinnitus Cognitions Questionnaire: Development and psychometric properties of a measure of dysfunctional cognitions associated with tinnitus. *International Tinnitus Journal, 4,* 23–30.

Wilson, P.H., Henry, J., Bowen, M., & Haralambous, G. (1991). Tinnitus reaction questionnaire: Psychometric properties of a measure of distress associated with tinnitus. *Journal of Speech, Language, and Hearing Research, 34,* 197–201.

World Health Organization. (1980). *International classification of impairments, disabilities, and handicaps—A manual of classification relating to the consequences of disease.* Geneva: Author.

World Health Organization. (1999). *International classification of impairments, activities, and functioning* [online]. Available Internet: www.who.int/msa/mnh/ems/icidh/index.html.

APPENDIX X-A

Abbreviated Profile of Hearing Aid Benefit (APHAB)

(Cox, R.M., & Alexander, G.C. [1995]. The Abbreviated Profile of Hearing Aid Benefit. *Ear and Hearing, 16,* 176–183 © Lippincott, Williams, & Wilkins. Reprinted with permission.)

The above-referenced Appendix can be found on the companion CD-ROM.

APPENDIX X-B

Hearing Performance Inventory (HPI)

(Giolas, T.G., Owens, E., Lamb, S.H., & Schubert, E.D. [1979]. Hearing Performance Inventory. *Journal of Speech and Hearing Disorders, 44,* 169–195. © American Speech-Language-Hearing Association. Reprinted with permission.)

The above-referenced Appendix can be found on the companion CD-ROM.

APPENDIX X-C

Hearing Aid Performance Inventory (HAPI)

(Walden, B.E., Demorest, M.E., & Hepler, E.L. [1984]. Self-report approach to assessing benefit derived from amplification. *Journal of Speech and Hearing Research, 27*, 49–56. © American Speech-Language-Hearing Association. Adapted with permission.)

The above-referenced Appendix can be found on the companion CD-ROM.

APPENDIX X-D

Shortened Hearing Aid Performance Inventory (SHAPI)

(Schum, D.J.[1992]. Responses of elderly hearing aid users on the Hearing Aid Performance Inventory. *Journal of the American Academy of Audiology, 3*, 308–314. © B.C. Decker. Reprinted with permission.)

The above-referenced Appendix can be found on the companion CD-ROM.

APPENDIX X-E

Client Oriented Scale of Improvement (COSI)

(Dillon, H., James, A., & Ginis, J. [1997]. Client Oriented Scale of Improvement. *Journal of the American Academy of Audiology, 8*, 27–43. © B.C. Decker. Reprinted with permission.)

The above-referenced Appendix can be found on the companion CD-ROM.

APPENDIX X-F

The Hearing Handicap Inventory for the Elderly (HHIE)

(Ventry, I.M., & Weinstein, B.E. [1982]. The hearing inventory for the elderly: A new tool. *Ear and Hearing, 3*, 128–134. © Lippincott, Williams, & Wilkins. Reprinted with permission.)

The above-referenced Appendix can be found on the companion CD-ROM.

APPENDIX X-G

The Hearing Handicap Inventory for the Adults (HHIA)

(Newman, C.W., Weinstein, B.E., Jacobson, G.P., & Hug, G.A. [1990]. The Hearing Handicap Inventory for Adults: Psychometric adequacy and audiometric correlates. *Ear and Hearing, 11,* 430–433. © Lippincott, Williams, & Wilkins. Reprinted with permission.)

The above-referenced Appendix can be found on the companion CD-ROM.

APPENDIX X-H

The Hearing Handicap Inventory for the Elderly—Screening Form (HHIE—S)

(Ventry, I.M., & Weinstein, B.E. [1982]. The hearing inventory for the elderly: A new tool. *Ear and Hearing, 3,* 128–134. © Lippincott, Williams, & Wilkins. Reprinted with permission.)

The above-referenced Appendix can be found on the companion CD-ROM.

APPENDIX X-I

The Hearing Handicap Inventory for Adults—Screening Form (HHIA—S)

(Newman, C.W., Weinstein, B.E., Jacobson, G.P., & Hug, G.A. [1990]. The Hearing Handicap Inventory for Adults: Psychometric adequacy and audiometric correlates. *Ear and Hearing, 11,* 430–433. © Lippincott, Williams, & Wilkins. Reprinted with permission.)

The above-referenced Appendix can be found on the companion CD-ROM.

APPENDIX X-J

Glasgow Hearing Aid Benefit Profile (GHABP)

(Gatehouse, S. [1999]. The Glasgow Hearing Aid Benefit Profile: Derivation and validation of a client-centered outcome measure for hearing aid services. *Journal of the American Academy of Audiology, 10,* 80–103. © B.C. Decker. Reprinted with permission.)

The above-referenced Appendix can be found on the companion CD-ROM.

APPENDIX X-K

Hearing Satisfaction Survey (HSS)

(Adapted from Kochkin, 1997)

The above-referenced Appendix can be found on the companion CD-ROM.

APPENDIX X-L

Satisfaction with Amplification in Everyday Life Scale (SADL)

(Cox, R.M, & Alexander, G.C. [1999] Measuring satisfaction with amplification in daily life: The SADL Scale. *Ear and Hearing, 20,* 306–320. © Lippincott, Williams, & Wilkins. Reprinted with permission.)

The above-referenced Appendix can be found on the companion CD-ROM.

APPENDIX X-M

Expected Consequences of Hearing Aid Ownership (ECHO)

(Cox, R.M., & Alexander, G.C. [2000]. Expectations about hearing aids and their relationship to fitting outcome. *Journal of the American Academy of Audiology, 11,* 368–382. © B.C. Decker. Reprinted with permission.)

The above-referenced Appendix can be found on the companion CD-ROM.

APPENDIX X-N

Hearing Aid Needs Assessment (HANA)

(Schum, D.J. [1999]. Perceived hearing aid benefit in relation to perceived needs. *Journal of the American Academy of Audiology, 10,* 40–45. © B.C. Decker. Reprinted with permission.)

The above-referenced Appendix can be found on the companion CD-ROM.

APPENDIX X-O

Assistive Listening Device (ALD) Selection Protocol

(Adapted from ASHA, 1997)

The above-referenced Appendix can be found on the companion CD-ROM.

APPENDIX X-P

Assistive Listening Device (ALD) Orientation and Fitting Checklist

(Adapted from ASHA, 1997)

The above-referenced Appendix can be found on the companion CD-ROM.

CHAPTER 11

Outcomes Measurement in Hearing Health-Care Networks

LEARNING OBJECTIVES

This chapter will enable readers to:

- Understand audiologists' participation in managed care through hearing networks
- Understand aural rehabilitation programming in a hearing network
- Describe methods of outcomes measurement in hearing networks
- Acknowledge the importance of outcomes measurement to hearing networks
- Comprehend the implementation and limitations of outcomes measurement in hearing networks

INTRODUCTION

Since the end of World War II, the American health-care system has generally operated under the traditional fee-for-service reimbursement model that provides little incentive for service-care providers to cut costs (ASHA, 1996). A disadvantage of fee-for-service reimbursement models is that they can monetarily reward unethical health-care providers who prescribe unnecessary treatment (Seppala, 1995). High volumes of unnecessary care have driven the cost of health care to higher and higher levels. In recent years, health-care costs have accounted for 1 out of every 6 to 7 dollars or 14% of the gross domestic product (GDP) (ASHA, 1996).

Managed care has been offered as a way to reduce the costs of health care by combining financing, clinical services, and management under a single system. More and more audiologists are participating in managed care through hearing plans. One of the advantages of managed care is the opportunity to participate in organized outcomes measurement and management systems (ASHA, 1996), assuming that health maintenance organizations (HMOs) use outcome measures and consider them a priority. These processes can help practitioners provide quality care and unify practice patterns.

Although it may run counter to some audiologists' experiences, the term "quality managed care" is not an oxymoron (Northern, 1997). Managed-care organizations must prove that they are meeting or exceeding rigorous accreditation standards by groups such as the National Committee on Quality Assurance (NCQA) (Casey, 1997). Furthermore, unification of practice patterns can establish standards of health care for patients. The purpose of this chapter is to discuss audiologists' participation in hearing networks, aural rehabilitation programming, and outcomes measurement in hearing networks.

AUDIOLOGISTS' PARTICIPATION IN HEARING NETWORKS

There are three major types of managed-care organizations (Griffin & Frazen, 1993):

- *Managed indemnity insurance programs—* are traditional fee-for-service plans that reimburse providers based on their billed charges for medical-care services in return for payment of a monthly premium by the enrollee.
- *Preferred provider organizations* (PPOs)— are organized by either insurers or providers themselves who have agreed to provide health-care services on a negotiated-fee schedule.
- *Health Maintenance Organizations* (HMOs)—provide a defined, comprehensive set of health services to a group of enrollees. There are four types of HMOs (ASHA, 1996):
  - ⇒ *Staff model*—requires that all health-care providers are employees of the HMO and work at the same facility.
  - ⇒ *Group model*—involves health-care provider groups contracted with the HMO to provide services either in their own offices or company facilities.

- ⇒ *Individual Practice Associations* (IPAs)—involve a group of health-care practitioners with whom an HMO has contracted to provide services in their own offices.
- ⇒ *Networks contract*—with HMOs are multi-speciality groups of individual practitioners in a wide geographic area who service a large population of enrollees.

The most common HMO arrangement for audiologists is the network (Johnson & Danhauer, 1999). There are two types of networks: (1) *vertically integrated networks* and (2) *horizontally integrated networks* (Klontz, 1997). Vertically integrated networks involve different types of associated providers (e.g., physical therapists, speech-language pathologists) who provide a continuum of care (Klontz, 1997). Horizontally integrated networks are formed when providers in the same profession combine over a geographic area (Klontz, 1997). Audiologists have affiliated with horizontally integrated networks such as *HEARx*, *National Ear Care Plan*, and *Sonus*. The corporate structure of these entities have changed and will continue to do so over time.

Physicians were introduced to managed care nearly 20 years ago (Casey, 1995). Dental and vision plans have been included as benefits by HMOs to entice individuals to enroll in their organizations (Casey, 1995). For quite some time, HMOs have been applying to the Health Care Finance Administration (HCFA) to provide Medicare services to the elderly population, which sometimes includes benefits such as "hearing plans" through subcontracting with networks of audiologists who provide an array of managed products and services (Casey & Grimes, 1997). Besides HMOs, other organizations that purchase hearing plans include: (1) employers, (2) multi-employer trust funds, (3) group-purchasing coalitions, and (4) consumer-discount organizations (Casey & Grimes, 1997). Audiology networks can be found from coast-to-coast. Hearing networks work with benefit administrators to design plans that: (1) contain overall program costs, (2) provide allowance for testing and hearing aids, (3) reduce patients' out-of-pocket expenses, (4) minimize patient costs for network development and administration, and (5) assure that audiologists deliver quality services (Charles D. Spencer & Associates, 1997).

Casey (1995) outlined the characteristics of hearing plans that ensure high quality professional care and products, as well as those plans that may be questionable. High quality hearing plans provide:

- A credentialed provider network
- Reimbursement for hearing assessments only when performed by licensed and/or certified audiologists
- A reasonable allowance toward the purchase of hearing aids
- Flexible hearing aid pricing to account for differing technologies while still providing significant discounts
- Freedom for enrollees and audiologists to select appropriate technologies, regardless of brand

Questionable hearing plans may include:

- "Free" hearing testing by individuals whose qualification may vary widely
- Use of "mail order" hearing aid companies
- Use of single-brand dispensers
- Little or no allowance for purchasing hearing aids
- Managing hearing aid costs through discounts from overly inflated "suggested retail" prices
- Limiting patients to the least expensive hearing aid circuitry and features

Increasingly, managed care is having an impact on private-practice audiologists (Johnson & Danhauer, 1999). As a result,

many audiologists view managed care with caution, suspicion, and fear (Casey, 1995). Private-practice audiologists face the dilemma of either affiliating with a network or remaining independent practitioners (Danhauer, 1998). Affiliated audiologists should expect to discount their products and services, face restrictions on testing (e.g., billable codes), and deal with lots of paperwork (Casey & Grimes, 1997). On the other hand, they should not have to tolerate unethical practices, an inability to do basic testing, being asked to provide services "for free," or the placement of severe restrictions on hearing aid technology (Casey & Grimes, 1997). Ormsby, Sawyer, and Benziger (1997) stated that good networks provide audiologists the following allowances:

- Negotiation for professionals
- Education of the managed-care organization (MCO) regarding audiology as a profession
- Recognition of the importance of patient satisfaction
- Explanation of laws and MCO requirements
- Automation of systems necessary for efficient outcome reporting, utilization of information, standardization of services, and diagnostic capabilities
- Automation of third-party administrative services
- Freedom to take risks
- Involvement in the process of change

HEARING NETWORKS AND AURAL REHABILITATION

As discussed in Chapter 7, although more traditionally associated with aural rehabilitative audiology, outcomes measurement is important in diagnostic audiology as well. For example, through assessment of the accuracy of diagnostic test results, one hearing network was able to determine that masking and air-bone gap issues had reduced the validity of results, which was then remedied by the use of insert earphones in all affiliated centers (Northern, 2000). However, it is fundamental to the outcomes measurement process that audiologists must understand aural rehabilitation programming issues in hearing networks.

Many HMOs want audiologic testing to be capitated under the primary-care physician and to contract only for the purchase of hearing aids (Johnson & Danhauer, 1999). Indeed, many affiliated audiologists who have already discounted their products and services do not want and should not have to provide aural rehabilitation for free. The realities of today's health-care arena mandate the development of innovative aural rehabilitation support programs that are consistent with the principles of managed care across service-delivery sites (Johnson & Danhauer, 1999). We have provided in-depth treatment of this topic in our earlier text, and readers are encouraged to refer to it for further information.

Some hearing networks are just beginning to include aural rehabilitation programming for their enrollees. For example, the *HEARx* network with over 78 hearing centers in four states (i.e., Florida, New Jersey, New York, and southern California) has established a network model aural rehabilitation support program called the Hearing Education and Listening Program (H.E.L.P) that has 20,000 patients participating each year (Beyer & Northern, 2000a). In addition, during 1998, *HEARx* served 30,000 patients and dispensed more than 24,000 hearing instruments (Northern & Beyer, 1999). Over 150 *HEARx* hearing professionals function under specific clinical protocols established to ensure consistent, high quality care for all patients (Northern & Beyer, 1999). *HEARx* adheres to a 30-day, return-for-refund period for hearing instruments, which is extended to

60 days for patients who participate in the H.E.L.P. classes that consist of extensive patient education and counseling in a one-on-one tutorial environment which is then reinforced in a group orientation setting (Beyer & Northern, 2000a; Northern & Beyer, 1999). Although many audiologists may not necessarily endorse *HEARx*, we use it as an example here because it is one of few that have published information regarding both its aural rehabilitation and system-wide outcomes measurement programs.

Patient Counseling

Patients' entry into *HEARx's* H.E.L.P. begins with the hearing aid delivery, typically, a one-hour appointment in which audiologists fit and provide orientation about the care and use of the hearing aids. Duration of the appointment and/or scheduling of additional appointments depend on patients' prior experience with hearing aids and unique amplification needs. Verification of the fitting is accomplished through real-ear probe-tube microphone measurements ensuring that the hearing aids provide adequate audibility of speech signals and are comfortable for the patient (Beyer & Northern, 2000a). The client-centered (patient-centered) counseling approach is educational in focus, involving the basic care and maintenance of the instrument, individual instructions for using and acclimating to hearing aid use, and discussion about patients' identified needs and expectations (Beyer & Northern, 2000a). Patients practice basic hearing aid skills (e.g., insertion and removal) and receive a detailed user guide, operation manual, and tips on listening and adjusting to the new hearing aids (Beyer & Northern, 2000a). Approximately 48 hours after the hearing aid fitting, audiologists contact patients by telephone to discuss any patients' questions and/or problems, and either schedule an immediate appointment for necessary troubleshooting or, if all is well, a meeting for final adjustment for fit and comfort and in two-weeks a recommendation to join the *HEARx* group rehabilitation program, Hearing Education and Listening Program (H.E.L.P.) (Beyer & Northern, 2000a).

Group Aural Rehabilitation

The Hearing Education and Listening Program (H.E.L.P.), designed to assist patients optimize their hearing through the use of hearing instruments, consists of a series of three 60 to 90 minute classes with specific objectives and activities (Beyer & Northern, 2000a):

1. Class One: Getting to Know Your Hearing Aids

   Learning Objectives are to:
   a. Demonstrate an understanding of hearing loss and the goals of amplification
   b. Identify realistic expectations of hearing aids
   c. Identify the limitations of hearing aids
   d. Understand the importance of binaural amplification
   e. Initiate a comfortable and satisfying hearing aid orientation period
   f. Demonstrate an ability to insert the hearing aids, change batteries, clean the hearing aids, and utilize the telephone effectively

   During the first meeting, audiologists spend time with the new hearing aid users who are just learning about the basics of how their hearing aids work, the use of the controls, the day-to-day care and use of their instruments (e.g., general warnings about moisture, sprays, extreme temperature, and safety, as well as demonstration of

cleaning different styles of hearing aids, changing batteries, and using the telephone), and the characteristics of different types of hearing aids (e.g., different controls, switches, and knobs, as well as advantages/disadvantages of different styles), such that much of the time is spent answering questions and providing hands-on activities (Beyer & Northern, 2000a). Other discussion focuses on different types of hearing loss and handicap resulting from hearing impairment, which is facilitated by patients' review and comparison of participants' audiograms and discussion of limitations based on their personal stories involving all areas of life, in addition to goals, benefits, and limitations of amplification (Beyer & Northern, 2000a). Patients are also given workbooks that include a troubleshooting chart reviewed in class and articles that are assigned as homework (Beyer & Northern, 2000a). Although most simple difficulties of hearing aid use can be overcome during this initial meeting, patients in the hearing network system are directed back to the dispensing audiologist for solving their more complex problems and for further counseling (Beyer & Northern, 2000a).

2. Class Two: Overcoming Hearing Loss

   Learning objectives are to:
   a. Identify the psychologic ramifications of hearing loss
   b. Promote the importance of accepting hearing loss as a (usually) permanent, yet treatable condition
   c. Introduce positive and assertive coping behaviors that can assist listeners in overcoming communication hardships
   d. Provide tips and strategies for family members of hearing aid users that

will assist in overcoming communication hardships

e. Identify listening strategies that can improve communication situations

The second class begins with audiologists' review of previous class material, discussion of assigned homework (e.g., psychological response to personal testimonials), patients' and significant others' own stories of adjustment to hearing loss (e.g., stages of denial, projection, anger, depression, and acceptance), and reasons why amplification does not immediately solve all communication problems (e.g., acclimatization, poor listening habits, adverse listening environments) creating a platform for positive action rather than negative attitudes toward hearing aid use (Beyer, & Northern, 2000a). Positive action results from patients' realization that they must adopt assertive communication behaviors, including accepting responsibility for communication difficulties by openly acknowledging their hearing losses, and either directly requesting or cueing partners to change their speaking patterns to facilitate communication within an interaction (Beyer & Northern, 2000a). Participants are also taught that communication is a two-way street. Therefore, spouses and significant others are provided with their own strategies about what to do (e.g., use "clear speech" [Schum, 1997]), speak slowly, be patient, develop an understanding and empathy for those with hearing problems, and maintain a sense of humor), and what not to do (e.g., do not speak from another room, while eating or chewing, walking away, or in competition with a TV or radio) for successful communication (Beyer & Northern, 2000a).

3. Class Three: Total Communication

Learning objectives are to:

a. Identify conditions within a listening environment that can impact communication ability either positively or negatively

b. Utilize positive and assertive listening strategies to overcome communication barriers

c. Identify and utilize visual cues that will assist in communication settings

d. Promote awareness of assistive listening devices and their applications

e. Provide additional resources on hearing losses and hearing aids

The goal is for most participants to achieve a level of comfort such that they can discuss their communication difficulties with ease by the third class which focuses on individual and group exercises heightening awareness of enhancing the visual aspects of communication (e.g., utilizing situational cues in restaurants, classrooms, and homes through identification of optimal environmental conditions for communication through use of carpeting, adequate lighting, close speaker-to-listener distances, and so forth) and finer details of speechreading, facial expressions, and the contributions of non-verbal cues to understanding various speakers (e.g., comparing auditory-only with auditory-plus-visual presentations in quiet and noise) (Beyer & Northern, 2000a). In addition, audiologists demonstrate the benefits of using various assistive listening and alerting devices in the home (e.g., watching T.V. at home with the family) and in public places (i.e., coupling hearing aids to an infrared receiver at the theater) as explained in their workbook which contains additional information on the Americans with Disabilities Act (ADA, 1990). At the end of the third week, the audiologist collects data using an 8-item questionnaire, the *Hearing Aid Satisfaction Survey*, which addresses the degree of improvement in a variety of listening conditions (e.g., small group, large group, and distance) plus an overall satisfaction and comfort rating for social situations (Beyer & Northern, 2000a). The *Hearing Aid Satisfaction Survey* is an example of outcomes measurement used by hearing networks.

METHODS OF OUTCOMES MEASUREMENT IN HEARING NETWORKS

Hearing networks employ several methods of outcomes measurement. The challenge of outcomes measurement within this service-delivery model is to analyze data patterns strategically to glean assumptions regarding the network's ability to provide a system of care that results in improved communication ability and satisfied hearing aid users (Beyer, 2001). Some of the methods used by *HEARx* involving patient satisfaction include:

1. The *Hearing Aid Satisfaction Survey*
2. The exit survey
3. Analysis of patient inquiries and complaints
4. Analysis of hearing aid exchange and return rates

The Hearing Aid Satisfaction Survey

As stated earlier, the *Hearing Aid Satisfaction Survey* is a 10-item questionnaire that is administered to new hearing aid wearers. Eight items involve satisfaction in specific lis-

tening situations, while 2 questions relate to overall comfort and satisfaction (Beyer, 2001). These outcome data are important because they provide immediate feedback regarding patients who may need additional counseling or hearing aid modifications and are aggregated at the corporate office for analysis so that strategies for improved patient satisfaction can be developed (Beyer & Northern, 2000a). In addition, the corporate database allows for analysis of improvement/satisfaction ratings according to hearing aid make and technology, degree of hearing loss, and other patient-specific information in order to understand how the hearing aid dispensing protocols are working and what types of post-hearing aid training would be of most benefit (Beyer, 2001; Northern, 2000).

Beyer and Northern (2000b) analyzed the results of the *Hearing Aid Satisfaction Survey* for 1,332 patients, including 767 (58%) males and 565 (42%) females with an average age range of 70 to 79 years) (Beyer, 2001). The investigators found that 88% of the respondents reported overall satisfaction with their hearing aids and that 90% reported improved comfort in social situations. In addition, they found the highest improvement/satisfaction ratings for one-on-one conversation and listening to the TV or radio. However, lower ratings were obtained for listening on the telephone and in large groups. Furthermore, respondents showed little difference in improvement ratings based on their degree of hearing loss. Some surprising findings from the survey included lower satisfaction ratings for digital instruments compared to other programmable hearing aids. In addition, lower than expected satisfaction differences were obtained between monaural and binaural hearing aid users. Behind-the-ear and in-the-ear styles received the greatest amount of improvement with smaller styles, particularly the mini-canal versions, resulting in smaller amounts of benefit (Beyer, 2001). Hearing networks can use the results of this type of investigation for improving patient improvement/satisfaction. For example, *HEARx* increased its counseling emphasis regarding telephone and noise-related listening strategies by scheduling a 6-hour continuing education course for affiliated audiologists on improving hearing aid performance in noise (Northern, 2000).

In Chapter 10, the use of various outcome measures in aural rehabilitation was discussed without regard to the constraints of "real world" service-delivery. The most widely used outcome measures are available on the companion CD-ROM to this text. Recall that some of these measures are short, while others are extremely long requiring the use of special software for data analysis and interpretation. Readers may be wondering, "OK, so when do I get to use my COSI or APHAB as a network-affiliated audiologist?" Such measures may not be entirely feasible in these types of service-delivery models for several reasons. First, hearing networks may have hundreds of dispensing professionals who operate high-volume, active centers in which traditional hearing outcome measures add little practical benefit to their hearing aid fitting protocols in comparison to their own methods (Northern, 2000). Second, many elderly patients may not have the attentiveness to complete most self-assessment scales such as the APHAB (Northern, 2000). Third, Northern (2000) found that the COSI was too open-ended to meet the reporting requirements for managed care. Thus, although this text has advocated the use of comprehensive self-assessment scales as outcome measures, we caution that readers need to weigh the "real world" limitations of the service-delivery sites and the needs of their patients in selecting the most appropriate instruments. Private practitioners have the flexibility of using any tool appropriate for unique clinical situations. Affiliated audiologists may have to use whatever measures are specified by the corporate headquarters.

Exit Survey and Analysis of Patient Inquiries and Complaints

Hearing networks may need to design their own outcome measures as brief, pointed surveys that can be completed quickly and easily and are more efficient for use in a busy office setting. For example, the *HEARx* exit survey is a postage-paid postcard that asks patients 7 questions about their overall impression of the facility, professional staff attitudes and helpfulness, appointment-waiting time, and if they would purchase hearing aids from *HEARx* and whether they would recommend their services to others if asked (Northern, 2000). *HEARx* routinely reviews the results of the exit survey and incorporates changes suggested by the data (Northern, 2000).

HEARx has a corporate-based customer-service department that ideally responds to patient inquiries and complaints within 24 hours, with resolution occurring within 4 working days (Northern, 2000). Patient complaints are written in logs and/or called in on an 800 number (Beyer, 2001). The inquiries and complaints are tracked carefully and are analyzed for trends in training and performance issues (Northern, 2000). Data on patient complaints are reported at the dispenser, center, regional, and corporate levels so that *HEARx* can identify issues that negatively affect patient outcomes (Beyer, 2001). Unfortunately, these data are difficult to evaluate because no national or published benchmarks are available with which to compare (Beyer, 2001).

Analysis of Hearing Aid Exchange and Return Rates

Another method of outcomes measurement in hearing networks is analyzing hearing aid exchange and return rates. A *hearing aid exchange* is defined as when a patient exchanges one hearing aid for another one, whereas a *hearing aid return* is defined as a hearing aid that is delivered to a patient who later returns it for a refund. The main purpose of analyzing these data is to gain insight into factors that may influence hearing aid outcomes and understand why patients do not keep the hearing aids they purchase (Northern & Beyer, 1999).

Northern and Beyer (1999) reviewed the records from a large cohort of hearing aid sales (N = 8,372) (i.e., those who ordered and accepted delivery of hearing aids during a 4-month period in 1998) to identify characteristics about those who returned at least one hearing aid during the trial period. Analysis of the data for 634 patients (or 7.6% of the cohort) were conducted on seven factors: age, gender, degree of hearing loss, previous hearing aid use, configuration of hearing aid fitting (i.e., monaural versus binaural fitting), style of hearing aid, and technology.

Most of the hearing aid purchasers in this sample were in the 70 to 79 and 80 to 89-year-old age groups who also happened to be those patients who had the highest return rates of 39% and 36%, respectively. Northern and Beyer (1999) found that the greater the degree of hearing loss, the greater the likelihood that patients would return their hearing aid(s). In addition, 56% of the sample represented previous hearing aid users who had a return rate of 9% as compared to 7% for new hearing aid users (44% of the sample). Surprisingly, those patients fit binaurally had a return rate of 10% compared to 5% for those with monaural fittings. Regarding style, the largest percentage of returns was for in-the-ear (ITE) (32%) and in-the-canal (ITC) (30%) styles, a direct result of the proportion of those styles sold. However, when return rates were compared to total sales, Northern and Beyer (1999) found that completely-in-the-canal (CIC) styles were twice as likely to be returned (15%) as behind-the-ear (BTE) (9%), ITC (8%), and ITE

(6%) styles. Similarly, analysis of return rates by technology showed that the more "high-tech" programmable/digital hearing aids accounted for 62% of the returns, followed by compression (AGC and K-AMP) (27%), and linear (11%) circuits. Northern and Beyer (1999) advised that these results must be interpreted with two caveats in mind. First, *HEARx* has a large number of managed-care contracts that require no co-pay for linear hearing aids, making them essentially free for enrollees. Thus, it was not likely that patients would return something given for free. Second, the high return rates for the high-technology circuitry resulted more from total sales rather than inherent limitations of the circuitry. For example, the highest return rates were found for programmable/digital instruments, the most popular technology dispensed by *HEARx*. It is important to note that not all networks or private practitioners would agree with these return rates and the causes posited here. It should be noted though that several other factors might have contributed to higher returns for the high-technology hearing aids. One possibility may relate to the particular type of products sold; not all digital devices are the same, for example. Another possibility may relate to the skill of those fitting the devices or possible limitations in service delivery in a hearing network. Through outcomes measurement, hearing networks can analyze these data as part of a corporate-wide quality improvement program.

What value is the analysis of hearing aid return rates as outcomes measurement? The study of hearing aid return rates can be useful to hearing networks for at least three reasons. First, return rates of hearing aids can serve as an overall quality indicator for network benchmarks. For example, patients may respond favorably on the exit and *Hearing Aid Satisfaction Surveys*, yet return one or both hearing aids. Therefore, the ultimate measure of satisfaction may be whether patients keep their hearing aids. Second, hearing networks should compare their return rates to those reported within the industry. For example, Northern and Beyer (1999) compared their results to return rates reported by manufacturers to the Hearing Industry Association (HIA) and found similar results regarding return rates by style of hearing aid reported in a recent *Hearing Journal* review (Kirkwood, 1999). Third, analysis of return rates provides networks with insights into areas in need of service-delivery improvement. For example, in response to high return rates for programmable instruments, Northern and Beyer (1999) hypothesized that counseling patients regarding realistic expectations of hearing aid use, improving methods of adjustment, and reducing the co-pay may reduce these return rates.

IMPORTANCE OF OUTCOMES MEASUREMENT TO HEARING NETWORKS

Many states require hearing networks, as other managed-care groups, to obtain national accreditation from independent organizations, such as the Joint Commission on the Accreditation of Healthcare Organizations (JCAHO) or the National Committee for Quality Assurance (NCQA) (Northern & Beyer, 1999). JCAHO is one of the major private health-care standards setting organizations (Gallagher, 1998) and has standards for and conducts surveys of (Hicks, 1998):

- Hospitals
- Non-hospital based psychiatric and substance abuse organizations
- Long-term care organizations
- Home-care organizations
- Ambulatory-care organizations
- Pathology and clinical laboratory services
- Health-care networks

JCAHO (1996) has established performance-based, functionally organized standards that provide a framework for providing optimal care and continuous quality improvement requiring outcomes measurement (Hicks, 1998). Hearing networks must keep abreast of current accreditation standards of JCAHO and other bodies, such as the NCQA which was formed nearly 10 years ago with the assistance of HMOs to examine, rate, and compare plans emphasizing continuous quality review and collection of outcome data (Gallagher, 1998). Although accreditation with the NCQA is voluntary, hearing networks that achieve the NCQA's highest rating can obtain a favorable position when competing with other networks for managed-care contracts (Gallagher, 1998). Accreditors such as JCAHO and NCQA stress assessment of adverse outcomes, and response to patient complaints and management of hearing aid returns and exchanges (Northern, 2000). Another important entity is the Health Care Financing Administration (HCFA), a division of the U.S. Department of Health and Human Services, which oversees the operations of Medicare HMOs and requires organizations to submit performance data regularly and demonstrate continued concern for quality improvement (Gallagher, 1998; Northern, 2000).

IMPLEMENTATION AND LIMITATIONS OF OUTCOMES MEASUREMENT IN HEARING NETWORKS

In previous chapters, we addressed the role of local, state, and national mechanisms for outcomes measurement in various areas of practice, such as early hearing detection and intervention (EHDI) programs. Effective and efficient hearing networks must find a way to collect outcome data and use the results to improve service delivery for their patients.

Readers may be wondering why Chapter 10 devoted so much discussion to the appropriate use of outcomes measurement in aural rehabilitation in terms of the selection of the most appropriate tools, psychometric criteria, and so forth. At that point, our discussion of outcomes measurement in various areas of practice was more general and without regard to limitations of specific service-delivery sites and models. Yet for the sake of practice in the real world, the type of practitioner, the populations served, and the constraints imposed by the specific service-delivery site dictate the use of outcome measures. Obviously, the use of traditional outcome measures may not be conducive for every clinical situation. It may be better to collect some data that are corporate-specific than to not participate in outcomes measurement at all. For example, *HEARx*, has all but abandoned many, if not all, the instruments presented in previous chapters. Regardless of its motivation, *HEARx* found a way to incorporate outcomes measurement for its purposes. Therefore, a discussion of the implementation and limitations of outcomes measurement in hearing networks for readers who may practice under other service-delivery models is warranted.

The implementation of outcomes measurement usually requires a quality assurance program, computer-based data management system, and a commitment of resources. As part of an overall quality assurance program, an accreditation team or committee is needed to (Hicks, 1998):

- Review standards of accrediting agencies on an ongoing basis to keep up-to-date
- Conduct self-assessments to determine the organization's accreditation readiness
- Develop plans for areas needing remediation and follow-up until those areas have improved
- Search the marketplace for information on outcomes measurement

- Provide input on accrediting agencies' requests for standards development and outcomes measurement
- Identify new accreditation organizations and their requirements

For example, *HEARx* has a quality assurance department that aggregates information from each of its outcome measures (e.g., *Hearing Aid Satisfaction Survey* and other assessments) that would not be possible without a full commitment of the network's time, money, and computer-based data management system (Northern, 2000). In Chapter 5, we discussed the important role of computer-based data management systems in outcomes measurement processes requiring collecting, manipulating, analyzing, and interpreting data from hundreds of thousands of patients on an on-line and ongoing basis from coast-to-coast. For example, *HEARx* monitors activities from all its centers via computer into the proprietary data management system which is downloaded to the corporate office daily (Northern, 2000). The quality assurance department, having access to a large patient sample, can ask questions for impromptu quality improvement studies (Northern, 2000). The computer-based data management system is dynamic and permits necessary modifications for moving forward with the network. Many of the processes have been designed to meet managed-care and health-care requirements that can be disseminated through quarterly performance reports developing training plans and insight into clinical protocols (Northern, 2000).

Aside from the positive aspects, outcomes measurement in hearing networks can have some limitations. Unfortunately, fewer than 20% of patients bother to complete even a short questionnaire or call in to register a complaint (Beyer, 2001). Furthermore, because networks such as *HEARx* conduct their own outcomes measurement, there may be little or no opportunity for peer review of service delivery, which can cast doubt on the credibility of reported results. However, similar problems exist with manufacturer-generated investigations of device efficacy. Patients must trust that *HEARx* and other hearing networks' primary impetus for outcomes measurement is to provide the best patient care possible through appropriate application of valid data. Similarly, comparison of specific networks' outcome data to those of outside organizations, consumer groups, manufacturers, or other suppliers may be difficult because of different sampling procedures, questions asked, and terminology used by other groups (Northern, 2000). For example, if a network tracks a cancelled hearing aid differently from a returned hearing aid, then comparisons to manufacturers' data may be problematic because these activities may be perceived as being separate events (Northern, 2000). Successful outcomes measurement requires at least some standardization of all aspects of audiologic practice (from training programs to the forms used by the practitioner) and widespread patient participation in the outcomes measurement process. For example, if some network-affiliated audiologists disregard the use of outcome measures in their specific offices because patients do not like filling-out forms, then the entire quality assurance program can be compromised. Thus, a network's quality assurance programs work only if affiliated hearing professionals believe in the process and make completion of these measures a priority. In order to increase compliance, some networks such as *HEARx* have not only reduced the length of their surveys, but also tried other techniques from telephone surveys to promising gifts for patient partici-

pation (Northern, 2000). Obviously, large networks have considerable leverage over their affiliated audiologists and can easily get them to participate in quality assurance efforts. In summary, in spite of some obvious limitations, hearing networks can include outcomes measurement as part of their ongoing quality assurance programs. Doing so shows that outcome measures can be implemented in the real world to enhance performance for the network, affiliated audiologists, and patients. In this way, outcomes measurement is a "win-win" situation.

SUMMARY

This chapter is the first in this section of this textbook concerned with outcomes measurement across service-delivery sites. In reality, outcomes measurement in hearing networks does not often occur exactly as described in the more theoretically based chapters of this book. Nevertheless, readers can benefit from understanding audiologists' participation in hearing networks, considering aural rehabilitation programming in hearing networks, learning about methods of outcomes measurement in a specific hearing network, acknowledging the importance of outcomes measurement to hearing networks, and comprehending the implementation and limitations of outcomes measurement in hearing networks. The most important point for readers to take from this chapter is that outcomes measurement is valuable only if the results are used to improve patient satisfaction and quality of life regardless of the service-delivery model.

LEARNING ACTIVITIES

- Contact all hearing networks and inquire about their quality assurance programs and use of outcome measures.

RECOMMENDED READINGS

Beyer, C.M. (2001). Tools of the trade: How to obtain meaningful patient data and outcomes. *Advance for Audiologists, 3*(2), 54, 56, & 78.

Beyer, C.M., & Northern, J.L. (2000). Audiologic rehabilitation support programs: A network model. *Seminars in Hearing, 21*(3), 257–265.

Northern, J.L. (2000). Page ten: Patient satisfaction and hearing aid outcomes. *The Hearing Journal, 53*(6), 10, 12, 14, & 16.

Northern, J.L., & Beyer, C.M. (1999). Hearing aid returns analyzed in search for patient and fitting patterns. *The Hearing Journal, 52*(7), 46, 48–49, & 52.

REVIEW EXERCISES

Fill-in-the-Blank

Instructions: Please fill-in-the-blanks with the correct terms from the word bank below.

1. _____ _____ _____ provide a defined, comprehensive set of health services to a group of enrollees.

2. _____ _____ requires that all health-care providers are employees of the HMO.

3. _____ _____ involves health-care provider groups contracted with the HMO to provide services either in their own offices or company facilities.

4. _____ _____ _____ involve a group of health-care practitioners with whom an HMO has contracted to provide services in their own offices.

5. _____ contract with HMOs and are multi-specialty groups of individual practitioners in a wide geographic area who service a large population of enrollees.

6. _____ _____ _____ involve different types of associated providers (e.g., occupational therapists, physical therapists, and speech-language pathologists) who provide a continuum of care.

7. _____ _____ _____ are formed when providers in the same profession combine over a geographic area.

8. A _____ _____ _____ is defined as when a patient exchanges one hearing aid for another one.

9. A _____ _____ _____ is defined as a hearing aid that is delivered to a patient who later returns it for a refund.

Word Bank:
Group model
Health maintenance organizations
Hearing aid exchange
Hearing aid return
Horizontally integrated networks
Networks
Staff model
Vertically integrated networks
Individual practice associations

ANSWERS

Fill-in-the-Blank:
1. Health maintenance organizations
2. Staff model
3. Group model
4. Individual practice associations
5. Networks
6. Vertically integrated networks
7. Horizontally integrated networks
8. Hearing aid exchange
9. Hearing aid return

REFERENCES

American Speech-Language-Hearing Association. (1996). *Curriculum guide to managed care.* Rockville, MD: Author.

Americans with Disabilities Act. (1990). Americans with Disabilities Act of 1990. Public Law 101-336, 42, U.S.C. 12101 et seq: *U.S. Statutes at Large, 104*, 327–378 (1991).

Beyer, C.M. (2001). Tools of the trade: How to obtain meaningful patient data and outcomes. *Advance for Audiologists, 3*(2), 54, 56, & 78.

Beyer, C.M., & Northern, J.L. (2000a). Audiologic rehabilitation support programs: A network model. *Seminars in Hearing, 21*(3), 257–265.

Beyer, C.M., & Northern, J.L. (2000b). *Hearing aid satisfaction by hearing aid technology.* Poster presentation at the Twelfth Annual Convention of the American Academy of Audiology, Chicago, IL.

Casey, P. (1995). Viewpoint: Managed care and dispensing audiology ... To play or not to play. *Audiology Today, 7*(3), 17–18.

Casey, P. (1997). Meeting the challenges of managed care. *The Hearing Journal, 50*(6), 32–34.

Casey, P., & Grimes, A.M. (1997*). Enhancing your audiologic practice.* A preconvention workshop of the Ninth Annual Convention of the American of the Academy of Audiology, Ft. Lauderdale, FL.

Charles D. Spencer & Associates, Inc. (1997, January). Managed hearing care plan offers employers low-cost way of enhancing health benefits. *Employee Benefit Plan Review,* January, 1997.

Danhauer, J.L. (1998). Who are those major multi-office audiology groups moving in on us, and—Is this town big enough for the both of us? *Audiology Today, 10*(2), 47–51.

Gallagher, T.M. (1998). National initiatives in outcomes measurement. In C.M. Frattali (Ed.), *Measuring outcomes in speech-language pathology* (pp. 527–557). New York, NY: Thieme.

Griffin, K.M., & Frazen, M. (1993). A managed care strategy for practicioners. In C.M. Frattal; (Eds.), *Quality improvement digest; Current information on issues related to managed care.* (pp. 1–7). Rochville, MD: American Speech-Language-Hearing Association.

Hicks, P.L. (1998). Outcomes measurement requirements. In C.M. Frattali (Ed.), *Measuring outcomes in speech-language pathology* (pp. 28–49). New York, NY: Thieme.

Johnson, C.E., & Danhauer, J.L. (1999). *Guidebook for support programs in aural rehabilitation.* Clifton Park, NY: Delmar Thomson Learning.

Joint Commission on Accreditation of Healthcare Organizations. (1996). *Comprehensive accreditation manual for hospitals.* Oakbrook, IL: Author.

Kirkwood, D.H. (1999). In '98 hearing aid market hit new highs, but growth slowed. *The Hearing Journal, 52*(1), 21–31.

Klontz, H. (1997). Managed care 101: A primer on whats, whys, and hows. *The Hearing Journal, 50*(6), 26, 28–29.

Northern, J.L. (1997). Quality managed care: It's not an oxymoron. *The Hearing Journal, 50*(6), 35, 38, & 40.

Northern, J.L. (2000). Patient satisfaction and hearing aid outcomes. *The Hearing Journal, 53*(6), 10, 12, 14, & 16.

Northern, J.L., & Beyer, C.M. (1999). Hearing aid returns analyzed in search for patient and fitting patterns. *The Hearing Journal, 52*(7), 46, 48–49, & 52.

Ormsby, M., Sawyer, D., & Benziger, L. (1997). Managed care: Open the window of opportunity! *The Hearing Journal, 50*(6), 42, 43–44.

Schum, D.J. (1997). Beyond hearing aids: Clear speech training as an intervention strategy. *The Hearing Journal, 50*(10), 36–38, 40.

Seppala, T. (1995). Health-care reform: Issues for audiologists. *Audiology Today, 7*(3), 19–20.

CHAPTER 12

Outcomes Measurement for Health- and Long-Term Residential Care Facilities for the Elderly

LEARNING OBJECTIVES

This chapter will enable readers to:

- Recognize the types of housing available for the elderly
- Define aural rehabilitation support programs
- Discuss the importance of and methods for outcomes measurement in long-term residential care facilities for the elderly and rehabilitation hospitals

INTRODUCTION

The number of individuals aged 65 years and older is expected to increase dramatically during the next 30 years, intensifying the need for access to affordable housing and health care. In many communities, housing for the elderly seems to be expanding, preparing for the change in demographics of the population. Senior citizens and their families have several (although all may not be equally attractive) options for *independent* (e.g., senior apartments, retirement hotels, subsidized housing, small group/supportive housing, and matched housing), *semi-independent* (e.g., assisted living facilities),

and dependent (e.g., nursing homes, skilled nursing facilities, extended-care homes, and continuing-care retirement communities) living. In addition, senior citizens need easy access to quality health care.

Unfortunately, in the past few years, elderly persons with shrinking HMO coverage and increased premiums have been frequent topics for sad stories in the newspapers and on nightly television news. More and more, we are witnessing conflicts between profit margins and quality of care for the elderly, regardless of whether facilities are managed by private, corporate, or non-profit structures. For example, several long-term residential care facilities for the elderly in Santa Barbara County, California were recently monitored for numerous infractions of standards of quality care for residents. Lawsuits and inquisitions about the alleged neglect of the elderly made the daily headlines and prompted investigation of every facility in the county resulting in closure in some cases.

One local newspaper article noted that a recent federal report was (Kienzel, 2001; p. 25), "... enough to scare you out of getting old. Surprisingly, it doesn't matter how rich you are, it doesn't matter which facility you pick ... you really can't escape the systematic problems that beset the long-term care industry: Not one of the nursing homes in our area was found to be in substantial compliance with regulations."

Facility administrators cite low profits, high costs, and the lack of qualified staff as reasons for a declining quality of care. However, the average wage for nursing-home staff is only about $9.00 per hour without benefits, and meals for residents cost about $2.84 per day. Moreover, present state and federal programs pay long-term residential care facilities approximately $180.00 per day per resident, regardless of the level of care required for the resident. A nationally known corporation that reported recent annual earnings of $1.97 billion owns several of the targeted facilities. Thus, if the $94 billion long-term care industry is so lucrative, why are the standards of care so low (Kienzel, 2001)?

Medicare caps on rehabilitation services experienced in the 1990s might be just a preview of the future limitations of these services as an over-extended health-care system attempts to provide for an unprecedented number of senior citizens (Johnson & Danhauer, 2000). Indeed, in order to provide quality hearing health-care services to the elderly in the new millennium, audiologists must take a proactive approach by develop-

ing innovative service-delivery models and demonstrating their effectiveness through outcomes measurement. For example, Johnson and Danhauer (1999) advocated the use of aural rehabilitation support programs in residential facilities for the elderly. Accreditation of these facilities requires documentation of continuous quality improvement of all relevant services including aural rehabilitation support programs. The purpose of this chapter is to describe the importance and methods of outcomes measurement of aural rehabilitation support programs in long-term residential care facilities for the elderly.

HEALTH- AND LONG-TERM RESIDENTIAL CARE FACILITIES FOR THE ELDERLY

(Adapted from Careguide Available Internet: www.careguide.com)

Elderly persons may find themselves in various health-care facilities and housing situations during their "golden years." Health-care facilities and housing are not mutually exclusive entities, but are merged in some situations to meet the needs of their residents. For example, a healthy, vibrant couple in their early 80s may choose to live in a golf community surrounded by much younger neighbors. On the other hand, another couple of the same age may require living in a continuing-care community that can accommodate their increasing health-care needs. Therefore, the level of independence of the residents who may be completely self-sufficient or need semi-dependent or dependent care can best describe housing for the elderly. In addition, many elderly persons may find themselves admitted to a rehabilitation hospital for a short period of time after some traumatic injury or cerebral vascular accident (CVA). Housing options for the elderly and rehabilitation hospitals are described below.

Housing Options for the Elderly

Independent Living Options

Independent living options include: senior apartments, retirement hotels, subsidized housing, small group/supportive housing, or matched housing.

Senior apartments—provide homes for individuals or couples, offering residents meals, housekeeping, and a variety of social, recreational, and cultural programming. Medications for residents may be dispensed on a case-by-case basis. However, no hospital or 24-hour-care facility is available on the premises. Requirements for residents include mobility and self-care skills. Often, monthly fees cover rent only, with an extra charge for meals and other services. Seniors and their families should consider that a prolonged illness or an inability to care for oneself necessitates moving to another facility offering a greater level of care. Obviously, the quality of facilities varies along with the types of services provided requiring a thorough investigation of all options.

Retirement hotels—provide furnished or unfurnished rooms with private or shared baths with the possibility of meals, maid, and/or linen services. Retirement hotels have few if any social programming. Dispensing of medications and other medical services varies by facility. Like the senior apartments, requirements for residents include mobility and self-care skills. Monthly fees cover rent only, with an extra charge for additional services. Again, seniors and their families should consider that a prolonged illness or inability to care for oneself requires moving.

Subsidized housing—provides state or federally funded low-income apartments for individuals or couples. Subsidized housing facilities usually provide between one-to-three meals a day, housekeeping, and some social, recreational, and cultural programs. Unfortunately, there are usually no hospitals or 24-hour-care facilities on the premises. Requirements for residents include being at least 62 years of age, specified income level, and ability to care for oneself. A monthly fee covers rent, meals, and programs. Considerations for seniors and their families are the existence of long waiting lists and no medical care.

Small group/supportive housing—usually sponsored by religious or advocacy groups, provides a shared home for 5 to 20 residents who do all of the cooking and housekeeping chores under the direction of full-time, live-in housekeeping managers. Requirements for residents include mobility, self-care skills, and the ability to do some household chores. Rent is paid monthly and residents must share in household expenses (e.g., power and phone bills). Considerations for seniors and their families involve, at first, living with strangers, which can be challenging, but residents often take care of each other once acquainted. Furthermore, a prolonged illness or the inability to care for oneself necessitates moving.

Matched housing—involves seniors staying in their own homes and providing room and board to a younger individual in exchange for assistance with household help. These situations are arranged privately and must be approached cautiously. For example, seniors and their families must consider that it may be difficult locating and trusting an individual to share one's home; however, if an appropriate match can be made, such arrangements can be beneficial to both parties. It is always wise for family members to monitor how the match works over time.

Semi-independent Living

Assisted living facilities—are licensed facilities that range from large private homes to converted hotels with apartments with shared dining rooms, with nurses on the premises. These facilities provide rooms with a private or shared bath, all meals, house-keeping, social programming, assistance with daily living needs (e.g., bathing, dressing, and other routine functions), and varying medical services. Requirements for residents include a monthly fee and the ability to live without skilled nursing or 24-hour care. Seniors and their families should be relieved to know that if the need for personal assistance increases, help is available on site. However, a prolonged illness may require moving to a nursing home. They should also consider that Medicare or Medicare funding does not pay for these living facilities, but that Medicaid may be available for a few facilities in some states.

Dependent Care

Nursing homes—(e.g., skilled facilities and extended-care homes) are licensed to provide private or semi-private rooms with a bath, skilled nursing care 24 hours a day, all meals, and social and cultural programming. In addition, assistance with eating, bathing, and grooming is provided, and medications are dispensed. Requirements for residents include a need for 24-hour skilled nursing care or rehabilitative services. Seniors and their families must consider that this housing option is expensive (i.e., daily fee that is billed monthly), but that Medicaid or Medicare generally takes over the payments for individuals who no longer can afford to pay.

Continuing-care retirement communities—provide rental or condominium apartments for individuals or couples in a community where residents may remain for the rest of their lives with hospital and nursing-home-care facilities and 24-hour care, as needed. Requirements for residents include good health when entering the community, and payment of a high entrance fee and monthly maintenance. Seniors and their families should consider that although very expensive, this option provides the most flexibility with no need of moving because of a prolonged ill-

ness or inability to care for oneself. In addition, as seniors' needs change, all levels of care are available. For example, couples can maintain their apartment in case one spouse falls and breaks a hip requiring occupational therapy and 24-hour nursing care.

Rehabilitation Hospitals

Traumatically injured adults are usually sent to acute-care hospitals until their conditions stabilize, and then are admitted to rehabilitation hospitals for therapy. Rehabilitation begins when a nurse liaison visits patients and their families in the acute-care hospitals to assist in the transition for admission to the rehabilitation hospital, where the elderly can stay for up to several weeks. Patients stay in private or semi-private rooms and undergo rigorous therapies (e.g., speech-language pathology, occupational therapy, and/or physical therapy) in preparation for returning home and to work. Aural rehabilitation support programs can assist in maximizing patients' benefit from these therapies.

AURAL REHABILITATION SUPPORT PROGRAMS

Aural rehabilitation support programs are innovative service-delivery models that meet the hearing health-care needs of patients in long-term residential care facilities for the elderly and rehabilitation hospitals in a cost-efficient manner that is consistent with many of the principles of managed care (Johnson & Danhauer, 1999; 2000). Discussion of the implementation of these programs is beyond the scope of this textbook, but readers are referred to Johnson and Danhauer (1999) for a detailed description of and materials for that purpose. Nevertheless, an understanding of the characteristics and limitations of these programs is a prerequisite for acknowledging the importance of and developing a program for outcomes measurement.

Regardless of the setting, aural rehabilitation support programs have several common characteristics. First, support programs assist in meeting the daily hearing needs of the elderly within residential health-care facilities that usually do not have an audiologist employed on site (Johnson & Danhauer, 1999; 2000). Second, audiologists usually contract with these facilities to meet direct hearing health-care needs of patients and to manage these support programs; they either bill the facility, patients' insurance, or the patients and/or their families themselves for services provided (Johnson & Danhauer, 1999; 2000). Third, support programs are consistent with many of the principles of managed care and can fit easily within the continuum of activities and/or medical services of these facilities (Johnson & Danhauer, 1999; 2000). For example, support programs should coordinate among practitioners, be applied at the appropriate consistency, adhere to practice guidelines, cost the least amount possible, be monitored under resource management, and achieve positive patient outcomes (ASHA, 1996). Fourth, successful support programs undergo a continuous cycle of development, planning, and evaluation requiring ongoing data collection, analysis, and interpretation as part of a comprehensive quality assurance program (Johnson, Benson, & Seaton, 1997; Johnson & Danhauer, 1999; 2000). Fifth, audiologists require at least 3 types of skills to manage all aspects of successful support programs (Bodenhemier, 1994; Johnson, et al., 1997; Johnson & Danhauer, 1999; 2000):

1. Technical skills
   a. Knowledge of preferred practices and guidelines for care across service-delivery sites
   b. Knowledge of state and federal laws mandating communication accessibility
   c. Knowledge of administrative issues specific to service-delivery site including budgeting
   d. Clinical expertise in effective service delivery across settings

2. Human-relations skills
   a. "Personality skills" needed to work effectively with administrators, other professionals, and support personnel to execute short-term and long-term goals
   b. Leadership skills
   c. Support-personnel policy development skills
   d. Ability to gain respect of support personnel
   e. Good communication skills (written, oral, and listening)
   f. Flexibility

3. Conceptual skills
   a. Ability to perform a systematic analysis of service-delivery sites to specify program needs
   b. Ability to understand the importance of support-program components for prioritization of needs
   c. Ability to predict future program needs (i.e., visioning)
   d. Ability to stress the importance of support programs to administrators, other professionals, and support personnel
   e. Ability to market support programs

Support programs also have several limitations. First, support programs should augment, not substitute for, ongoing comprehensive diagnostic and rehabilitative audiologic service delivery. Second, support programs are not to be provided "free of charge." Audiologists should be wary about administrators of facilities who are not at least willing to provide some "start-up" support. Third, once established, support programs are not completely self-sustaining and require ongoing support to cover patient-related costs, replace necessary materials, and meet human-resource requirements.

Aural Rehabilitation Support Programs in Long-Term Residential Facilities for the Elderly

Many audiologists choose not to practice in long-term residential care facilities for the elderly because services often must be provided on site, in less than pleasant conditions, with no guarantee of reimbursement, and with little cooperation or assistance from administrators, nursing staff, residents, or family members (Johnson & Danhauer, 1999). Unpleasant sights, sounds, and smells, and cries of pain and loneliness often greet the audiologist at the door (Johnson & Danhauer, 1999). However, carefully planned aural rehabilitation support programs can go a long way toward improving the quality of life for these patients.

Aural rehabilitation support programs in these facilities can be simple with only a few components, or complex, offering (Shultz & Mowry, 1995):

- Comprehensive patient services
  - ⇒ Screening programs and documentation
  - ⇒ Hearing evaluations
  - ⇒ Hearing aid evaluations, fitting, repairs, and monitoring
  - ⇒ Selection, fitting, and orientation of assistive listening devices (ALDs)
  - ⇒ Cerumen management
  - ⇒ Direct consultation with residents, physicians, families, social workers, and nursing staff
  - ⇒ Weekly in-house visits and emergency services
- Facility services
  - ⇒ Ombudsman Reconciliation Act: Receptive Communication Classification-Minimum Data Set (MDS)
  - ⇒ Screening report for medical records
  - ⇒ Inservice training for nursing administrative staff and ancillary personnel
  - ⇒ Americans with Disabilities Act (ADA) recommendations and compliance verification
  - ⇒ Family lecture night series
- Special services
  - ⇒ Hospice-patient care
  - ⇒ Fundraising
  - ⇒ Hearing aid safety cords

The extent of programming depends on the type of facility and patients' (residents') needs. For example, audiologists may make monthly visits to retirement hotels to perform hearing aid checks for active, independent seniors. Alternatively, audiologists may be hired by continuing-care retirement communities to provide patient, facility, and special services to residents. However, all aural rehabilitation support programs often have the same key components. First, comprehensive screening and audiologic evaluation programs are needed to identify patients with hearing loss. Second, hearing aid monitoring programs should be in place to ensure that patients' hearing instruments do not end up lost in the laundry or in denture cups. Furthermore, levels of assistance should be established to account for patients' abilities to function with their hearing aids: independent, partial, and full assistance, and supervised use (see Johnson & Danhauer, 1999 for further explanation). Third, facilities should be communicatively accessible to patients with hearing impairment and their families. Audiologists can make simple suggestions that can enhance communication for all. Fourth, an ongoing, comprehensive inservice program ensures that all staff are prepared to serve as audiologic support personnel and communicate appropriately with residents. Fifth, audiologists need to make frequent on-site visits to these facilities and maintain communication with administrators regarding the support program and the audiologic needs of residents.

Aural Rehabilitation Support Programs in Rehabilitation Hospitals

Rehabilitation-hospital patients cannot maximally benefit from any type of therapy unless they can communicate with staff. Furthermore, patients who have a physical loss of function from accidents or CVAs may feel overwhelmed and experience some emotional reactions to their disability including, but not limited to, sadness, fear, and denial (Johnson & Danhauer, 1999). Moreover, patients may experience even greater emotional discomfort if they have sensorineural hearing loss that causes increased feelings of isolation, frustration, and disappointment, and that is associated with a higher incidence of heart arrhythmia, ischemic heart disease, hypertension, and osteoarthritis (Crandell, 1998). Clearly, undetected and unmanaged hearing loss can drive up the cost of health care and warrants the establishment of aural rehabilitation support programs in this setting.

As stated earlier, admission to the rehabilitation hospital begins with a visit from the nurse liaison to prepare patients and their families for the transition to rehabilitative care (Griffin, Clark-Lewis, & Johnson, 1997; Johnson, Clark-Lewis, & Griffin, 1998). Patients are asked about their hearing status and use of hearing aids. Those patients who believe that they have a hearing loss are identified and scheduled for a hearing screening upon admission (Johnson & Danhauer, 1999; 2000). Patients confirming existence of a hearing loss and use of hearing aids are scheduled for a hearing evaluation and hear-

ing aid check as part of their intake physicals (Johnson & Danhauer, 1999; 2000). In addition, the nurse liaison reminds patients to bring along important personal items, such as workout clothes, sneakers, and their hearing aids, for their rehabilitation programs (Griffin, et al., 1997; Johnson, et al., 1998).

Upon admission, patients with confirmed hearing loss should complete an informed-consent form prior to participation in the support program, which involves hearing screenings; audiologic evaluations; staff notification of hearing status and needs; hearing aid evaluations, fittings, checks, and monitoring; ALD and communication accessibility information; and short-term aural rehabilitation (Johnson & Danhauer, 1999; 2000). Patients can agree to participate in one or all aspects of the program. Although some patients may be sensitive, those consenting to staff notification of their hearing loss have signs placed over their beds or on their doors declaring their communication needs (Griffin, et al., 1997; Johnson, et al., 1998; Johnson & Danhauer, 1999; 2000). Thus, the staff needs training in 4 areas on how to (Johnson & Danhauer, 1999; 2000):

1. use appropriate communication tips and strategies,
2. assist with insertion/removal of patients' hearing aids,
3. check/troubleshoot patients' hearing aids, and
4. obtain an ALD for patient use during the day.

In this way, patients' immediate hearing health-care needs should be met during their rehabilitation-hospital stays, which rarely last more than two months. Long-term aural rehabilitation can begin on an outpatient basis upon discharge to home or a long-term residential care facility (Johnson & Danhauer, 1999; 2000).

IMPORTANCE OF OUTCOMES MEASUREMENT FOR AURAL REHABILITATION SUPPORT PROGRAMS

Kricos and Lesner (2000) stated that two reasons for outcomes measurement of aural rehabilitation support programs are to:

1. determine efficient allocation of health-care resources, and
2. evaluate the effectiveness of programming so that improvements in the quality of services can be made.

Audiologic services have yet to receive the same recognition as other professions (e.g., occupational therapy, physical therapy, and speech-language pathology services) in the rehabilitation industry. Without documentation, there is little or no chance for reimbursement for services by third-party payers. What must audiologists do in order to achieve this status? Some audiologists have jumped on the managed-care bandwagon by either forming or affiliating with hearing networks. Chapter 11 discussed how hearing networks, such as *HEARx*, have implemented outcomes measurement as a requirement for accreditation by important health-care organizations, a precursor to reimbursement by third-party payers. Similarly, rehabilitation hospitals and long-term residential care facilities for the elderly must also be accredited by comparable agencies.

Although different, rehabilitation hospitals and long-term residential care facilities for the elderly are often accountable to meet the outcomes-measurement requirements of the same accreditation bodies (Johnson & Danhauer, 1999). The Rehabilitation Accreditation Commission, formerly the Commission on Accreditation of Rehabilitation Facilities (CARF), is a national, non-profit organization founded in 1996 (Hicks, 1998). It is the preeminent standard-setting body that promotes the delivery of quality services to people with disabilities and those in need of rehabilitation (Hicks, 1998). The organization has placed increased importance on outcome-based program evaluations, outcome measures, and evidence of patient involvement in treatment planning (Gallagher, 1998). The accreditation standards are "national consensus standards," meaning that a wide variety of individuals (e.g., providers, consumers, and so forth), including audiologists, have a chance to provide input (Hicks, 1998).

The Joint Commission on Accreditation of Healthcare Organizations (JCAHO) was formed in 1951 as the Joint Commission on Accreditation of Hospitals by the American College of Physicians, the American Medical Association, the Canadian Medical Association, and the American Hospital Association (Gallagher, 1998). The JCAHO develops standards for hospitals, non-hospital-based psychiatric and substance abuse organizations, long-term care organizations, home-care organizations, ambulatory-care organizations, pathology and clinical laboratory services, and health-care networks (Hicks, 1998). Included in those standards are procedures for measuring quality of care and treatment outcomes (Gallagher, 1998). Although these outcome measures are not yet required for rehabilitation. ASHA has submitted measures to JCAHO's National Library of Healthcare Indicators (Gallagher, 1998). Other accreditation bodies require outcomes measurement pertaining to service delivery in these facilities, but are not discussed here.

Even more fundamental than accreditation of health-care facilities, outcomes measurement is needed to convince our own profession that aural rehabilitation support programs result in positive patient outcomes. Some audiologists believe that providing services in these facilities is a waste of time that could be better spent on patients who may show greater benefit (Schow, 1982). We need to prove that our services are effective and that we can improve the quality of life of our senior citizens in these long-term residential care facilities through aural rehabilitation? These services are valuable and worth the effort, as we have witnessed substantial improvements in patients' quality of life as a result of our efforts that have been confirmed by feedback from patients, their families, facility staff, and administrators. These programs can and do work, but outcomes measurement is critical for *proving* the effectiveness of aural rehabilitation support programs in these facilities.

OUTCOMES MEASUREMENT FOR AURAL REHABILITATION SUPPORT PROGRAMS

Kricos and Lesner (2000) stated that outcomes measurement begins with stipulating the goals of aural rehabilitation support programs. The goals of these support programs depend on the service-delivery site. For example, the goals or outcomes for patients of long-term residential care facilities for the elderly are different from those for rehabilitation-hospitals. Elderly patients often live the rest of their lives in long-term residential care facilities. The patient (resident) population is much more static and patient outcomes for support programs are to restore and maintain the highest possible level of functioning, preserve autonomy, and stabilize chronic medical conditions (ASHA, 1997; Kane, Ouslander, & Abrass, 1994). A positive outcome is one that enhances patients' quality of life through enhanced communication with the significant others in their lives. On the other hand, traumatically injured patients are admitted to rehabilitation hospitals for short periods of time with the ultimate outcome of returning to their lives in the outside world. The rehabilitation-hospital patient popula-

tion is constantly changing. In this case, the outcome of support programs is to maximize patients' communication potential so that they may optimally benefit from their individual therapy programs in a more effective and speedy fashion. Therefore, variations in patient outcomes for these facilities are reflected in their outcomes measurement programs.

Kricos and Lesner (2000) summarized 7 methods of evaluating aural rehabilitation support programs:

1. Observations by professional staff
2. Attendance patterns
3. Knowledge area tests
4. Customer-satisfaction surveys
5. Measures of hearing aid use
6. Measures of hearing aid benefit
7. Measures of hearing aid satisfaction

Observations by Professional Staff and Attendance Patterns

Observations by professional staff can be particularly useful for collecting outcome data in long-term residential care facilities for the elderly. In these facilities, hearing loss is often overlooked, undetected, or ignored. If staff members know the signs of hearing loss, patients can be targeted for screening and diagnostic procedures. Appendix XII–A, "*Nursing Home Hearing Handicap Index (NHHI),*" by Schow and Nerbonne (1977) on the companion CD-ROM has two versions:

1. Self Version (self-evaluation of hearing handicap)
2. Staff Version (evaluation of nursing-home resident's hearing handicap)

Respondents answer 10 questions, such as, "When you are with other people do you wish you could hear better?" by marking options on a 5-point scale ranging from

"Almost Never" (i.e., "1") to "Very Often" (i.e., "5"). Scores on the NHHI can range from 0 (no hearing handicap) to 100 (maximum hearing handicap). Similarly, nursing-home staff answer the same 10 questions about patients on the staff version. Observation of residents by staff using this instrument can be very useful for at least three reasons. First, nursing-home residents may have been isolated so long with a hearing impairment that they may not know the extent of their handicap. For example, the authors found that staff ratings correlated much better with patients' pure-tone averages than did the ratings by the residents themselves (McCarthy & Sapp, 2000). Second, comparisons of ratings made by residents to those of staff members can identify those patients in denial about their hearing loss. Third, the NHHI may be used as a pre- and postintervention measure following participation in the aural rehabilitation support program.

Observations by professional staff can also aid in assessing the effectiveness of hearing aid fittings and hearing aid orientation programs (HOPs). Appendix XII–B, "Hearing and Skills Checklist," found on the companion CD-ROM, is a series of questions developed by Kricos and Lesner (1997) that was adapted into a checklist by Johnson and Danhauer (1999), which staff can use when unobtrusively observing patients' ability to manage their hearing aids. For example, the checklist asks questions such as whether the patient's hearing aid is being worn and inserted into the ear correctly and so forth. Consistent with the patient outcomes for long-term residential care facilities for the elderly, effective hearing aid fitting procedures should ensure residents' independence in managing their hearing instruments. Alternatively, staff observations revealing patients' inability to manage amplification may indicate a need for participation group HOPs.

HOPs are easily implemented in long-term residential care facilities for the elderly

and have been shown to be an effective way of reducing return-for-credit rates and improving patient satisfaction with hearing aids (Abrahamson, 2000). The details of HOPs are beyond the scope of this textbook and readers are referred to Abrahamson (2000) for further information. HOPs can have two formats: instructional, and interactive groups.

Instructional groups are those in which audiologists teach participants about important topics or how to perform certain skills. For example, audiologists can use Appendix XII–B to assess whether patients can demonstrate new hearing aid management skills. *Interactive* groups are those in which group participants learn from and support each other. Assessment of the effectiveness of interactive groups is somewhat more elusive, but can be accomplished through staff use of Appendix XII–C, "Group Interaction Checklist" (Johnson & Danhauer, 1999; Kricos & Lesner, 1997) that can be found on the companion CD-ROM. For example, the checklist asks questions such as, "Is the audiologist doing no more than 30% of the talking, with 70% of the talking conducted by group participants?" to which staff respond by marking "yes" or "no." The more "yes" responses, the more effective the interactive group.

Staff observations can also be useful for assessing hearing aid benefit in patients with dementia or Alzheimer's disease. Recall in Chapter 3, it was stated that third-party payers might believe that purchasing hearing aids for patients with Alzheimer's disease (AD) is wasteful because these patients are considered to be difficult or even impossible to test (Palmer, Adams, Bourgeois, Durrant, & Rossi, 1999). Furthermore, large-scale randomized clinical trials would be difficult with this population because of the unique behavioral manifestations of the disorder within individuals and a lack of an organized health-care system to manage these patients. Thus, benefits provided by single-subject designs (flexibility across patients, behaviors, and service-delivery sites) are needed for efficacy studies of hearing aid treatment in patients with AD. Using a multiple-baseline single-subject design, Palmer, et al. (1999) demonstrated a reduction of caregivers' observations of negative behaviors (e.g., negative statements, forgetfulness, pacing) and an increase in patients' likelihood of participating in interactions, conversations, and awareness of environmental sounds after being fit with hearing aids. Therefore, professional staff can record both the number of social interactions and the number of problem behaviors before and after fitting hearing aids on Alzheimer's patients for outcome data.

Residents' attendance patterns to HOPs and facility-sponsored social events can also serve as outcome data for aural rehabilitation efforts. Staff can simply take attendance at all facility functions and tabulate totals for each patient at the end of each week. Pre- and postintervention attendance records at these events may be one measure of the effectiveness of aural rehabilitation support programs in reducing patients' hearing handicap. For example, a patient who shows a dramatic increase in the number of social events attended after the fitting of amplification may provide evidence that intervention reduces hearing handicap.

Knowledge Area Tests

Knowledge area tests for both audiologic support personnel and patients can serve as outcome data for aural rehabilitation support programs in both long-term residential care facilities for the elderly and rehabilitation hospitals. Because audiologists must rely on other professionals to serve important roles in their programs, inservice training is very important to teach necessary knowledge and skills to audiologic support personnel. For example, all staff need to be trained to observe residents' communication behaviors

and assist in the management of hearing aids. Outcome data are needed to assess the effectiveness of inservice training. Briefly, effective inservice programming has the following 11 components (Johnson & Danhauer, 1999; 2000):

1. Direction by licensed and/or certified audiologists
2. Implementation of specific support personnel selection criteria (American Academy of Audiology, 1997)
3. Definition of topics and behavioral objectives specific to assigned tasks
4. Verification that the scope and intensity of training encompass all assigned tasks
5. Confirmation that training is competency-based
6. Assurance of adequate equipment and materials
7. Provision of training in both formal and informal formats
8. Documentation in announcements, staff newsletters, letters to the administration, listing in quarterly support program reports, and so forth
9. Incorporation of the latest information and technology
10. Evaluation of inservice by participants
11. Evaluation of participants through knowledge area tests

Both evaluations by and of participants can serve as excellent outcome data for inservice programming. Participants' evaluation of inservices is important to administrators and to instructors. For example, administrators want to know if staff view inservices as worthwhile experiences. Audiologists must be cautioned that these assessments go far beyond the specific inservice experience and have much to do with the marketing of aural rehabilitation support programs from the "get-go" (readers are referred to Johnson and Danhauer [1999] for further discussion of this topic). For example, staff may negatively evaluate otherwise excellent inservices that they feel are irrelevant to their job responsibilities. In addition, participants' evaluations can provide very important information to audiologists about how to improve the inservices.

Evaluation using knowledge area tests motivates participants to pay attention and vary according to the type of inservice format. Johnson and Danhauer (1999; 2000) specified 3 inservice formats: informational, skill-based, and a combination of informational and skill-based. *Informational inservices* are those that present material in a lecture format (e.g., on topics of hearing, hearing loss, and how to communicate with residents with hearing impairment) and should be required of all staff who come into contact with residents who have hearing impairment. Knowledge area testing for this format can be accomplished via paper-and-pencil quizzes. *Skill-based inservices* are those that teach participants how to complete certain tasks using a supervised practicum format (e.g., visual and listening checks of hearing aids). Combined *informational/skill-based inservices* used both lecture and supervised practicum formats and are appropriate for those who perform visual/listening checks and troubleshoot hearing aids and ALDs. Testing for these formats should include both paper-and-pencil quizzes and demonstrations of newly learned skills. Knowledge area testing should have consequences that are enforced by administrators. For example, participants must achieve a passing mark of at least 70% or they must repeat the learning experience.

Customer-Satisfaction Surveys

Customer-satisfaction surveys are another source of outcome data for aural rehabilitation support programs in long-term residential care facilities for the elderly and rehabilitation hospitals. In health care, patients now have a major role in selection of both providers and facilities (Hicks, 1998). Therefore, documentation that facilities with aural rehabilitation support programs achieve better patient outcomes than those that do not bodes well for the future of the audiologic service provision in these service-delivery sites (Johnson & Danhauer, 1999). Indeed, today's health-care system has placed an unparalleled emphasis on meeting consumers' demands (Johnson & Danhauer, 1999). Facilities are held accountable to meet—or even exceed—consumer expectations (Rao, Blosser, & Huffman, 1998). Rao and Goldsmith (1991) identified 7 factors to compel providers, namely audiologists, to adopt consumer satisfaction as part of outcomes measurement of aural rehabilitation support programs:

1. Standards of accreditation bodies (e.g., JCAHO)
2. Industry dictate (e.g., consumer lobby)
3. Components of risk management
4. Components of institutional marketing programs
5. Components of program/service evaluation
6. Research on consumer needs/patient-care perspective
7. Components of the quality-improvement process

Audiologists must realize that consumers of aural rehabilitation support programs include not just patients, but their families, staff, administrators, and so forth. However, for patients and their families, Appendices XII–D and XII–E on the companion CD-ROM contain customer-satisfaction questionnaires for hearing support programs for both rehabilitation hospitals and long-term residential care facilities for the elderly, respectively. Audiologists can administer these questionnaires at periodic intervals in a continuous cycle of development, planning, and evaluation as part of a comprehensive quality assurance program.

Measures of Hearing Aid Use, Benefit, and Satisfaction

Measures of hearing aid use, benefit, and satisfaction can also be used as outcome data in measuring the effectiveness of aural rehabilitation support programs in long-term residential care facilities, more so than for those in rehabilitation hospitals. Recall that the fundamental patient outcomes for each of these types of facilities are different. Patients come to long-term care facilities for the "long haul" and often are there for the rest of their lives. Rehabilitation-hospital patients, on the other hand, stay for relatively short periods of time in the facility with the ultimate goal of returning home and to work. Therefore, hearing services in rehabilitation hospitals are usually short-term, perhaps first identifying the presence of hearing loss and then offering temporary solutions (e.g., ALDs) to facilitate communications between patients and their therapists. Therefore, once hearing aids are found to fit and work properly, measurements of patients' hearing aid use, benefit, and satisfaction may be more appropriate in long-term residential care facilities for the elderly than in rehabilitation hospitals.

The number of hours that appropriately fitted and functioning hearing aids are worn during the day is an indirect, yet effective, indicator of patient satisfaction (Kochkin, 1997). Patients who wear their hearing aids 4 hours or more a day for at least 1 year might be considered to be successful users (Kochkin, 1997). Direct measures of hearing disability were discussed in Chapter 10. The validity of those tools has more to do with their application rather than their inherent psychometric properties (Hyde, 2000). For example, most of these tools are more applicable to seniors who are non-institutionalized, active individuals (e.g., *Hearing Handicap Inventory for the Elderly* [HHIE: Ventry & Weinstein, 1982]). Furthermore, some of these measures may be too long (e.g., the *Communication Profile for the Hearing Impaired* [CPHI: Demorest & Erdman, 1987]) or require too much abstraction (e.g., the *Client-Oriented Scale of Improvement* [COSI: Dillon, James, & Ginis, 1997]) for use with some elderly individuals. Therefore, these measures may be more valid for facilities housing independent elderly persons living in condominiums or apartments.

SUMMARY

Audiologists have a long way to go in proving the worth of aural rehabilitation services in long-term residential care facilities for the elderly and rehabilitation hospitals. Indeed,

---

LEARNING ACTIVITIES

- Shadow audiologist who provide services in either long-term residential care facilities or rehabilitation hospitals and describe their current participation outcomes measurement, and then provide feedback regarding possible expansions in the quality assurance program.

- Review the literature and develop an outcomes measurement notebook of useful tools to use in the service-delivery sites discussed in this chapter.

that process must begin with convincing the profession that patients in these service-delivery sites can and do benefit from aural rehabilitation. As mentioned earlier, if we, as a group, do not believe in ourselves, how can third-party payers be convinced? Success requires two tasks: creativity in the development of innovative service-delivery models and outcomes measurement documenting the effectiveness of those efforts. This chapter has briefly discussed the implementation of aural rehabilitation support programs and various methods of collecting outcome data. We hope we have provided some "food-for-thought" toward accomplishing these goals.

RECOMMENDED READINGS

Johnson, C.E., & Danhauer, J.L. (1999). *Guidebook for support programs in aural rehabilitation.* Clifton Park, NY: Delmar Thomson Learning.

Johnson, C.E., & Danhauer, J.L. (2000). Aural rehabilitation support programs for adults. *Seminars in Hearing, 21,* 213–225.

Kricos, P.B., & Lesner, S.A. (2000). Evaluating the success of adult audiologic rehabilitation support programs. *Seminars in Hearing, 21,* 267–279.

REVIEW EXERCISES

Fill-in-the-Blank

Instructions: Please fill-in-the-blanks with the correct terms from the word bank below.

1. _____ _____ provide homes for individuals or couples, Ω offering residents meals, housekeeping, and a variety of social, recreational, and cultural programming.

2. _____ _____ provide furnished or unfurnished rooms with private or shared baths with the possibility of meals, maid, and/or linen services.

3. _____ _____ provides state or federally funded low-income apartments for individuals or couples.

4. _____ _____ / _____ _____ , usually sponsored by religious or advocacy groups, provide a shared home for 5 to 20 residents who do all of the cooking and housekeeping chores under the direction of full-time, live-in housekeeping managers.

5. _____ _____ involves seniors staying in their own homes and providing room and board to a younger individual in exchange for assistance with household help.

6. _____ _____ _____ are licensed facilities that range from large private homes to converted hotels with apartments with shared dining rooms and nurses on the premises.

7. _____ _____ are licensed facilities that provide private or semi-private rooms with a bath; skilled nursing care, 24 hours a day; all meals, and social cultural programming.

8. _____ - _____ _____ _____ provide rental or condominium apartments for individuals or couples in a community where residents remain for the rest of their lives with hospital and nursing-home-care facilities and 24-hour care, as needed.

9. _____ _____ are those in which audiologists teach participants about important topics or how to perform certain skills.

10. _____ _____ are those in which group participants learn from and support each other.

11. _____ _____ are those that present material in a lecture format.

12. _____ - _____
_____ are those that teach participants how to complete certain tasks using a supervised practicum format.

13. _____ / _____ -
_____ _____ use both lecture and supervised practicum formats.

Word Bank:
Assisted living facilities
Continuing-care retirement communities
Informational inservices
Informational/skill-based inservices
Instructional groups
Interactive groups
Matched housing
Nursing homes
Retirement hotels
Senior apartments
Skill-based inservices
Small group/supportive housing
Subsidized housing

ANSWERS

Fill-in-the-Blank:
1. Senior apartments
2. Retirement hotels
3. Subsidized housing
4. Small group/supportive housing
5. Matched housing
6. Assisted living facilities
7. Nursing homes
8. Continuing-care retirement communities
9. Instructional groups
10. Interactive groups
11. Informational inservices
12. Skill-based inservices
13. Informational/skill-based inservices

REFERENCES

Abrahamson, J. (2000). Group audiologic rehabilitation. *Seminars in Hearing, 21,* 227–233.

American Academy of Audiology. (1997). Position statement and guidelines of the consensus panel on support personnel in audiology. *Audiology Today, 9*(3), 27–28.

American Speech-Language-Hearing Association. (1996). *Curriculum guide to managed care.* Rockville, MD: Author.

American Speech-Language-Hearing Association. (1997). Guidelines for audiology service delivery in nursing homes. *ASHA, 39*(Suppl. 17), 15–29.

Bodenhemier, W.G. (1994). Managing a hearing conservation service. In D.M. Lipscomb (Ed.), *Hearing conservation* (pp. 273–286). Clifton Park, NY: Delmar Thomson Learning.

Careguide. (1998). Available Internet: www.careguide.com.

Crandell, C.C. (1998). Hearing aids and functional health status. *Audiology Today, 10*(4), 20–21, 23.

Demorest, M.E., & Erdman, S.A. (1987). Development of the communication profile for the hearing impaired. *Journal of Speech and Hearing Disorders, 52,* 129–139.

Dillon, H., James, A., & Ginis, J. (1997). Client-Oriented Scale of Improvement (COSI) and its relationship to several other measures of benefit and satisfaction provided by hearing aids. *Journal of the American Academy of Audiology, 8,* 27–43.

Gallagher, T.M. (1998). National initiatives in outcomes measurement. In C. Frattali (Ed.), *Measuring outcomes in speech-language pathology* (pp. 527–557). New York, NY: Thieme.

Griffin, D.J., Clark-Lewis, S., & Johnson, C. (1997). Rehabilitating patients with hearing impairments. *Outcomes: HealthSouth Corporation, 2*(4), 20–21.

Hicks, P.L. (1998). Outcomes measurement requirements. In C. Frattali (Ed.), *Measuring outcomes in speech-language pathology* (pp. 28–49). New York, NY: Thieme.

Hyde, M.L. (2000). Reasonable psychometric standards for self-report outcome measures in audiologic rehabilitation. *Ear and Hearing, 21*(Suppl. 4), 24S–36S.

Johnson, C.D., Benson, P.V., & Seaton, J.B. (1997). *Educational audiology handbook.* Clifton Park, NY: Delmar Thomson Learning.

Johnson, C.E., Clark-Lewis, S., & Griffin, D. (1998). Experience, attitudes, and competencies of audiologic support personnel in a rehabilitation hospital. *American Journal of Audiology: A Journal of Clinical Practice, 7*(2): 26–31.

Johnson, C.E., & Danhauer, J.L. (1999). *Guidebook for support programs in aural rehabilitation.* Clifton Park, NY: Delmar Thomson Learning.

Johnson, C.E., & Danhauer, J.L. (2000). Aural rehabilitation support programs for adults. *Seminars in Hearing, 21,* 213–225.

Kane, R., Ouslander, J., & Abrass, I. (1994). *Essentials of clinical geriatrics* (2nd ed.). New York, NY: McGraw Hill.

Kienzel, O.K. (2001). Not for sissies: A grim picture of our nursing homes. *The Santa Barbara Independent, 15*(741), 25–27, 29.

Kochkin, S. (1997). Subjective measures of satisfaction and benefit: Establishing norms. *Seminar in Hearing, 18,* 37–48.

Kricos, P.B., & Lesner, S.A. (1997). *Evaluating the success of hearing aid orientation programs.* Instructional course presented at the 9th Annual Convention and Exposition of the American Academy of Audiology, Ft. Lauderdale, FL.

Kricos, P.B., & Lesner, S.A. (2000). Evaluating the success of adult audiologic rehabilitation support programs. *Seminars in Hearing, 21,* 267–279.

McCarthy, P.A., & Sapp, J.V. (2000). Rehabilitative needs of the aging population. In J.G. Alpiner & P.A. McCarthy (Eds.), *Rehabilitative audiology: Children and adults* (3rd ed., pp.402–434). Philadelphia, PA: Lippincott, Williams & Wilkins.

Palmer, C.V., Adams, S.W., Bourgeois, M., Durrant, J.D., & Rossi, M. (1999). Reduction in caregiver-identified problem behaviors in patients with Alzheimer's disease after hearing aid fitting. *Journal of Speech, Language, and Hearing Research, 42,* 312–328.

Rao, P.R., Blosser, J., & Huffman, N.P. (1998). Measuring consumer satisfaction. In C. Frattali (Ed.), *Measuring outcomes in speech-language pathology* (pp. 89–112). New York, NY: Thieme.

Rao, P., & Goldsmith, T. (1991). How to keep your customer satisfied: Consumer satisfaction measure. Poster presented to the American Congress of Rehabilitation Medicine, Washington, D.C.

Schow, R.L. (1982). Success of hearing aid fittings in nursing homes. *Ear and Hearing, 3,* 173–177.

Schow, R.L., & Nerbonne, M.A. (1977). Assessment of hearing handicap by nursing home residents and staff. *Journal of the American Academy of Rehabilitative Audiology, 10,* 10–12.

Schultz, D., & Mowry, R.B. (1995). Older adults in long-term care facilities. In P.B. Kricos & S.A. Lesner (Eds.), *Hearing care for the older adult: Audiologic rehabilitation* (pp. 167–184). Boston, MA: Butterworth-Heinemann.

Ventry, I.V., & Weinstein, B.E. (1982). The hearing handicap inventory for the elderly: A new tool. *Ear and Hearing, 3,* 128–133.

APPENDIX XII-A

Nursing Home Hearing Handicap Index (NHH)

(Schow & Nerbonne, 1977)

The above-referenced Appendix can be found on the companion CD-ROM.

APPENDIX XII-B

Hearing Aid Skills Checklist

(Johnson & Danhauer, 1999; Kricos & Lesner, 1997)

(Johnson, C.E., & Danhauer, J.L. [1999]. *Guidebook for support programs in aural rehabilitation* [pp. 326]. Clifton Park, NY: Delmar Thomson Learning. © Delmar Thomson Learning. Reprinted with permission.)

The above-referenced Appendix can be found on the companion CD-ROM.

APPENDIX XII-C

Group Interaction Checklist

(Johnson & Danhauer, 1999; Kricos & Lesner, 1997)

(Johnson, C.E., & Danhauer, J.L. [1999]. *Guidebook for support programs in aural rehabilitation* [pp. 327]. Clifton Park, NY: Delmar Thomson Learning. © Delmar Thomson Learning. Reprinted with permission.)

The above-referenced Appendix can be found on the companion CD-ROM.

APPENDIX XII-D

Customer Satisfaction Questionnaire for Rehabilitation Hospital Hearing Support Programs

(Johnson, C.E., & Danhauer, J.L. [1999]. *Guidebook for support programs in aural rehabilitation* [pp. 342]. Clifton Park, NY: Delmar Thomson Learning. © Delmar Thomson Learning. Reprinted with permission.)

The above-referenced Appendix can be found on the companion CD-ROM.

APPENDIX XII-E

Customer Satisfaction Questionnaire for Hearing Support Programs in Long-Term Residential Care Facilities for the Elderly

(Johnson, C.E., & Danhauer, J.L. [1999]. *Guidebook for support programs in aural rehabilitation* [pp. 343]. Clifton Park, NY: Delmar Thomson Learning. © Delmar Thomson Learning. Reprinted with permission.)

The above-referenced Appendix can be found on the companion CD-ROM.

CHAPTER 13

Outcomes Measurement in the Public Schools

LEARNING OBJECTIVES

This chapter will enable readers to:

- Discuss the importance and challenges of outcomes measurement in the public schools
- Understand the possible effects of service-delivery model on outcomes measurement
- Implement outcomes measurement in various aspects of educational audiology

INTRODUCTION

Nightly news reports state that our public schools are in chaos. Metal detectors, police officers in the hallways, drugs, and drive-by shootings on playgrounds are all pitifully part of the reality of today's school children. Simply surviving in urban public school systems is an accomplishment in itself. Above and beyond the crime in today's schools are shrinking school budgets, teacher shortages, and the continued erosion of educational programs.

Daily visual and listening checks on children's hearing aids, while important to educational audiologists, may not be the top priority of school principals trying to keep their children in school and alive. Of course, not all school systems are in such peril and current realities of American society do not necessarily preclude the provision of adequate services to children with disabilities, including those with hearing impairment.

However, the realities of service provision to school children with hearing loss are not exactly rosy either. For example, there is a nationwide shortage of educational audiologists, and the current average audiologist-to-child (aged 3 to 21 years) ratio of 1:68,804 far exceeds the recommended ratio of 1:12,000

(Johnson, Benson, & Seaton, 1997). One wonders how the hearing health-care needs of children are being met, if at all. Audiologists providing services in this service-delivery site must be clever in devising programs that can do more with less. Effective programming requires program development, evaluation, and management. Outcomes measurement in public schools involves program evaluation, but is a waste of time unless the results are used in program development and management. The purpose of this chapter is to discuss the importance and challenges of outcomes measurement in the public schools, and the possible effects of service-delivery model on outcomes measurement and its implementation in educational audiology.

IMPORTANCE AND CHALLENGES OF OUTCOMES MEASUREMENT IN THE PUBLIC SCHOOLS

Outcomes measurement was non-existent in the schools of yesterday because public education was just assumed to be good (Eger, 1998). At that time, the school populations were fairly homogeneous and the enrollment of students with special needs was low (Eger, 1998). However, today regular education is not adequate, as evidenced by state seizure of failing local school systems and calls for widespread educational reforms, particularly in some of our largest urban areas (Amiot, 1998).

The passage of legislation, such as Public Law 94-142 or the Education for All Handicapped Children's Act of 1975, was the beginning of formal outcomes measurement in special education. Accountability has been emphasized in the business world, in the health-care arena, and now more than ever in the public schools. A focus on data-based education has prompted the development of the National Center on Educational Out-comes (NCEO) conceptual model of outcomes, which is consistent with state-identified goals and national data collection programs (Eger, 1998). Beyond the state level, an increasing national presence in policy reform is establishing Washington as a major stakeholder in education (Amiot, 1998). Furthermore, the interfacing of schools and health care has necessitated clinicians' participation in outcomes measurement through managed care, because third-party payers are interested in demonstrable functional results in relation to their costs (O'Brien & Huffman, 1998).

During the past 10 years, Congress has had some of its most spirited debate concerning students' with disabilities rights to special education services, which eventually evolved into the passage of the 1997 Amendments of the Individuals with Disabilities Education Act (IDEA, 1990) in June, 1998. That act advanced the old concept of this law (i.e., the right to an education for students with disabilities) to a new emphasis on the performance of students and accountability for their outcomes (Amiot, 1998). The American Speech-Language-Hearing Association (ASHA) has responded to these mandates for accountability through establishment of outcome and clinical trials projects in the public schools. For example, ASHA established the Task Force on Treatment Outcomes and Cost-Effectiveness (TOCE) to develop the National Outcomes Measurement System for Speech-Language Pathology and Audiology (NOMS) (see Chapters 2 and 6). NOMS is currently under the direction of ASHA's Department of Science and Research and consists of four components (Gallagher, Swigert, & Baum, 1998). Four of the components involve speech-language pathology: adults, kindergarten–12th grade (K–12: Health), kindergarten–12th grade (K–12: Education), and pre-kindergarten.

The fourth component of NOMS is the only direct application to audiology and involves universal newborn hearing screening programs (UNHS) as discussed in Chapters 5 and 6.

NOMS represents an attempt to measure outcomes at the national level in several areas of practice. School-based clinicians who participate in NOMS receive periodic reports from ASHA summarizing their data, in addition to an aggregation of data from all participating programs (Gallagher, et al., 1998). With these data, clinicians can:

- Demonstrate functional changes following receipt of speech-language pathology and/or audiology services
- Negotiate with policymakers on a more informed basis
- Meet accreditation standards that demand national comparative data
- Benchmark with local, state, regional, and national trends
- Facilitate program planning and evaluation
- Predict accurate resource utilization and impacts of program changes

Regardless of the many benefits of this system, NOMS provides some formidable challenges for outcomes measurement in the public schools. First, clinicians find that filling out all the necessary paperwork is time consuming, particularly during two peak periods of school year activity: the beginning and end (Gallagher, et al., 1998). For example, at the beginning of the school year, Entrance Forms must be completed on all children who are to receive services. Second, methods of streamlining data entry must be continually refined to meet time constraints (Gallagher, et al., 1998). Refinement of data-entry fields to a minimum data set (MDS) would reduce the time commitment for clinicians (Gallagher, et al., 1998). Third, paperwork requirements imposed by some school districts are not compatible with participation in NOMS (Gallagher, et al., 1998). For

example, unless participation in NOMS is a priority for both participating clinicians and their supervisors, outcome measurement efforts are doomed for failure. Therefore, as discussed in Chapter 11 concerning hearing networks, outcome data collection must be done effectively and efficiently within standard service delivery in the public schools (Gallagher, et al., 1998; Northern, 2000). Fourth, tracking continuity of care may be difficult when students move into or out of the school district (Gallagher, et al., 1998). If families abruptly move out of the school district, it may be difficult to evaluate the effectiveness of service delivery for those children. Fifth, the diversity of service-delivery models (e.g., numbers, variations, and combinations) in the provision of speech-language and audiology services is greater in school systems than in any other setting. In particular, the types of service-delivery models used in educational audiology can have a great effect on outcomes measurement in the public schools.

EFFECT OF SERVICE-DELIVERY MODEL ON OUTCOMES MEASUREMENT IN EDUCATIONAL AUDIOLOGY

The effect of service-delivery model on outcomes measurement in hearing conservation programs was discussed in Chapter 8. Johnson, et al. (1997) described two service-delivery models for audiologists in the public schools: *school-based* and *contract-for-service*. Some of the same issues involving hearing conservation are applicable when considering the variation in services provided by school-based and contract-for-service audiologists in the public schools. School-based audiologists are permanent employees of the school district or educational agencies in which they (Johnson, et al., 1997):

- are relatively autonomous;
- provide comprehensive services as stipulated by a job description;
- are peers to other school employees;
- are often considered as "insiders" by other school personnel;
- have very large caseloads;
- use equipment purchased and maintained by the district;
- may be more costly to the school district; and
- may be more efficient for larger school districts than smaller, rural school districts.

Alternatively, contract-for-service audiologists are hired to provide specific services by school districts or educational agencies for a specified period of time (e.g., school year) in which they (Johnson, et al., 1997):

- are completely autonomous;
- provide limited services as specified by a contract;
- are often considered as "outsiders" by other school personnel;
- have caseloads specified in a contract;
- use their own equipment (i.e., district not responsible);
- may be more cost-effective for the school district; and
- may be more efficient for smaller, rural school districts than larger school districts.

Regarding outcomes measurement, school-based audiologists may have an easier time collecting data than contract-for-service audiologists for at least four reasons. First, school personnel may cooperate with school-based audiologists (i.e., "insiders") more easily than contract-for-service audiologists (i.e., "outsiders"). School-based audiologists are more likely to enlist the participation of teachers in outcome data collection (e.g., filling out forms) than contract-for-service audi-

ologists. Second, school-based audiologists are more likely to be employed by school districts over longer periods of time, permitting year-to-year program evaluation activities that are not possible for contract-for-service audiology services which may be provided by different clinicians from year to year. Third, school-based audiologists can use outcome data for comprehensive program evaluation, whereas contract-for-service audiologists are limited to the specific services to be provided. For example, school-based audiologists can assess the effectiveness of a new amplification-monitoring program on children's classroom functioning much more easily than contract-for-service audiologists. Fourth, school-based audiologists are often employed by school districts that have adequate resources for outcomes measurement, whereas contract-for-service audiologists are usually used by smaller, rural districts to save money. For example, school-based audiologists may have a computer-based data management system available for their use, while contract-for-service audiologists may find little support from administrators for developing an outcomes-measurement system. Clearly, school-based audiologists are in a better position for participating in outcomes measurement than are contract-for-service audiologists.

Regardless of service-delivery model, outcomes measurement is still difficult because of the current realities facing educational audiologists (Johnson, et al., 1997):

- A large in-school population
- A large out-of-school population
- An increasing percentage of children and youth with disabilities requiring special education and related services
- An alarming shortage of educational audiologists
- Administrators and other educational personnel who know little or nothing about the auditory needs of students

- Limited financial resources
- Limited time for adequate service provision as mandated by federal legislation
- Federal legislation that is interpreted differently from state-to-state, district-to-district, and from professional-to-professional
- Variable commitment toward audiology services across the country
- Adaptation of a traditionally medical model of audiology that is not always cohesive in the educational milieu

Furthermore, although ASHA's NOMS K–6 educational component is reported to be assessing the effectiveness and efficiency of both speech-language pathology and audiology services, the inconsistency in service-delivery models and the challenges facing educational audiologists prevent little, if any, meaningful collaborative outcomes measurement efforts between the two professions (Gallagher, et al., 1998). How can national benchmarking occur when service delivery is so inconsistent from district to district? Moreover, how can the effects of speech-language pathology and audiologic service delivery be validated separately when measured by the same quality indicators? Thus, if any headway is to be made in improving service delivery to children and youth with hearing impairment in the public schools, audiologists must play a leadership role outcomes measurement.

OUTCOMES MEASUREMENT IN EDUCATIONAL AUDIOLOGY

How can educational audiologists champion outcomes measurement despite the realities and challenges of service delivery in today's public schools? Educational audiologists face an uphill battle when fighting for adequate service provision as mandated by federal law.

However, outcomes measurement is an integral part of that process. Acknowledging the importance of outcomes measurement is not enough. Unless involved in outcomes measurement, educational audiologists should not complain about their caseloads or the inadequacy of resources that preclude providing optimum care for school-aged children with hearing impairment. Audiologists must listen to questions posed by students, their parents, administrators, third-party payers, and other stakeholders, and provide data for those individuals having the power to make funding decisions impacting the well-being of our nation's children (Baum, 1998). In previous chapters, we have discussed the "power of one" and found that one audiologist can make a difference. The remainder of this chapter focuses on outcomes-measurement techniques in some key areas of educational audiology: program adequacy, student outcomes, amplification systems, and hearing support programs.

Program Adequacy

Chapter 8 on hearing conservation reviewed two different approaches for outcomes measurement: *outcome-based* and *prescriptive*.

The *outcome-based* approach involves assessing the efficiency, effectiveness, and/or efficacy of audiologic service delivery in the public schools. The *prescriptive* approach involves assessing the comprehensiveness of services by inventorying effectiveness indicators in key areas of educational audiologic programming. On the companion CD-ROM, Appendix XIII-A, "*IEP Checklist: Recommended Accommodations and Modifications for Students with Hearing Impairment*," (Johnson, et al., 1997) can be used to inventory critical services for students with hearing impairment in the following areas: amplification options, assistive devices, communication accommodations, physical environment accommodations, instructional accommodations, curricular modifications, evaluation modifications, and other needs and considerations. Audiologists simply check-off which accommodations are being provided and acknowledge those yet to be developed. Similarly, the companion CD-ROM contains Appendix XIII-B, "*Self-Assessment: Effectiveness Indicators for Audiology Services in the Schools*," which can be used in program assessment and planning in the following areas of practice: community/family collaboration, prevention, identification, assessment, amplification, management and habilitation/rehabilitation, and program management/development. Audiologists simply assess service provision in these areas by determining if each of the effectiveness indicators has been accomplished, is emerging, is targeted as a goal, or is not applicable. In addition, space has been provided for use during team planning meetings, for taking notes on actions (i.e., past, present, or future), planning, or for documenting any pertinent comments.

At this point, some audiologists may be wondering how these comprehensive outcomes measurement tools apply to those who provide very specific services through a contract. Are only applicable sections of these instruments to be used? For example, should contract-for-service audiologists managing amplification programs for schools only be concerned with the sections concerned with amplification in Appendices XIII-A and XIII-B? Yes, those sections are most applicable if concerned with amplification only. However, the answer is no if audiologists want to make a difference through the "power of one." As stated earlier, contract-for-service situations frequently are used by smaller, rural school districts that do not have the resources to hire a full-time audiologist. If all children with hearing impairment are ever to receive adequate services, clinicians should seize every opportu-

nity to educate administrators and school personnel on the importance of appropriate accommodations and comprehensive educational audiologic programming. Moreover, audiologists may be professionally liable if they do not at least document their attempts to advocate for better services for students in these school districts. Audiologists should not only convey the status of specific contracted services, but also document recommendations to administrators on the development of comprehensive audiologic programming ensuring appropriate accommodations and modifications for students with hearing impairment.

Student Outcomes

The IDEA stipulates that each student enrolled in special education has an Individualized Education Program (IEP) which is the contract or written record of the decisions made regarding a child's overall educational program (Eger, 1998; Johnson, et al., 1997). Details regarding federal laws and audiologists' roles in developing IEPs are not presented here and readers are referred to Johnson, et al. (1997) for further explanation. Briefly, the IEP document is a(n) (Johnson, et al., 1997):

- record of the commitment of resources for a child with a disability to receive special education and related services;
- management tool to ensure that the child's education and related services are appropriate for the student's unique learning needs;
- compliance/monitoring document used by authorized personnel from local, state, and federal levels to determine whether children with disabilities are receiving a free and appropriate public education (FAPE) as agreed by the public agency and parents; and

- evaluation device to assess whether a child is making appropriate progress toward goals.

The Colorado Department of Education has developed annual goals and short-term objectives to be used in the IEPs of children with hearing impairment so that they may develop skills that maximize their use of residual hearing (Johnson, et al., 1997). *Annual goals* are outcomes for students to achieve over the span of a school year. *Short-term objectives* are intermediary aims to be achieved toward the ultimate accomplishment of an annual goal. Table 13-1 shows some recommended annual goals and examples of related short-term objectives.

For example, students must achieve short-term goals of insertion/removal and self-monitoring of hearing aids prior to accomplishing an annual goal of independent use of amplification. In addition, short-term goals must have specific criteria (e.g., correct insertion/removal of hearing aids 8 out of 10 times) and contexts (e.g., as observed by the teacher in the classroom setting) for achievement. For example, the short-term objectives listed in Table 13–1 are incomplete without specific criteria and contexts for achievement that must be tailored to meet the needs and circumstances of each student.

With the development of EHDI programs summarized by the Joint Committee on Infant Hearing Position 2000 Statement (JCIH, 2000), audiologists must be very familiar with the requirements of Part H of the IDEA regarding services for infants with hearing impairment and their families (Roush, 2000). Similar to the IEP for older children, the Individual Family Services Plan, (IFSP) defines services for infants and toddlers (birth through age 2 years) and their families, and should (Johnson, et al., 1997):

- be flexible, focused on the family, and non-intrusive;

- involve a variety of services and supports that provide different service-delivery options for families; and
- support, enable, and empower families to use local community resources.

Part C of the IDEA states that an interdisciplinary developmental evaluation be undertaken to determine the child's level of functioning in the following areas: cognitive, physical, communicative, social/emotional, and adaptive development (JCIH, 2000). An interdisciplinary team must develop an IFSP within 45 days of receipt of a referral (Roush, 2000). The IFSP developed by the family and the service coordinator specifies needs, outcomes (i.e., annual goals and short-term objectives), intervention components, and anticipated developmental progress (JCIH, 2000). Every 6 months, the family and service coordinator review progress made toward objectives to determine the need for any modification in outcomes (JCIH, 2000). The outcomes for early intervention suggested by the JCIH (2000) were discussed in Chapters 6 and 9. Recall that the JCIH's Year 2000 Position Statement specified that infants should be enrolled in a family-centered, early-intervention program by age 6 months with qualified service providers using the family's preferred mode of communication (Roush, 2000). Except for general benchmarks regarding language development for deaf and hard-of-hearing infants identified through UNHS programs, examples of appropriate annual goals and short-term objectives for these families are rare because previously, hearing loss was rarely, if ever, identified at birth. Outcomes measurement is a critical aspect of developing practice guidelines in working with these children and their families. As discussed in Chapter 6, outcomes measurement at local, state, and national levels must be coordinated to monitor and develop realistic quality indicators for early intervention benchmarks. Existing systems

Table 13-1. Examples of annual goals and short-term objectives for IEPs of students with hearing impairment (Colorado Department of Education, 1996; Johnson, et al., 1997).

GOAL 1: THE STUDENT WILL DEMONSTRATE INDEPENDENT USE OF AMPLIFICATION (HEARING AIDS, COCHLEAR IMPLANTS, FM DEVICE, OR OTHER SYSTEM)
Short-term Objectives:
The student will:
- Arrive at school properly wearing amplification
- Correctly insert and remove amplification
- Monitor his/her own amplification
- Notify appropriate personnel when amplification is not functioning properly
- Demonstrate basic knowledge, and/or care of assistive listening device utilization
- Be responsible for the use of his/her FM system in all appropriate education situations

GOAL 2: THE STUDENT WILL DEVELOP OR IMPROVE HIS/HER AUDITORY SKILLS
Short-term Objectives:
The student will :
- Develop/improve sound awareness skills in a variety of listening situations (e.g., quiet, noise, close, distant, etc.)
- Develop/improve suprasegmental listening skills (e.g., pitch, duration, intensity, rate, etc.)
- Develop/improve vowel discrimination and identification
- Auditorally discriminate his/her name
- Develop/improve consonant discrimination and identification
- Develop/improve auditory comprehension of directions
- Discriminate common phrases
- Identify familiar language patterns
- Increase ability to answer questions about auditorally presented information

GOAL 3: THE STUDENT WILL DEMONSTRATE APPROPRIATE COMPENSATORY STRATEGIES (ACCOMMODATIONS AND MODIFICATIONS).
Short-term Objectives:
The student will:
- Explain his/her need for preferential seating
- Independently choose or request to sit in an appropriate seat
- Ask for repetition/clarification
- Utilize available clues (e.g., visual, contextual, lipreading, etc) to aid in comprehension

GOAL 4: THE STUDENT WILL DEMONSTRATE KNOWLEDGE OF HIS/HER HEARING LOSS AND RESULTING NEEDS.
Short-Term Objectives:
The student will:
- Describe the type, amount, and cause of his/her hearing loss
- Demonstrate an understanding of the benefits/limitations of amplification as they relate to his/her hearing loss

GOAL 5: THE STUDENT WILL ADVOCATE APPROPRIATELY FOR HIS/HER NEEDS.
Short-term Objectives:
The student will:
- Inform teachers of his/her hearing loss and resulting needs
- Request appropriate visual and/or supplementary materials as needed (i.e., copy of notes, film script, captioning, and so forth)
- Demonstrate and make use of appropriate assistive technology (e.g., TTY, captioner, and so forth)

---

must persevere in outcomes measurement beyond UNHS programs through to diagnosis and intervention efforts involving public school systems. For example, the UNHS component of NOMS (the only strictly audiology component) could be coordinated with the existing pre-kindergarten component of NOMS in establishing a national outcomes measurement system for early intervention programs.

Amplification Systems

FM Systems

Outcomes measurement is of little value unless incorporated into a comprehensive plan of audiologic care. Appendix XIII-C (Johnson, et al., 1997), appearing on the companion CD-ROM, includes outcomes measurement as part of the comprehensive *FM Fitting Protocol* that includes:

- Pre-selection Considerations
- Teacher Pre-evaluation
- Student Questionnaire (Pre-evaluation)
- Feature Matching
- Selection and Comparison of Devices
- Evaluation Process
- Management and Monitoring
- Teacher Post-Evaluation
- Student Question (Post-Evaluation)

Audiologists should use the *FM Fitting Protocol* (Johnson, et al., 1997) in conjunction with the new, *Guidelines for Fitting and Monitoring FM Systems* (In press), a revision of an earlier version (ASHA, 1994) completed by the ASHA Ad Hoc Committee on FM Systems. The revised version includes the latest guidelines for the fitting and monitoring of FM systems for school-aged children. In particular, these guidelines have recommendations for the latest verification methods (e.g., fitting goals for remote/local microphones) and speech perception validation methods (e.g., monitored-live-voice assessment). The "*FM Fitting Protocol*" (Johnson, et al., 1997) includes both pre-evaluation and post-evaluation student and teacher questionnaires. The teacher questionnaire inquires about auditory and behavioral concerns regarding the student. Alternatively, the student questionnaire asks about difficulty in understanding the teacher, or classmates, in noise, at far distances, or when speakers turn away. Use of these questionnaires before and after the fitting is ideal for validation of the effectiveness of the FM system from both the student's and teacher's perspectives. The *FM Fitting Protocol* has a checklist to ensure that the outcomes for the evaluation process (e.g., functional gain, probe-tube microphone measurements, 2-cc coupler measurements, and so forth) are completed, including the documentation on children's IEP regarding their present level of performance with the FM system (e.g., student uses FM system approximately 80% of the school day, 5 days a week) and a descriptive statement of the important features of the FM system (e.g., An FM system is used to provide an appropriate signal-to-noise ratio necessary for learning with hearing impairment.) under accommodations, modifications, and/or assistive technology (Johnson, et al., 1997). Audiologists must acknowledge evaluation as an ongoing process and continuously reconsider student preferences and changes in educational environment and programs. Audiologists must be sensitive to the fact that older students may insist on behind-the-ear FM receivers, instead of more cumbersome and cosmetically unappealing body-worn instruments.

The *FM Fitting Protocol* also has a management and monitoring section inventorying the orientation (e.g., hands-on demonstration) and training for the troubleshooting of minor problems for students, teachers, and classroom paraprofessionals. Additional opportunities for outcomes measurement exist in these areas, including the evaluation of inservices by participants and assessment of their knowledge and skills after training. These actions involve others in the service-delivery site in the outcomes measurement process, establishing students, parents, teachers, and other educational personnel as stakeholders in the success of audiologic programming. Moreover, audiologists should consider using outcomes measures for children as discussed in Chapter 9 such as the *Listening Inventory for Education (L.I.F.E.)* (Anderson & Smaldino, 1998) to measure the effectiveness of FM systems for students with hearing impairment.

Sound-Field FM Amplification Systems

Outcomes measurement is also important in marketing sound-field FM amplification systems. Preparation is the key to successful marketing of these systems and should include the following steps:

- Identification of a receptive school with an administration that is excited about innovations
- Selection of (a) teacher(s) who want(s) to try out the equipment
- Selection of the appropriate equipment to suit the needs of the targeted classroom
- Training of the teacher(s) and aides in the care and use of the equipment

The details of these processes are beyond the scope of this textbook but are discussed at length in Crandell, Smaldino, and Flexer (1995). Nevertheless, data collection and outcomes measurement are fundamental to both marketing and assessing the effectiveness of these amplification systems in the classroom.

Initial outcomes measurement assessing the effectiveness of sound-field FM amplification systems in classrooms should be made after a brief trial period of the equipment in selected classrooms involving different procedures. Verification procedures should be implemented prior to the trial period, using measures such as the, "*Classroom Acoustics*

Documentation Form" (Appendix XIII-D) (Smaldino & Crandell, 1995) found on the companion CD-ROM. Using a sound-level meter, audiologists can measure the level of the teacher's voice in the unamplified and amplified conditions in various locations (usually at students' desks) in the classroom. The levels of the teacher's voice can be compared to the level of the background noise for determination of signal-to-noise ratio (S/N) in both the unamplified and amplified classroom conditions. For example, if the background noise level is 65 dB-A and the unamplified teacher's voice level is 65 dB-A as compared to an amplified level of 75 dB-A, the S/N has improved from 0 dB in the unamplified condition (i.e., 65 dB-A speech level − 65 dB-A ambient noise level = 0 dB S/N) to +10 dB A (i.e., 75 dB-A speech level - 65 dB-A ambient noise level = +10 dB S/N). Two important points must be made regarding classroom acoustics measurements. First, remember that the minimum S/N for classrooms to be used by children under 13 years of age is +15 dB. Second, verification procedures are made by audiologists to determine the proper adjustment and placement of equipment for maximum benefit, but also can be used in reports to school officials providing they understand the concept of S/N and have experienced a demonstration of challenging listening situations simulating different S/Ns.

Validation of sound-field FM amplification systems includes participation of administrators (e.g., principals), trained teachers, and students in the outcomes measurement process through completion of evaluation forms that can be found on the companion CD-ROM in Appendices XIII-E, XIII-F, and XIII-G, respectively. The subjective feedback gleaned from these evaluation forms can be very meaningful to school superintendents, Parent Teacher Association (PTA) members, and local service organizations that may supply funding for programs (Allen & Anderson, 1995).

Other important data include the cost effectiveness of sound-field FM classroom amplification systems. Administrators may have difficulty conceptualizing the cost effectiveness of these systems when all of them must be purchased at once, especially if funds are low. To avoid this situation, Allen and Anderson (1995) suggested a minimal to modest expansion in which only a few classrooms per year receive equipment, spreading the costs over a longer period of time. Another strategy is to use the statistics from the literature to develop savings projections by weighing the costs of equipment in relation to the decrease in special education costs (Allen & Anderson, 1995). Still another strategy is to use a "single-child approach" (Allen & Anderson, 1995) by targeting a student in the pilot-study classroom and assessing pre- and post-intervention classroom functioning using outcome measures such as the *Listening Inventories for Education (L.I.F.E.)* (Anderson & Smaldino, 1998), discussed in Chapter 9. Outcome data demonstrating improved functioning in the classroom for a known student after placement of sound-field FM amplification equipment can be particularly convincing for educational personnel. Audiologists may elect to use one or all of these strategies to document the effectiveness of sound-field FM amplification on the front end. However, audiologists must be clever in developing outcomes measurement programs to demonstrate long-term effectiveness and

efficiency of these devices to warrant continued technical support and investment.

Hearing Support Programs

Johnson and Danhauer (1999) advocated the development of aural rehabilitation or hearing support programs in service-delivery settings that traditionally have a shortage of audiologists such as rehabilitation hospitals, long-term residential care facilities for the elderly, and the public schools. School-based and contract-for-service audiologists establish hearing support programs as a strategy to do more with less given the realities of shrinking budgets and constant cutbacks. Hearing support programs necessitate the use of support personnel to help "fill-in-the-gaps" to unserved and underserved populations. Audiologists providing services with less than adequate resources have little or no time for outcomes measurement. Therefore, Johnson and Danhauer (1999) developed a single "*Customer-Satisfaction Questionnaire for Educational Hearing Support Programs*" (Appendix XIII-H on the companion CD-ROM) that can be completed by parents, teachers, and other educational personnel who indicate their degree of agreement to various evaluative statements regarding program effectiveness. As mentioned in Chapter 11, outcome measures that are quick and simple, yet comprehensive and conducive for use

---

LEARNING ACTIVITIES

■ Interview audiologists who are either employed by or provide services through a contract with a local school district about their opinions of and participation in outcomes measurement.

■ Make a list of how ASHA's NOMS could be used for outcomes measurement for all components of EHDI programs.

in today's complex world have the greatest likelihood for success.

SUMMARY

This chapter discussed the importance/challenges of outcomes measurement for audiologists providing services in the public schools. In addition, two different service-delivery models were reviewed in terms of their effects on outcomes measurement involving various areas of educational audiology. Recently, federal funding for special education and related services has increased, in addition to increases in funds for EHDI programs. Audiologists must seize the opportunity and demonstrate program efficiency, effectiveness, and/or efficacy to warrant continued support.

RECOMMENDED READINGS

Crandall, C.C., Smaldino, J.J. & Flexer, C. (1995). *Sound-field FM amplification: Theory and practical applications.* Clifton Park, NY: Delmar Thomson Learning.

Johnson, C.D., Benson, P.V., & Seaton, J.B. (1997). *Educational audiology handbook.* Clifton Park, NY: Delmar Thomson Learning.

REVIEW EXERCISES

Fill-in-the-Blank

Instructions: Please fill-in-the-blanks with the correct terms from the word bank below.

1. The _____ - _____ audiologist is a permanent employee of the school district or educational agency.

2. The _____ - _____ - _____ audiologist is hired to provide specific services by the school

district or the educational agency for a specified period of time (e.g., school year).

3. The _____ - _____ approach involves assessing the efficiency, effectiveness, and/or efficacy of audiologic service delivery in the public schools.

4. The _____ approach to outcomes measurement involves assessing the comprehensiveness of services by inventorying effectiveness indicators in key areas of educational audiologic programming.

5. _____ _____ are outcomes for students to achieve over the span of a school year.

6. _____ - _____ _____ are intermediary aims to be achieved toward the ultimate accomplishment of an annual goal.

Word Bank:
Annual goals
Contract-for-service
Outcome-based
Prescriptive
Short-term objetives
School-based

REFERENCES

Allen, L., & Anderson, K. (1995). Marketing sound-field amplification systems. In C.C. Crandell, J.J. Smaldino, & C. Flexer (Eds.), *Sound-field FM amplification: Theory and practical applications* (pp. 201–221). San Diego, CA: Singular Publishing Group.

American Speech-Language-Hearing Association. (1994). Guidelines for fitting FM systems. *ASHA, 36*(Suppl. 12), 1–9.

American Speech-Language-Hearing Association. (in press). Guidelines for fitting and monitoring FM systems. *ASHA Desk Reference.*

Amiot, A. (1998). Policy, politics, and the power of information: The critical need for outcomes and clinical trials data in policy-making in the schools. *Language, Speech, and Hearing Services in the Schools, 29,* 245.

Anderson, K., & Smaldino, J. (1998). *The Listening Inventories for Education (L.I.F.E.).* Tampa, FL: Educational Audiology Association.

Baum, H.M. (1998). Overview, definitions, and goals for ASHA's treatment outcomes and clinical trials activities (What difference do outcome data make to you?). *Language, Speech, and Hearing Services in the Schools, 29,* 246–249.

Colorado Department of Education. (1996). *Planning and preparing quality individual education programs.* Denver, CO: Author.

Crandall, C.C., Smaldino, J.J. & Flexer, C. (1995). *Sound-field FM amplification: Theory and practical applications.* Clifton Park, NY: Delmar Thomson Learning.

Education for all Handicapped Children Act of 1975, Public Law 94-142, 20, U.S.C. 1401–1461: *U.S. Statutes at Large, 89,* 773–779 (1975).

Eger, D.L. (1998). Outcomes measurement in the schools. In C.M. Frattali (Ed.), *Measuring outcomes in speech-language pathology* (pp. 438–452). New York, NY: Thieme.

Gallagher, T.M., Swigert, N.B., & Baum, H.M. (1998). Collecting outcomes data in schools: Needs and challenges. *Language, Speech, and Hearing Services in the Schools, 29,* 250–255.

Individuals with Disabilities Education Act of 1990 (IDEA), Public Law 101-476, 20, U.S.C. 1400 et seq: *U.S. Statutes at Large, 104,* 1103–1151 (1990).

Johnson, C.D., Benson, P.V., & Seaton, J.B. (1997). *Educational audiology handbook.* Clifton Park, NY: Delmar Thomson Learning.

Johnson, C.E., & Danahuer, J.L. (1999). *Guidebook for support programs in aural rehabilitation.* Clifton Park, NY: Delmar Thomson Learning.

Joint Committee on Infant Hearing (2000). Year 2000 position statement: Principles and guidelines for early hearing detection and intervention programs. *American Journal of Audiology: A Journal of Clinical Practice 9*(1), 9–29.

Northern, J.L. (2000). Patient satisfaction and hearing aid outcomes. *The Hearing Journal, 53*(6), 10, 12, 14, 16.

O'Brien, M.A., & Huffman, N.P. (1998). Impact of managed care in the schools. *Language, Speech, and Hearing Services in the Schools, 29,* 263–269.

Roush, J. (2000). What happens after screening? *The Hearing Journal, 53*(11), 56, 58–60.

Smaldino, J.J., & Crandell, C.C. (1995). Acoustic measurements in classrooms. In C.C. Crandell, J.J. Smaldino, & C. Flexer (Eds.), *Sound-field FM amplification: Theory and practical applications* (pp. 69-81). Clifton Park, NY: Delmar Thomson Learning.

APPENDIX XIII-A

IEP Checklist: Recommended Accommodations and Modifications for Students with Hearing Impairment

(Johnson, C.D., Benson, P.V., & Seaton, J.B. [1997]. *Educational audiology handbook* [pp. 448]. Clifton Park, NY: Delmar Thomson Learning. © Delmar Thomson Learning. Reprinted with permission.)

The above-referenced Appendix can be found on the companion CD-ROM.

APPENDIX XIII-B

Self-Assessment: Effectiveness Indicators for Audiology Services in the Schools

(Johnson, C.D., Benson, P.V., & Seaton, J.B. [1997]. *Educational audiology handbook* [pp. 468–474]. Clifton Park, NY: Delmar Thomson Learning. © Delmar Thomson Learning. Reprinted with permission.)

The above-referenced Appendix can be found on the companion CD-ROM.

APPENDIX XIII-C

FM Fitting Protocol

(Johnson, C.D., Benson, P.V., & Seaton, J.B. [1997]. *Educational audiology handbook* [pp. 392–400]. Clifton Park, NY: Delmar Thomson Learning. © Delmar Thomson Learning. Reprinted with permission.)

The above-referenced Appendix can be found on the companion CD-ROM.

APPENDIX XIII-D

Classroom Acoustics Documentation Form

(Smaldino, J., & Crandell, C. [1995]. Acoustic measurements in classrooms. In C.C. Crandell, J.J. Smaldino, & C. Flexer [Eds.], *Sound-field FM amplification: Theory and practical application* [pp. 71]. Clifton Park, NY: Delmar Thomson Learning. © Delmar Thomson Learning. Reprinted with permission.)

The above-referenced Appendix can be found on the companion CD-ROM.

APPENDIX XIII-E

Sound-Field Classroom Amplification Teacher Questionnaire

(Allen, L.A., & Anderson, K.L. [1995]. Marketing sound-field amplification. In C.C. Crandell, J.J. Smaldino, & C. Flexer [Eds.], *Sound-field FM amplification: Theory and practical application* [pp. 219]. Clifton Park, NY: Delmar Thomson Learning. © Delmar Thomson Learning. Reprinted with permission.)

The above-referenced Appendix can be found on the companion CD-ROM.

APPENDIX XIII-F

Sound-Field Classroom Amplification Administrator Questionnaire

(Allen, L.A., & Anderson, K.L. [1995]. Marketing sound-field amplification. In C.C. Crandell, J.J. Smaldino, & C. Flexer [Eds.], *Sound-field FM amplification: Theory and practical application* [pp. 220]. Clifton Park, NY: Delmar Thomson Learning. © Delmar Thomson Learning. Reprinted with permission.)

The above-referenced Appendix can be found on the companion CD-ROM.

APPENDIX XIII-G

Sound-Field Classroom Amplification Student Questionnaire

(Allen, L.A., & Anderson, K.L. [1995]. Marketing sound-field amplification. In C.C. Crandell, J.J. Smaldino, & C. Flexer [Eds.], *Sound-field FM amplification: Theory and practical application* [pp. 221]. Clifton Park, NY: Delmar Thomson Learning. © Delmar Thomson Learning. Reprinted with permission.)

The above-referenced Appendix can be found on the companion CD-ROM.

APPENDIX XIII-H

Customer-Satisfaction Questionnaire for Educational Hearing Support Programs

(Johnson, C.E., & Danhauer, J.L. [1999]. *Guidebook for support programs in aural rehabilitation* [pp. 341]. Clifton Park, NY: Delmar Thomson Learning. © Delmar Thomson Learning. Reprinted with permission.)

The above-referenced Appendix can be found on the companion CD-ROM.

CHAPTER 14
Outcomes Measurement in University Training Programs

LEARNING OBJECTIVES

This chapter will enable readers to:

- Define the participants, process, mediums, modes, and reasons for outcomes measurement in university training programs
- Understand critical issues for outcomes measurement in Au.D. programs

INTRODUCTION

By the year 2012, the required entry-level degree for the Certificate of Clinical Competence in Audiology from the American Speech-Language-Hearing Association (ASHA) will be a doctoral degree. In response to this mandate, university training programs have either already upgraded to offer the doctor of audiology degree (Au.D.), have closed their master's degree programs, or are in a transition from master's to doctoral-level education. The transition to a doctoral level profession has sent the field into a state of flux. The profession has done well in answering some, but not all of the following questions: Is the

expansion necessary? How will Au.D. programs compare with traditional master's degree programs? What admission criteria should be used? What courses should be taken? Who should be teaching these courses? Can currently practicing audiologists be "grand-fathered" in? Can seasoned audiologists with master's degrees be called "doctor" by virtue of a portfolio review?

Some answers to these questions came after careful study; others were evident only after a painful trial and error process. For example, expansion of the scope of practice in audiology led the Council on Professional

Standards (Standards Council) in 1995 to modify audiology certification standards to require a doctoral degree and to draft proposed audiology standards available for public review. Alternatively, closely patterned after a medical-school model, the program at Baylor College of Medicine (the first to offer an Au.D.) closed its doors in part because many students could not meet the rigorous demands of the curriculum.

Today, many Au.D. programs are up-and-running to meet the needs of students just entering traditional university-based programs with bachelor's degrees as well as seasoned practitioners with master's degrees enrolling in distance-education Au.D. programs. Does the existence of these programs mean that the battle is over? No, now that these programs have matriculating students, the onus is on the profession to be accountable to stakeholders that the transition efforts to a doctoral-level profession are worth it. The stakeholders are the same as for other areas of outcomes measurement discussed in this textbook: faculty members, patients and their families, practitioners, third-party payers, taxpayers, and the list goes on. Besides accountability, outcomes measurement also provides opportunities for quality improvement of Au.D. programs to ensure that they are continuing to meet or exceed the rigorous standards to prepare students to meet the challenges of audiologic practice in the new millennium. The purpose of this chapter is to review some of the issues in outcomes measurement for university Au.D. training programs.

OUTCOMES MEASUREMENT IN UNIVERSITY TRAINING PROGRAMS

Administrators in higher education can get lost in the data routinely collected as part of outcomes measurement in colleges and universities. Rassi (1998) listed several areas of outcomes measurement for university training programs:

- Admissions:
  ⇒ Applicants: demographic distribution, characteristics, and entry qualifications
  ⇒ Process: criteria, procedural steps, and timelines
- Alumni: gift support
- Budget:
  ⇒ Funding: equipment and maintenance
  ⇒ External funding
  ⇒ Salary schedules
- Campus:
  ⇒ Campus life: dormitory life, faculty availability, and student housing
  ⇒ Campus size
  ⇒ Coordination and management of campus services: business office, campus police, building maintenance, parking, and registration
  ⇒ Staff views: library, computer center, and research office
- Curriculum:
  ⇒ Design: development and planning
  ⇒ Scope: topic coverage
- Facilities:
  ⇒ Classrooms
  ⇒ Laboratories
  ⇒ Space availability
- Faculty:
  ⇒ Characteristics: age, gender, rank, and tenure status
  ⇒ Individual teaching loads
  ⇒ Qualifications: teaching, publications, and research accomplishments
  ⇒ Size of faculty: number of full-time equivalents (FTEs)
- Financial assistance for students
- Mission:
  ⇒ Adherence to university mission
  ⇒ Adherence to program mission
- Research:
  ⇒ Grants funded
  ⇒ Funding for doctoral programs

- Resources:
  - ⇒ Financial
  - ⇒ Physical
- Service:
  - ⇒ Activities of the university in the community
  - ⇒ University relations with the community
- Students:
  - ⇒ Enrollment: full-time versus part-time
  - ⇒ Grades
  - ⇒ Graduate employment rates
  - ⇒ Retention rates
- Teaching:
  - ⇒ Class size
  - ⇒ Course design

Outcomes measurement is also complicated at the departmental level for heads of graduate programs in communication sciences and disorders. A clear perspective is needed of both the *participants* in and *processes* of outcomes measurement. Participants include those persons who provide the evaluative data (e.g., clinical supervisors, course instructors, lab instructors, employers, professional certification bodies, and licensure boards) and those individuals being evaluated (e.g., students, graduates, certificate applicants, and licensure applicants) (Rassi, 1998). Participants may include, but are not limited to, individuals within the department (e.g., undergraduate, graduate students, course instructors), those outside the department, but within the university (e.g., administrators), and those outside the university (e.g., patients and their families, practicum internship supervisors, clinical fellowship year [CFY] supervisors, and other employees or supervisors) (Rassi, 1998). The processes of outcomes measurement include the participants, *mediums*, *modes*, specific outcomes measures, and specific *reasons* for activities. *Mediums* are tools for outcomes measurement including both standardized and non-standardized examinations, surveys, questionnaires, and so forth. *Modes* of outcomes measurement are methods of administration and include interview, paper-and-pencil, and computer formats. *Reasons* for outcomes measurement include the specific uses for the data, including university and program accreditation, tenure and promotion of faculty, determination of student outcomes, and clinical operations.

Participants need to believe in the importance of outcomes measurement if it is to be successful. For example, students at the end of the semester may feel apathetic about completing instructor evaluation forms because, "No one ever reads them anyway." Alternatively, professors may not try as hard if student evaluations are meaningless in the long run. Students and faculty members must believe that these outcome data are important and have a significant effect on tenure and promotion decisions and on improving the quality of instruction. Furthermore, administrators must strategically optimize the mediums and modes for success in outcomes measurement. For example, students will be more likely to complete instructor evaluation forms (i.e., mode) if they are short and to-the-point, yet provide useful information. In addition, students may be more likely to provide candid responses via an on-line (i.e., medium) questionnaire as opposed to a paper-and-pencil method within the classroom setting.

CRITICAL AREAS FOR OUTCOMES MEASUREMENT IN AU.D. PROGRAMS

Although outcomes measurement is important to all facets of Au.D. programs, four critical areas are discussed here:

1. Accreditation
2. Distance learning
3. Promotion and tenure for clinical faculty
4. Student outcomes

Accreditation

As of January 1, 1996, the Educational Standards Board (ESB) was replaced by the Council on Academic Accreditation in Audiology and Speech-Language Pathology (CAA) which has the responsibility of overseeing the approval of graduate education programs that prepare entry-level professionals in audiology and speech-language pathology as recognized by the U.S. Department of Education (USDE) and the Council on Higher Education (CHEA) (ASHA, 1999). The specific purposes of the CAA are to (ASHA, 1999):

- formulate standards for the accreditation of graduate education programs that provide entry-level professional preparation in audiology and speech-language pathology,
- evaluate programs that voluntarily apply for accreditation,
- grant certificates and recognize those programs deemed to have fulfilled requirements for accreditation,
- maintain a registry of holders of such certificates, and
- prepare and furnish to appropriate persons and agencies lists of accredited programs.

Outcomes measurement is fundamental to accreditation based on the premise that all professions that provide services to the public be of the highest quality (ASHA, 1999). Therefore, public identification of training programs that meet or exceed accreditation standards is of importance to all stakeholders. The accreditation process encourages institutional freedom, ongoing quality assurance (e.g., teaching, learning, research, and professional practice), educational experimentation, and constructive innovation (ASHA, 1999). Programs are evaluated on the basis of their own training models, goals, and objectives (ASHA, 1999). The CAA requests

that the mission statements of the university, the college, and the program be included in re-accreditation applications.

The Self-Study

Prior to submission of any applications to the CAA, a program must undergo a self-study. Graduate programs that engage in continuous quality improvement (CQI) should not find the self-study for determining compliance with accreditation standards a chore. Achieving and maintaining compliance to the standards is a continuous cycle of quality assessment and improvement for strengthening programs. Figure 14-1 shows the cyclical nature of a self-study beginning with the formal initiation of a process, which should engage all stakeholders (e.g., higher administrators, faculty, off-campus supervisors, students, and so forth), and not just program directors (adapted from ASHA, 1999).

The second step is development of a statement of program objectives describing what the department wants students to know (cognitive), think (attitudinal), or do (behavioral), followed by the identification of the appropriate means of assessment of those objectives (Nichols & Nichols, 2000). The third step is development of a plan for data collection, including assignment of stakeholders' roles and establishment of mechanisms for determining program status. Program directors and departmental committees must decide who does what, when, and how. All participants, from clinical patients to the university administrators, must be "on the same page" and provide input to the mechanics of outcomes measurement. For example, stakeholders' suggestions may be critical for the seamless accommodation of data collection into departmental operations.

Data collection and evaluation, the fifth and sixth steps of a self-study, are facilitated through use of computer-based data management systems as discussed in Chapter 5.

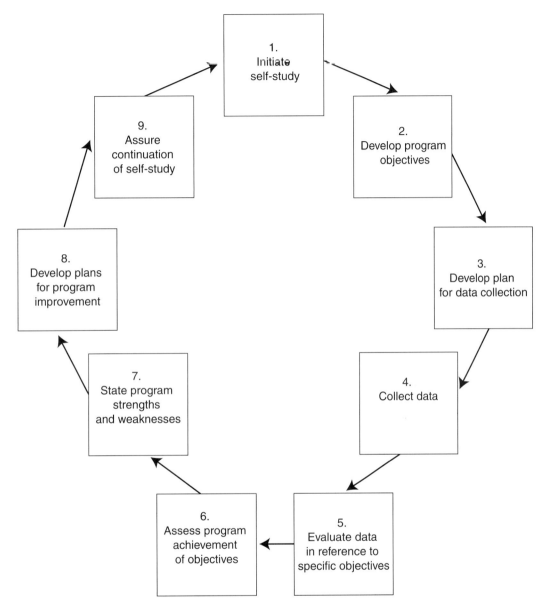

Figure 14-1. Cycle of self-study (Adapted from ASHA, 1999).

Program directors need to manipulate outcome data to suit their administrative needs. Annual PRAXIS scores must be a few mouse clicks away when assessing the effect of curriculum changes on students' performance on standardized tests, for example. More importantly, statistical software can be invaluable to department heads and faculty who must assess program attainment of stated objectives through analysis of outcome data, the sixth step of the self-study. From this process, departments can determine their strengths and weaknesses, develop plans for improvement, and ensure a continual process of quality assurance, the seventh through ninth steps of self-study respectively. The continual process of self-study is good for the evolution of a degree program, and is required for accreditation by the CAA.

The Accreditation Process

There are five steps in the accreditation process:

1. Initial evaluation
2. Site visit
3. CAA review and action on initial and re-accreditation applications
4. CAA review and action on annual reports
5. Application for re-accreditation

The initial evaluation begins with submission of either an initial or re-accreditation application which the CAA reviews to determine whether the program is in compliance with standards and, if so, a site visit is recommended. Any questions or concerns that the CAA has in the initial review of the document are relayed to the program and reviewed by its director and faculty who must decide collectively to continue on with the process or withdraw the application. The decision whether to proceed is based upon the program's ability to demonstrate compliance with the standards by the site visit, often requiring consideration of key outcome data. Whatever the decision, the program director has 30 days from the date of the letter of concern to notify the CAA of its decision. Programs electing to proceed on with the accreditation process must address the concerns of the CAA in writing at least 30 days before the site visit. If the site visit is not scheduled within 6 months of the date of the letter of concern, the program must submit updated information to the CAA.

The CAA and the program director decide both the length of the site visit (e.g., usually 2 days) and the size of the site-visit team (e.g., at least 2 people). Longer site visits and larger site-visit teams may be needed if the visit is with another accrediting agency or the program is on more than one campus. Individuals who cannot serve as site-visit team members are those who:

- live or work in the same state as or in close geographic proximity to the program under review,
- are former students/faculty,
- have served as consultants to the program for the program's preparation for accreditation, or
- cannot ensure impartiality/objectivity because of a potential conflict of interest.

Sometimes, observers may accompany the site-visitor team (e.g., site-visitor trainees or representatives from another accrediting agency). The program director submits a tentative site-visit agenda at least 30 days before the visit and announces, in a timely manner, the visit so that the public (e.g., faculty, administrators, students, clients/patients, and community professionals) has an opportunity to address the team.

Site visitors are responsible for a comprehensive review of programs and presenting documentation relative to all standards for CAA accreditation. The team:

- confers with the institution's administrators on attitudes toward and plans for the program verifying the administrative structure;
- reviews the physical facilities and library holdings;
- interviews the academic and clinical staff regarding the academic and clinical programs verifying instructional staff's allocation of time;

- selects and reviews materials and records on the curriculum and academic programs;
- selects and reviews materials and records on clinical education;
- selects and reviews student records of academic and clinical experiences;
- visits off-campus practicum sites and interviews off-campus practicum supervisors; and
- gathers information relative to concerns the CAA expressed while reviewing the application.

Communication between site visitors and administrators, faculty, and students is critical to obtaining information for the exit report. The site-visit team provides an exit report to the program director for clarification and verification of the information.

The chairman of the site-visit team submits a written report to the CAA within 30 days of the visit which includes a summary of the visitors' verifiable observations of standards, information contained within the application, and programs' strengths and limitations. Within 10 days of receipt, the chair of the CAA sends the site-visit report to the director of the program and the institution's president. Within 30 days of the postmark, the program director must provide a written response to the CAA that remarks on the accuracy of the report and any changes that have been made in the training program since the site visit. The report is shared with the site-visitors who have two weeks to add their comments to the CAA, who may contact team members for further clarification. The CAA reviews the application, the site-visit report, and the program's response to that report, and any additional comments from team members. Within 60 days, the CAA decides to award initial accreditation or re-accreditation, place the program on probation, or withhold or withdraw accreditation.

Accredited programs must submit an annual report to the CAA on or before the anniversary date of accreditation to document continuing compliance with current standards. Annual reports are reviewed by the CAA to determine if programs are within compliance of the standards and take one of 3 options: (1) continues the program's accreditation, (2) places a program on probation, or (3) withdraws accreditation.

A program is placed on probation when the CAA declares that its annual report clearly reveals a lack of compliance to the standards jeopardizing the capability of providing an adequate educational experience for students. Programs on probation must demonstrate compliance with the standards in their next annual report, or accreditation is withdrawn. An organized approach to outcomes measurement is vital to the survival of a marginal degree program that must decisively demonstrate compliance with accreditation standards. Probationary accreditation can be extended, but not for a period to exceed 2 years. The Secretary of the United States Department of Education (USDE) and the appropriate state post-secondary review entity are notified within 30 days of a decision to award a program's accreditation or re-accreditation. ASHA provides similar information on graduate programs in communication sciences and disorders through various mechanisms.

Many new Au.D. programs may have to go through a status of "Candidacy of Accreditation," which the CAA mandated for emerging educational programs in speech-language pathology and audiology. Programs meeting specified standards are designated, as a "Candidate" for CAA Accreditation in Audiology." A program cannot hold candidacy status for longer than 3 years. At the conclusion of candidacy status, programs must meet all the standards for CAA accreditation. Therefore, new programs must be proactive in outcomes measurement to develop plans for complying with CAA standards within three short years. Beginning with year one, a statement of program objectives must be developed with corresponding benchmarks and quality indicators. There is no time to waste. Candidate programs are required to submit progress reports every 6 months and a completed application for accreditation to the CAA by the second anniversary of the award of candidacy status. Although the accreditation process discussed here has been well defined by the CAA for traditional programs, a standard for distance-learning programs is a relatively new concept.

Distance-Learning Programs

The dominant educational model for the past 40 years in communication sciences and disorders has involved providing students with coursework and clinical practicum on traditional university campuses (Traylor, 2001). Today, many audiologists who are employed full-time come home and get onto the information superhighway to hook-up with fellow classmates in chat rooms to discuss the latest assignments in their distance-education Au.D. classes. Universities have developed on-line Au.D. programs, and the American Speech-Language-Hearing Association has launched on-line continuing education workshops (Traylor, 2001).

Why all this focus on distance-education programming? First, changing the requirements for the Certificate of Clinical Competence in Audiology (CCC-A) from earning a master's degree to a doctoral degree by 2012 has necessitated alternative means for gainfully employed audiologists with master's degrees to upgrade to a doctoral degree. Second, more and more non-traditional students—those over 35 years of age—are enrolling in post-secondary institutions, with the number expected to increase significantly in the next 15 to 20 years (Busacco, 2001).

Cost-cutting at major universities has prompted exploration of how digital technology can replace the more expensive traditional degree programs (Busacco, 2001). In fact, it is estimated that the number of traditional campuses will decrease by 50% during the next two decades to be replaced by virtual universities that can distribute educational programming at the time, place, pace, and in learning style of each student (Busacco, 2001).

Distance learning is providing alternative models of teaching and learning, new challenges for faculty, and new sources to obtain higher educations (Eaton, 2001). Eaton (2001) stated that distance learning has impacted three areas:

1. Growth of credit-bearing distance learning in accredited, degree-granting institutions (e.g., distance-learning Au.D. programs of the University of Florida and Central Michigan-Vanderbilt University/Bill Wilkerson Center)
2. Emergence of "new providers" of higher education (e.g., new stand-alone, degree-granting, on-line colleges and universities, degree-granting consortia, nondegree-granting on-line consortia, corporate universities, and unaffiliated on-line programs and courses)
3. Development of electronic service partnerships between institutions and the corporate sector (e.g., University of Florida Distance Education Au.D. Program partnership with Intellicus to provide on-line programming)

Distance learning has three key features (Eaton, 2001):

1. *Computer-mediated classrooms*—In these virtual classrooms, faculty and students communicate with each other through keyboards and monitors, rely-

ing heavily on the written word rather than face-to-face interactions.

2. *Separation in time between communications*—In Cyberspace, teachers and students must rely on asynchronous modes of communication, causing a separation in time between questions and answers posed in E-mails, for example.

3. *Availability of services on-line*—Students receive services such as advising, counseling, mentoring, and library services that are integrated with on-line teaching and learning environments.

These components offer some advantages and disadvantages for the stakeholders in higher education. Advantages include students having connectivity to information/ resources (e.g., on-line journals and consumer Web sites), and each other, faculty, and professionals via the Internet, E-mail, electronic bulletin boards, and chat rooms (Busacco, 2001). However, there are some disadvantages to distance-learning programs. First, distance learning decreases, or eliminates face-to-face interaction between faculty and students (Busacco, 2001). One-on-one interactions between supervisors and students are critical for both clinical practicum and research experiences in the laboratory. Students learn as much or more by what their mentors do in the clinic and the laboratory as by what they say in the classroom. Second, many colleges and universities may not be able to obtain the necessary start-up funding to purchase, maintain, and upgrade the hardware/software to deliver these educational services; hire staff to train faculty in how to use educational technology; and provide technical support to students (Busacco, 2001). Third, the proliferation of distance-learning opportunities is increasing, raising serious concerns about the accuracy, consistency, and quality of the educational experiences (Busacco, 2001). What are char-

acteristics of quality distance-learning programs? To what types of educational benchmarks should these programs aspire? What are some quality indicators for these benchmarks? To what standards should these programs be held accountable for accreditation? Should current standards for site-based education be modified for use with distance-learning programs?

Accrediting bodies, such as the CAA, must resolve many issues regarding the accreditation of distance-learning programs. Indeed, the accrediting community has at least five responsibilities to assist institutions and programs in traversing the uncertain topography of the distance-learning landscape (Eaton, 2001):

- Responsibility 1: Identify the distinctive features of distance-learning delivery; whether within traditional settings or supplied by one of the new providers
- Responsibility 2: Modify accreditation guidelines, policies or standards to assure quality within the distinctive environment of distance delivery
- Responsibility 3: Pay additional attention to student achievement and learning outcomes in the context of distance learning
- Responsibility 4: Work with government to adjust current policy understandings about the use of federal funds and quality assurance in a distance-learning setting, while sustaining shared commitment to self-regulation through voluntary accreditation and preserving the autonomy of institutions
- Responsibility 5: Assume more responsibility for addressing public interest in the quality of higher education as distance-learning opportunities and providers diversify and expand

To this end, drafts of two important documents were developed during the fall of

2000: (1) "*Statement of the Regional Accrediting Commissions on the Evaluation of Electronically Offered Degree and Certificate Programs*," and (2) "*Guidelines for the Evaluation of Electronically Offered Degree and Certificate Programs*." An important part of these documents deals with the evaluation and assessment of student achievement and the overall program by using such measures as (CHEA, 2001):

- The extent to which student learning matches intended course outcomes (e.g., evaluations of student performance, review of student work and archive of student activities)
- The extent to which student intent is met
- Student retention rates (e.g., number of students who enroll to those who successfully complete the program)
- Student satisfaction (e.g., regular end-of-course and end-of-program surveys)
- Faculty satisfaction (e.g., regular surveys, formal/informal peer review processes, and discussion groups)
- Student access (e.g., enrollment records and student surveys)
- Students' use of library and learning resources (e.g., instructor assignments)
- Student competence in fundamental skills
- Cost-effectiveness of the program (e.g., survey of cost for students and institution's analyses that relate costs to goals of the program)

In addition, distance-learning evaluation must be part of the institution's continual self-evaluation and outcomes measurement toward continuous quality improvement for more effective use of technology in education, advances in student achievement of learning outcomes, improved retention rates, effective use of resources, and demonstrated improvements in the institution's service to the community. Furthermore, the evaluation of distance-learning programs should take place within the context of the regular evaluation of all programs. The CAA has sent representatives to important conferences on these topics to obtain important information to develop accreditation standards for distance-learning programs in communication sciences and disorders. Recently the CAA stated that distances learning programs must meet the same accredidation standards as do traditional programs.

Department heads and faculty ask how should audiologists instructing in distance-learning programs assess the effectiveness of their courses? Should they wait for standards of performance to come from the CAA or start outcomes measurement programs of their own? Again, instructors should exercise the "power of one," where one audiologist can be a pioneer and make a difference. However, peer-reviewed publications regarding the outcomes of distance-learning programs are practically non-existent. What should be measured? What type of experimental design should be used in these studies?

English, Rojeski, and Branham (2000) investigated the effectiveness of a distance-learning course in achieving the outcome of teaching counseling skills to 23 master's level practicing audiologists (7 male; 16 females) enrolled in a counseling course via distance-learning to fulfill requirements for the doctor of audiology degree (Au.D.), jointly offered by Central Michigan University and Vanderbilt Bill Wilkerson Center. Specifically, the experimental questions were (English, et al., 2000):

- Do practicing audiologists provide technical information to patients' personal adjustment comments?
- Does an Internet course in counseling result in a decrease in technical responses and a corresponding increase in affective responses to personal adjustment comments?

English, Mendel, Rojeski, and Hornak (1999) found that audiologists typically provided technical responses (e.g., "There are no research studies to confirm this assertion") to patients' personal adjustment comments (e.g., "My family says our daughter was born deaf because I worked until the last week of the pregnancy") rather than affective responses (e.g., "You seem very worried that this might be true"). Effective counseling requires expanding audiologists' role beyond the transfer of information (e.g., technical) to more closely resembling traditional models of counseling (e.g., affective) (English, et al., 2000).

English, et al., (2000) administered 5-items from an instrument developed in an earlier study to assess practitioners' ability to recognize and respond appropriately to patients' expressions of personal adjustment concerns (English, et al., 1999) as a pre- and post-course measure to the 23 students (i.e., 10 randomly selected students completed pre- and post-course measures and 13 students completed post-course measures only) enrolled in a course and to a control group of 10 doctoral students (i.e., all completed pre- and post-course measures) enrolled in a distance-learning course on another topic. The distance-learning counseling course covered the following topics and did not provide specific instructions on how to respond to the dependent variable for the study (English, et al., 2000):

- Psychosocial implications of hearing loss
- The "Hearing Aid Effect" and other external stressors
- Self-concept and hearing loss
- Counseling approaches
- Building patient relationships
- Conveying diagnostic information
- Counseling families
- Pediatric counseling
- Counseling adults
- Counseling elderly persons and their families
- Helping people cope
- Counseling efficacy

Statistical analyses of the pre- and post-course measures revealed no significant differences between the pre- and post-measures of the control group, indicating little or no history, maturation, or Hawthorne effects (English, et al., 2000). Similarly, no significant differences were found between the pre- and post-course measures of students enrolled in the counseling course, indicating minimal pretest effects. However, significant differences were found between the pre- and post-course cohorts of students enrolled in the distance-learning counseling course, indicating that instruction was effective in reducing students' technical responses and increasing their affective responses to patients' personal adjustment concerns (English, et al., 2000). More well-controlled studies are needed to assess the effectiveness of distance-learning programs.

Promotion and Tenure for Clinical Faculty

Chapter 2 discussed important issues regarding the training of Ph.D. and Au.D. students. The development of Au.D. programs has raised important questions regarding appropriateness of Ph.D. audiologists teaching in Au.D. programs. Traditional graduate programs in communication sciences and disorders primarily use Ph.D.-level professionals to teach academic courses and employ master's level clinicians to supervise students in their practica. Are Ph.D.-level audiologists trained for careers in university teaching, research, and service clinically competent to teach in Au.D. programs? Are current master's level clinicians qualified to supervise and/or teach Au.D. students? Typically, universities hire and retain Ph.D.-level audiologists primarily for their ability to develop independent research programs, capable of attracting extramural funding and secondarily for their ability to teach students.

Will this attract the "best and brightest" faculty to teach in Au.D. programs? Similarly, clinical instructor positions in university training programs are often low paying with little or no chance for advancement. Ideally, audiologists with Au.D.s should teach in Au.D. programs. However, universities must address several issues before this model can become a reality. First, universities must develop faculty positions that can attract new graduates into pursuing careers in teaching and direct-service delivery in academic settings. For example, why would an Au.D.-level audiologist elect to work in a low-paying teaching job over a lucrative position in private practice? Second, communication sciences and disorders programs, along with other professional degree programs (e.g., nursing, occupational therapy, pharmacy, and physical therapy), must develop professional tracks that provide opportunities for promotion and tenure of clinical faculty. Some "academic" faculty may balk at this proposal stating that, "I had to get 50 publications for full professor, and so should 'clinical' faculty." Separate, but equal criteria or outcomes must be designated for tenure and promotion of clinical faculty. For example, in 2000, Auburn University developed a Clinical Title Series that established a career ladder for clinical faculty consisting of three tiers with established outcomes of achievement for promotion.

There are 3 levels of appointment in the Clinical Trial Series:

1. Assistant Clinical Professor. This rank is the usual entry-level rank for a candidate who has completed the appropriate terminal degree or has the equivalent in training, ability, and experience, and has been judged to:
   a. Have a current independent capability of having a reliable clinical practice,
   b. Have a potential for significant professional growth in the area of clinical practice, and
   c. Hold the professional degree including licensure/certification appropriate to the field.
2. Associate Clinical Professor. This rank is a rank of distinction that is attained through performance of assigned duties, and has been judged to have:
   a. Demonstrated mastery of the subject matter in the field;
   b. Continuous improvement and contribution in clinical practice supported through contracts, grants, generated income, or other designated funds; and
   c. Emerging stature as a regional or national authority.
3. Clinical Professor. This rank requires professional peer-recognition of the individual as an authority in the field, and be judged to be:
   a. Nationally and perhaps internationally recognized by associates as a clinician; and
   b. Outstanding in practice and education or other creative activity supported through contracts, grants, generated incomes, or other designated funds.

Four important areas of activity are used in the evaluation of individuals for appointment, performance review, and promotion:

1. Documented evidence of effective clinical practice
2. National and international professional status and activity as indicated by evaluation statements from external peer review
3. Ability to initiate and maintain a program of clinical practice supported by contracts, grants, or generated income
4. Collegiality

Career ladders and criteria for continuation of appointment are often met with mixed feelings by clinical faculty. Initially, some clinicians may fear the concept and wonder how they can ever live up to the "publish or perish" outcomes of their colleagues with traditional tenure-track appointments. However, if clinical faculty members are included in the development of benchmarks and quality indicators defining successful professional accomplishment, then most should welcome clinical career ladders and appreciate opportunities for promotion and commensurate salary increases.

Student Outcomes

"If you build it, they will come ..." This phrase, originating from the motion picture industry, seems applicable to the current development of new Au.D. programs. University administrators and faculty are confident that qualified students will seek out their programs, apply for admission, matriculate, and eventually graduate with their Au.D. and go on to earn salaries justifying the cost of their degrees (e.g., time, effort, and money) in positions of leadership. Is this too much to hope? What can the profession do to ensure positive outcomes for Au.D. programs for all stakeholders, including students, faculty, patients, the public, and so forth. Measuring student outcomes for Au.D. programs is a good starting place.

Students' outcomes begin prior to their entry into the Au.D. program. Selecting the best students for admission to Au.D. programs requires consideration of many issues. For example, which pre-admission criteria are most predictive of success as a graduate student and ultimately as an audiologist? Are undergraduate grade-point averages (UGPAs) or scores on the Graduate Record Examination (GRE) predictive of success? How should student success be measured?

One outcome measure that has been used to gauge graduate student success has been scores on the PRAXIS examination, formerly known as the National Examination in Speech Pathology and Audiology. In order to assess the predictability of traditional admission criteria, Ryan, Morgan, and Wacker-Munday (1998) quantified the relationship between UPGA and GRE to communication disorders graduate student success as measured by performance on the PRAXIS and the graduate grade-point average (GGPA). Ryan, et al. (1998) chose the PRAXIS score as the outcome measure for graduate student success because it is the "gold standard" against which all certified clinicians are compared, is the only quantitative value used by the American Speech-Language-Hearing Association, and substitutes for traditional comprehensive examinations in many graduate programs. Ryan, et al. (1998) submitted data obtained from the records of 96 graduate students who completed their degrees between 1993 and 1997 to a step-wise multiple regression analysis in which PRAXIS scores and GGPA were regressed on the independent variables consisting of various combinations of GRE area scores and UGPA. In agreement with the results of similar studies in other disciplines, GRE scores failed to predict PRAXIS score or GGPA (accounting for less than 16% of the variance). Furthermore, UGPA was no better than chance at predicting either PRAXIS scores or GGPA. The authors concluded that traditional pre-admission criteria presently in use are of little predictive value on selected measures of success (Ryan, et al., 1998).

Au.D. programs need to assess the value of pre-admission criteria in predicting graduate student success. Should current master's degree programs in audiology raise the bar with regard to the traditional pre-admission criteria? Should expanded degree programs require a higher caliber of student with higher UGPAs and GREs? However, there is no evidence to suggest that these pre-admission criteria will be any more effective in predicting student success. Academicians at the *Academic Town Meeting* at the 2000 ASHA Convention in San Francisco, CAA suggested other admission criteria useful for all graduate programs in communication sciences and disorders including (Tullos, 2000):

- Interview (e.g., including several applicants at one time who must read an article and are evaluated on how well they work together, follow up on others' comments, and give others credit for previous comments)
- Letters of recommendation
- Written statement
- Resume (e.g., including jobs, memberships, and other responsibilities)

Admissions committees must find ways to quantify these qualitative pre-admission criteria in terms of their utility in predicting success as an audiologist. How should the profession define success and when should it be measured? Is "success" defined differently depending on the stakeholder? For example, audiologists may define their professional success by their annual incomes. Alternatively, patients may define successful audiologists as those who are instrumental in achieving positive outcomes for their problems.

The profession must determine if transitioning to a doctoral-level profession has been worthwhile for all stakeholders. From the student's perspective, will undergraduates find a rewarding and lucrative career justifying the time, effort, and expense of completing a 4-year post-baccalaureate professional Au.D. program? Will seasoned master's degree-level audiologists achieve professional outcomes commensurate with the time, effort, and expense of enrolling in distance-learning Au.D. programs? From the patient's perspective, will higher quality services be delivered by Au.D.-level audiologists versus audiologists with master's degrees? Indeed, the onus is on the profession to prove through outcomes measurement that raising the educational level for practicing as an audiologist has indeed been worth it.

SUMMARY

The next decade is going to be one of tremendous change for the profession of audiology. Outcomes measurement should play a paramount role in defining and shaping the training programs of the future. Professional growth requires change. Training programs must change to meet the growing demands of the field. However, change is not easy, nor does it occur overnight. To be effective, change must be gradual and driven by a cycle of continuous quality improvement (CQI) through outcomes measurement.

LEARNING ACTIVITIES

- Conduct a focus group to identify the participants and processes of outcomes measurement regarding the current standards of the Council on Academic Accreditation in Audiology and Speech-Language Pathology (CAA).

- Interview Au.D. program directors regarding outcomes measurement in their academic units.

- Conduct a survey of Au.D. students regarding their role in outcomes measurement in their degree program.

RECOMMENDED READINGS

American Speech-Language-Hearing Association. (1999). *Accreditation handbook for the Council on Academic Accreditation in Audiology and Speech-Language Pathology.* Rockville, MD: Author.

English, K., Rojeski, T., & Branham, K. (2000). Acquiring counseling skills in mid-career: Outcomes of a distance-learning course for practicing audiologists. *Journal of the American Academy of Audiology, 11,* 84–90.

Nichols, J.O., & Nichols, K.W. (2000). *The departmental guide and record book for student outcomes assessment and institutional effectiveness* (3rd ed.). New York, NY: Agathon Press.

REVIEW EXERCISES

Fill-in-the-Blank

Instructions: Please fill-in-the-blanks with the correct terms from the word bank below.

1. _____ in outcomes measurement include those persons who provide the evaluative data and those individuals being evaluated.

2. _____ of outcomes measurement include the participants, mediums, modes, specific outcome measures, and specific reasons for activities.

3. _____ are tools for outcomes measurement (e.g., standardized and nonstandardized examinations, surveys, and questionnaires).

4. _____ of outcomes measurement are methods of administration and include interview, paper-and-pencil, and computer formats.

5. _____ for outcomes measurement include the specific uses for the data including university and program accreditation, tenure and promotion of faculty, determination of student outcomes and clinical operations.

Word Bank:

Mediums	Processes
Modes	Reasons
Participants	

ANSWERS

Fill-in-the-Blank:
1. Participants
2. Processes
3. Mediums
4. Modes
5. Reasons

REFERENCES

American Speech-Language-Hearing Association. (1999). *Accreditation handbook for the Council on Academic Accreditation in Audiology and Speech-Language Pathology.* Rockville, MD: Author.

Commission on Higher Education. (September, 2000). *Draft: Statement of the Regional Accrediting Commissions on the Evaluation of Electronically Offered Degree and Certificate Programs and Guidelines for the Evaluation of Electronically Offered Degree and Certificate Programs.*

Busacco, D. (2001). Learning at a distance—Technology and the new professional. *The ASHA Leader, 6*(2), 4–5, 9.

Eaton, J.S. (2001). Distance learning: Academic and political challenges for higher education accreditation. *Council for Higher Education (CHEA) Monograph Series 2001, 1,* 1–18.

English, K., Mendel, L.L., Rojeski, T., & Hornak, J. (1999). Counseling in audiology, or learning to listen: Pre- and post-measures from an audiology counseling course. *American Journal of Audiology: A Journal of Clinical Practice, 8,* 34–39.

English, K., Rojeski, T., Branham, K. (2000). Acquiring counseling skills in mid-career:

Outcomes of a distance education course for practicing audiologists. *Journal of the American Academy of Audiology, 11,* 84–90.

Nichols, J.O., & Nichols, K.W. (2000). *The departmental guide and record book for student outcomes assessment and institutional effectiveness,* (3rd ed.). New York, NY: Agathon Press.

Rassi, J.A. (1998). Outcomes measurement in universities. In C. Frattali (ed.), *Measuring outcomes in speech-language pathology* (pp. 477–502). New York, NY: Thieme.

Ryan, W.J., Morgan, M., & Wacker-Munday, R. (1998). Pre-admission criteria as predictors of selected outcome measures for speech-language pathololgy graduate students. *CICSD, 5,* 54–61.

Traylor, V.S. (2001). Diving into the data stream: Access to on-line learning expands in 2001. *The ASHA Leader, 6*(2), 1–21.

Tullos, D.C. (2000). *Moving beyond the numbers.* Papers presented at the Annual Meeting of the Council of Graduate Programs in Communication Sciences and Disorders, San Diego, CA.

C H A P T E R   1 5

Future of Outcomes Measurement in Audiology

L E A R N I N G   O B J E C T I V E S

This chapter will enable readers to:

- Recognize the importance of outcomes measurement to the future of early hearing detection and intervention (EHDI) programs
- Identify obstacles to outcomes measurement in audiology
- Understand the benefit of using outcomes measurement in private practice
- Consider preparation for a future of evidence-based practice

INTRODUCTION

We have discussed outcomes measurement from many angles. Starting with outcomes measurement and the audiologist, we discussed outcomes measurement in specific areas of practice and in some selected service-delivery sites. The chapters on outcomes measurement for specific areas of practice tended to focus on "pie-in-the-sky" approaches while those addressing specific service-delivery sites focused on "real-world" limitations. In writing this textbook, we had little or no idea of how it would be received or used within the field. Should students, particularly in Au.D. programs, have a

course in outcomes measurement? Would the topic be met with disdain from students who want to be "clinicians," and not "researchers?" One goal of this textbook was to try to demonstrate how outcomes measurement is critical to the survival of the profession and the achievement of positive patient outcomes.

It is difficult to tell what the future will bring for outcomes measurement in audiology. Will it be a passing fancy fueled by the pendulum swing of accountability in health care in the 1990s? Or will it achieve a permanent place in standard clinical practice? It is difficult to predict what will become of the urgency of outcomes measurement. However, this chapter will focus on the future and importance of 4 critical needs areas in outcomes measurement: early hearing detection and intervention programs (EHDI), breaking down barriers to outcomes measurement, outcomes measurement in private practice, and preparing for a future of evidence-based practice.

MAKING GOOD ON A HEAD START PROVIDED BY EARLY HEARING DETECTION AND INTERVENTION (EHDI) PROGRAMS

Chapter 6 discussed successful outcomes measurement in early hearing detection and intervention (EHDI) that requires mechanisms for and interrelationships between and among local, state, and federal data management systems. Achievement of the benchmarks and respective quality indicators mentioned in the Joint Committee on Infant Hearing Year 2000 Position Statement (JCIH, 2000) is just the start of demonstrating that the benefits of the universal newborn hearing screening (UNHS) component of EHDI programs goes beyond the identification of the relatively small number of newborns and infants who are congenitally deaf and hard-of-hearing (Hayes & Downs, 2000). Is the cost of UNHS programs worth the price?

Although wholeheartedly supporting the ultimate goal of early diagnosis and intervention for newborns and infants with hearing loss, some audiologists believe that the UNHS model is neither cost-effective nor does it guarantee universal early diagnosis of hearing loss (Kileny & Jacobson, 2000). From data of recently published studies by the New York Hearing Screening Project assessing 69,671 newborns using otoacoustic emissions (OAEs) and automated auditory brainstem response (AABR) protocols, Kileny and Jacobson (2000) found the following when reviewing the outcomes of 43,311 newborns screened during the first 2 years of the 3-year project:

- 85 newborns were diagnosed with hearing loss (0.2 of 1% of the total sample).
- 52 of those 85 newborns would have been identified in a neonatal intensive care unit (NICU) screening program.
- 10 of the remaining 33 newborns had risk factors for hearing loss that would have been identified by a focused high-risk screening program
- Only 8 of the remaining 23 newborns were fit with amplification; the other 15 either had unilateral or hearing losses too mild to be aided.

Kileny and Jacobson (2000) concluded that 23 of 85 (i.e., 27%) of the babies with hearing loss would have been missed if it were not for the UNHS program, which is significantly below the estimated 50% possibly undetected as estimated in the UNHS literature. Furthermore, in only 8 of 85 (i.e., 9%) cases did identification of hearing loss culminate in immediate intervention (Kileny & Jacobson, 2000).

Kileny and Jacobson (2000) stated that three types of costs must be considered when calculating the total costs of UNHS programs:

1. *Variable direct costs*—are expenses associated with disposable supplies (e.g., electrodes, earpieces, and tubing) used to carry out hearing screenings (e.g., $15 per baby).
2. *Fixed direct costs*—involve allocated unit overhead associated with UNHS, including salaries and benefits for program personnel.
3. *Indirect expenses*—comprise the allocated hospital overhead for the proportion of administrative costs of the UNHS program.

Total costs (i.e., total costs = variable direct costs + fixed direct costs + indirect expenses) for each baby screened can range from $50 to $60, resulting in an estimated cost of $100,000 to $300,000 per diagnosis for UNHS model programs, as compared to only $3,000 per diagnosis for targeted screening programs that are coupled with increased physician training on hearing loss (Kileny & Jacobson, 2000).

Hayes and Downs (2000) contended that society's decision regarding the value of UNHS cannot be made on the basis of financial costs alone, but must be considered within the context of improved language skills in deaf and hard-of-hearing children and decreased costs to society for special education training and earnings support. Their argument is supported by three undeniable facts regarding the effectiveness of UNHS and outcomes for children:

1. UNHS programs result in early identification and intervention.
2. Language outcomes for early-identified deaf and hard-of-hearing infants are significantly better than those for later-identified children.
3. Techniques other than those used for UNHS programs do not result in identification and intervention by age 6 years.

Furthermore, the benefits of improved child development, and enhanced family interaction and communication, and greater educational and career opportunities for individuals who are deaf or hard-of-hearing, are priceless (Hayes & Downs, 2000). Unfortunately, health-care policy makers are interested in data, not sentiment. For example, the United States Preventative Service Task Force (USPSTF) stated that sufficient evidence does not exist to either support or refute the efficacy of UNHS programs improving long-term language outcomes for children (Thomson, et al, 2001).

The future of UNHS programs must include developing short-term and long-term plans for outcomes measurement in meeting the challenges of demonstrating the effectiveness, efficiency, and efficacy of all components (i.e., identification, confirmation of hearing loss, and intervention) of EHDI programs. Short-term plans for outcomes measurement should include developing benchmarks and quality indicators for confirmation of hearing loss and early intervention components of EHDI programs through the aggregation of data using local, state, and national mechanisms. Long-term plans should include prospective studies regarding the academic and socioeconomic achievement of early-identified children who are deaf or hard-of-hearing and have benefited from EHDI programs. The future will judge the profession on whether we made good on the head start provided by UNHS.

BREAKING DOWN BARRIERS TO OUTCOMES MEASUREMENT

In each chapter of this textbook, we have discussed obstacles to outcomes measurement in audiology in specific areas of practice and in various service-delivery sites. For example, in Chapter 6, we stated that the lack of interconnections between local, state, and national computer-based data management systems presents significant obstacles to the aggregation of data necessary for establishment of universal benchmarks and quality indicators for EHDI programs. We will describe just three barriers recently discussed in the literature, including those to establishing a uniform set of measures for hearing aid benefit, executing clinical trials in "real world" environments, and garnering an international cooperation in outcomes measurement.

Establishing a Uniform Set of Measures for Hearing Aid Benefit

One major frustration is wading through the results of clinical trials and trying to compare findings across studies for particular hearing aid technologies. After receiving numerous consumer complaints in the late 1980s and early 1990s, the Federal Trade Commission (FTC) and Food and Drug Administration (FDA) demanded that hearing aid manufacturers submit for review their advertising benefit claims, substantiated by clinical data, prior to public release (Walden, 1999). In response, hearing aid manufacturers implemented clinical trials with a wide variation of dependent variables and testing conditions measuring hearing aid benefit that led to results which are difficult to interpret and compare across instruments (Walden, 1999).

Walden (1997) believed that a uniform set of test measures would enable consumers to evaluate different hearing aid technologies prior to purchase. Furthermore, manufacturers could benefit from consumer feedback for improving the amount of benefit in everyday life provided by their product lines (Walden, 1997). However, Byrne (1998) argued that a uniform protocol design could not accommodate all testing purposes. Walden (1999) believed, however, that a consensus on how to measure hearing aid benefit in everyday living could be developed from a cooperative effort of clinical scientists and industry representatives. He cautioned that such measures would have to be realistic from the manufacturers' point-of-view. For example, the in-depth protocol utilized in the National Institute of Deafness and other Communicative Disorders (NIDCD)/ Department of Veteran's Affairs (DVA) hearing aid clinical trial is probably too involved to be adopted universally by hearing aid manufacturers (Larson, et al., 2000). Nevertheless, collaboration must continue toward development of univer-

sally accepted protocols for use by clinicians, researchers, and manufacturers.

Executing Clinical Trials in "Real World" Environments

Similarly, clinical trials of hearing aid efficacy must move out of the laboratory setting to include patients' significant other persons within "real world" contexts to increase the external validity of these studies. Clinical trials regarding the efficacy of fitting high-technology amplification on young children must occur within the classroom environment and involve educational personnel rating students' listening behaviors, for example. Furthermore, participation in clinical trials has advantages for all stakeholders in the educational milieu (e.g., students, parents, administrators, and clinicians) (O'Toole, Logemann, & Baum, 1998). For example, students benefit from the availability of state-of-the-art treatment, educational personnel can access objective data on students' performance, and the school system has heightened visibility for participating in research (O'Toole, et al., 1998).

Clinical trials involving difficult-to-test populations in "real life" contexts using alternate experimental designs are needed to assess the potential efficacy of amplification for *all* patients. For example, third-party payers may believe that purchasing hearing aids for patients with Alzheimer's disease (AD) is wasteful because they are considered to be difficult or even impossible to test (Palmer, Adams, Bourgeois, Durrant, & Rossi, 1999). Furthermore, large-scale randomized clinical trials would be difficult with this population because of the unique behavioral manifestations of the disorder within individuals and a lack of an organized health-care system to manage these patients. Thus, benefits provided by single-subject designs that permit flexibility across patients, behaviors, and service-delivery sites are needed for efficacy studies of hearing aid treatment in patients with AD. Using a multiple-baseline single-subject design, Palmer, et al. (1999) demonstrated a reduction of caregivers' reports of negative behaviors (e.g., negative statements, forgetfulness, pacing) and an increase in patients' likelihood of participating in interactions and conversations, and an awareness of environmental sounds in patients in their natural environments after being fit with hearing aids.

Garnering International Cooperation in Outcomes Measurement

Walking through the corridors of the convention hall during the annual conventions of the American Academy of Audiology and overhearing a variety of languages, audiologists agree that our profession has achieved a global community. Audiologists from all over the world come to these meetings to share their knowledge and learn the latest in state-of-the-art audiologic service delivery. Unfortunately, cultural, ethnic, and other non-audiologic variables affect comparing the outcome of services across countries (Arlinger, 2000). For example, it is becoming increasingly important to compare hearing health-care systems across national borders and even to pool results from multi-center clinical trials performed in different countries (Arlinger, 2000). Obstacles to adopting universal "gold standards" for outcomes measurement include national variations in (Arlinger, 2000):

- Target populations (e.g., different countries may vary regarding the varieties of genetic disorders, diseases, industries, and age distributions)
- Speech communication patterns (e.g., different cultures use languages that may

vary in the degree of understandability by persons with hearing impairment)
- Public activities (e.g., countries differ on the types of religious ceremonies or vary as to the degree of access [e.g., assistive listening devices] to movies and theatres to those with hearing loss)
- Public environments (e.g., countries may vary in the acoustic conditions regarding levels of street noise, urban versus rural environments, and so forth)

Arlinger (2000) believed that a universal outcome measure could be developed, but that consideration of the above factors would reduce the number of useful items to a limited number of situations and would require an international consortium of experts meeting to discuss issues related to outcomes measurement.

Recently, an international group of experts convened at the Eriksholm Workshop on "*Measuring Outcomes in Audiologic Rehabilitation Using Hearing Aids,*" to develop a universal outcome measure to promote data comparison across different social, cultural, and health-care delivery systems (Cox, et al., 2000). The second goal of the workshop involved designating four common goals of self-report outcome measures:

1. Goal 1: To assess the rehabilitative outcomes for an individual person with hearing impairment
2. Goal 2: To assess the effectiveness of the services provided by a particular clinical unit or agency
3. Goal 3: To assess the effectiveness of new technology
4. Goal 4: To evaluate the effectiveness of hearing rehabilitation services on quality of life

A third goal of the workshop was to direct international research initiatives by ranking the most pressing research needs in outcome measurement (only top 5 of 10 are listed):

1. Explore the relationship between expectation and outcome, especially including satisfaction
2. Determine the relationship of the *Client Oriented Scale of Improvement* (COSI) to other outcome measures in multiple countries
3. Delineate the effects of extra-audiologic factors in outcomes measurement
4. Determine the generic components of quality of life that are affected by a hearing problem
5. Develop a client oriented instrument that specifically evaluates both disability and handicap

Similar meetings of experts from all over the world are needed to overcome international barriers to outcomes measurement in other areas of audiologic practice.

OUTCOMES MEASUREMENT IN PRIVATE PRACTICE

Many audiologists participate in outcomes measurement because someone (e.g., their employer) or something (e.g., quality assurance department of a hospital) requires them to. The true test for outcomes measurement is if private-practice audiologists believe it is worth their time and effort. Unfortunately, these audiologists do not use many of the outcome measures found on the companion CD-ROM in validating their patients' hearing aid fittings because of the length and complexity of the instruments, and the necessity of pre- and post-fitting administrations (Hosford-Dunn & Halpern, 2000). These audiologists believe that the use of subjective measures of benefit are not justified because they do not validly predict successful hearing aid fittings nor do they identify problem areas

beyond aided improvement in speech understanding (Hosford-Dunn & Halpern, 2000). The validity of these instruments lies in their inherent psychometric properties, and also their intended use with the appropriate populations and in specific service-delivery sites (Hyde, 2000). Universal utility of these instruments requires validation with a variety of patient populations, hearing aid fittings, and fitting environments (Hosford-Dunn & Halpern, 2000). For example, Hosford-Dunn and Halpern (2000; 2001) completed a two-part investigation of the clinical applicability of the *Satisfaction of Amplification in Everyday Life* (SADL) (Cox & Alexander, 1999) in private-practice settings. Hosford-Dunn and Halpern (2001) concluded that with its good construct validity and psychometric properties, the SADL could serve as a gold standard for satisfaction outcomes and as a basis for development of a predictive model of hearing aid success for use in private practice.

Unfortunately, many private practitioners will not engage in outcomes measurement unless the results directly relate to their costs, reimbursement rates, and revenue. Recently, Cunningham, Lazich, Guerreiro, and Toppel (2000; 2001) published a two-part article on how to grow a private practice. The articles present a common sense approach to success in practice management that is grounded in the basic principles, methods, and importance of outcomes measurement. For example, patients are primed for problem solving in the "here and now" when asked to complete a short hearing-loss questionnaire upon arrival to a "seamless" hearing evaluation that includes a brief experience with amplification immediately following diagnosis of hearing loss. For example, patients often experience a "wow" effect when programmable hearing aids are inserted into their ears, inducing a personal amplification epiphany. During the brief amplification experience, patients and their significant others complete the *Amplification Response and*

Recommendation Form (ARRF), using a 5-point Likert scale to answer questions such as: Is the sound comfortable and clear? Can the significant other communicate more easily? Does the patient perceive benefit? Is the patient motivated to pursue amplification? The "seamless" hearing evaluation and completion of the ARRF reduces resistance to obtaining amplification and can be sent to patients' physicians and to their homes to stimulate scheduling of a hearing aid evaluation. In this way, outcomes measurement can stimulate sales.

Cunningham, et al. (2000) stated that successful practices give patients more than they expect through continuous quality improvement in services at all levels and in product lines. For example, staff members are encouraged to make each patient visit a pleasant experience by greeting them immediately and providing coffee/soft drinks when operating behind schedule. Furthermore, patients are encouraged to complete "Patient Comment/Complaint" forms which are taken very seriously by all staff who work in synchrony endorsing the practice's mission statement and objectives. All staff work together to set measurable goals for each facet of the practice and for each group of clinicians. Management plots income and expenses each month and shares this information with the team who earn bonuses if targets are achieved. At first glance, priorities seem to be on profit through the selling of hearing instruments, but, in reality, attention is focused on meeting patients' needs. Profit is a by-product of achieving positive patient outcomes. Moreover, if private practitioners can connect profit to positive treatment outcomes, they will be more likely to use self-assessment instruments, such as the Client Oriented Scale of Improvement in identifying and fulfilling patients' needs (Dillon, James, & Ginis, 1997).

Cunningham and his colleagues work in a professional service corporation (PSC) composed of faculty and staff of the Au.D. program at the University of Louisville School of Medicine. Cunningham, et al. (2000) operate hearing clinics in three major teaching hospitals, a community speech and hearing clinic, a retail dispensary, an outpatient department, a multispeciality practice, and a special needs program in which students are an integral part of service-delivery, learning the synergism between outcomes measurement and the business aspects of practice management. Direct participation in outcomes-based practice is not enough, however. Practical experience must be coupled with providing future clinicians with a sound foundation in scientific inquiry—one of the most formidable challenge facing the profession.

PREPARING FOR A FUTURE OF EVIDENCE-BASED PRACTICE

Gagne (2000) stated that although the ultimate goal of professional training programs is to prepare students to be competent clinicians, they must also be taught to evaluate treatment effectiveness research. However, who is going to do the research? Will future audiologists sit back and merely observe the research process expecting someone else to conduct investigations on the effectiveness of their intervention efforts? Professional training must be based in the sciences in order to develop the critical thinking skills of clinical audiologists.

Ryals, Hunter, and Roush (2001) stated that at the 12th Annual Convention and Exposition of the American Academy of Audiology (AAA) in Chicago, Illinois in 2000, Past-President Bob Glaser announced at his Opening Address a need to focus attention and efforts on preserving the research base of the profession and support the scientific education of audiologists. Ryals, et al. (2001) stated that the AAA developed a task force to study this problem and recommend ways that the Academy can promote and strengthen the scientific and research bases of the profession. To this end, the task force sent out a survey to gather opinions about where to begin and most respondents agreed that the process must begin with students in the initial stages of their academic careers.

Most graduate students in audiology dread the research methods course, and at its conclusion, are thankful for a passing grade. Comments on course evaluations range from, "the teacher really tried to make a boring topic interesting," to "the course had absolutely nothing to do with what I'll be doing as a professional." The few students who elect to do master's theses receive huge amounts of peer pressure to quit their research endeavors in favor of taking comprehensive examinations. Indeed, waiting until post-graduate training to involve students in research is much too late. The process must begin much earlier than that.

Faculty members may contribute to erosion of the scientific education of audiologists by inadvertently not considering undergraduate students' participation in the research process. For example, well-meaning faculty members may only invite graduate students to participate in their research programs while discouraging seemingly average undergraduate students who may become frustrated by extra challenges. Even more injurious are those academicians who only want to work with the "best and the brightest" students who require minimal investiture of time for faculty to reap publication after publication. What is the immediate pay-off for those who spend enormous amounts of precious time and effort in mentoring "average" students whose only asset for success may be their enthusiasm? Unfortunately, in research mentoring, there are no guaranteed future "pay-offs" except for the hope of turning students onto science and the joy in the process of discovery.

In Chapter 14 regarding outcomes measurement in university training pro-grams, we discussed the need for identifying pre-admission criteria that predict success in graduate school and professional practice. Many faculty are discouraged at the academic skill level of those students currently applying to their graduate programs. Some talk of the "good old days" when students were clearer thinkers and writers, and were more motivated ... Faculty members wonder how they can possibly train students into being the next pioneers on the cutting-edge of evidence-based practice when these young people enter their classrooms unable to write a coherent paragraph. Faculty need not be discouraged, however, and must give credence to Hillary Rodham Clinton's observation that, "it does take a village" to nurture students into becoming the best professionals and people they can be. The profession is strengthened and enriched by this process, one student at a time. We all know the professors who have made a difference for us. We wonder how we can ever repay them for their efforts. We can pass it onward. Over the course of a career, faculty members have scores of students who take their classes and seek their advice. Seemingly meaningless things that teachers say and do can have a huge impact on the values that students have as practitioners. The most important value that teachers can instill in their students is a standard of excellence in professional practice requiring an evidence-based approach. Students must expect the best out of themselves, others, and the profession to "get along" in the increasingly competitive healthcare arena in the years to come.

In October 1999, *Audiology Today* published a special issue about audiology in the new millennium. Leaders in the field were asked to look into their crystal balls and write short articles on selected topics regarding the future of the profession. Beck (1999) stated that, in the past, scientists and researchers, clinicians, academicians, engineers, technology and industry experts working in laboratories, hospitals and clinics, universities, and the business communities have worked hard to establish a scientific and technologic foundation for our field. As the torch of responsibility is passed to the next generation of professionals, they must be prepared to meet, and exceed the standards of service delivery dictated by various accrediting agencies, such as the Joint Committee on the Accreditation of Healthcare Organizations (JCAHO) and the National Committee on Quality Assurance (NCQA). Beck (1999) stated that audiologists must be prepared to practice within the context of evidence-based health care, which requires data to demonstrate the necessity for treatment. Moreover, Beck (1999) believed that, as time goes on, audiologists must demonstrate the efficacy of their treatments and develop practice guidelines that recommend or exclude specific procedures through rigorous investigation. In other words, the scientific foundation of our profession, the barometer of our credibility, must be estab-

lished through evidence-based practice and the use of outcomes measurement.

SUMMARY

We end this textbook at the same place that we started; that is, in discussing the training needs of future generations of audiologists. In that same prophetic issue of *Audiology Today*, Danhauer (1999) wrote about how the future of the profession lies in its, "roots and seeds." He stated that audiology needs to get back to its roots: aural rehabilitation and research that were germinal to our discipline and vital to our future. He believed that we must nurture both our Au.D. and Ph.D. degrees; clinicians need to know research and researchers need clinical insights. Moreover, Danhauer (1999) stated that seeds are essential for any crop; they are for audiology too. He believed that the profession must cultivate new minds in the field, one student at a time.

LEARNING ACTIVITIES

- Initiate a telephone survey on private-practice audiologists' use of outcomes measurement.

- Develop a class consensus on the role of research training in Au.D. programs.

- Write a prediction on the future use of outcome measures in audiologic practice.

RECOMENDED READINGS

Cox, R., Hyde, M., Gatehouse, S., Noble, W., Dillon, H., Bentler, R., Stephens, D., Arlinger, S., Beck, L., Wilkerson, D., Kramer, S., Kricos, P., Gagne, J.P., Bess, F., & Hallberg, L. (2000). Optimal outcomes measures, research priorities, and international cooperation. *Ear and Hearing, 21*(Suppl. 4), 106–115.

REVIEW EXERCISES

Fill-in-the-Blank

Instructions: Please fill-in-the-blanks with the correct terms from the word bank below.

1. _____ _____ _____ are expenses associated with disposable supplies (e.g., electrodes, earpieces, and tubing) used to carry out hearing screenings (e.g., $15 per baby).

2. _____ _____ _____
   involve allocated unit overhead associated with UNHS, including salaries
   and benefits for program personnel.

3. _____ _____ comprise
   the allocated hospital overhead for the
   proportion of administrative costs of
   the UNHS program.

Word Bank:
Fixed direct costs
Indirect expenses
Variable direct costs

ANSWERS

Fill-in-the-Blank:
  1. Variable direct costs
  2. Fixed direct costs
  3. Indirect expenses

REFERENCES

Arlinger, S. (2000). Can we establish internationally equivalent outcome measures in
audiological rehabilitation? *Ear and Hearing, 21*(Suppl. 4), 97–99.

Beck, L.B. (1999). Audiology service delivery
in the new millennium: Are you ready?
*Audiology Today, Special Issue: Audiology
and the New Millennium, 11*(10), 28.

Byrne, D. (1998). Hearing aid clinical trials:
Specific benefits need specific measures.
*American Journal of Audiology: A Journal
of Clinical Practice, 7*, 17–19.

Cox, R.M., & Alexander, G.C. (1999). Measuring satisfaction with amplification in daily
life: The SADL. *Ear and Hearing, 20*,
306–319.

Cox, R., Hyde, M., Gatehouse, S., Noble, W.,
Dillon, H., Bentler, R., Stephens, D.,
Arlinger, S., Beck, L., Wilkerson, D.,
Kramer, S., Kricos, P., Gagne, J.P., Bess,
F., & Hallberg, L. (2000). Optimal out-
comes measures, research priorities, and
international cooperation. *Ear and Hear-
ing, 21*(Suppl. 4), 106–115.

Cunningham, D.R., Lazich, R.W., Guerreiro,
S.M., & Toppel, K. (2000). Cover story:
Growing a successful practice. *Advance for
Audiologists, 2*(5), 50–54.

Cunningham, D.R., Lazich, R.W., Guerreiro,
S.M., & Toppel, K. (2001). Growing a successful practice: Part II. *Advance for Audiologists, 3*(1), 63–64.

Danhauer, J.L. (1999). Roots and seeds for
audiology's success. *Audiology Today,
Special Issue: Audiology and the New Millennium, 11*(10), 13.

Dillon, H., James, A., & Ginis, J. (1997).
Client Oriented Scale of Improvement
(COSI) and its relationship to several other
measures of hearing aid benefit and satisfaction provided by hearing aids. *Journal
of the American Academy of Audiology, 8*,
27–43.

Gagne, J.P. (2000). What is treatment evaluation research? What is its relationship to
the goals of audiological rehabilitation?
Who are the stakeholders of this type of
research? *Ear and Hearing, 21*(Suppl. 4),
60–73.

Hayes, D., & Downs, M.P. (2000). Counter-
point: Value of UNHS is price. *The Hearing
Journal, 53*(11), 61, 62, 64–67.

Hosford-Dunn, H., & Halpern, J. (2000).
Clinical application of the Satisfaction
with Amplification in Daily Life Scale in
private practice I: Statistical, content, and
factorial validity. *Journal of the American
Academy of Audiology, 11*, 523–539.

Hosford-Dunn, H., & Halpern, J. (2001).
Clinical application of the SADL scale in
private practice II: Predictive validity of fitting variables. *Journal of the American
Academy of Audiology, 12*, 15–36.

Huch, J.L., & Hosford-Dunn, H. (2000).
Inventories of self-assessment measurements of hearing aid outcome. In R. Sandlin (Ed.), *Textbook of hearing aid
amplification* (pp. 489–521). Clifton Park,
NY: Delmar Thomson Learning.

Hyde, M.L. (2000). Reasonable psychometric standards for self-report outcomes measures in audiological rehabilitation. *Ear and Hearing, 21*(Suppl. 4), 24–36.

Joint Committee on Infant Hearing. (2000). Year 2000 position statement: Principles and guidelines for early hearing detection and intervention programs. *American Journal of Audiology: A Journal of Clinical Practice, 9,* 9–29.

Kileny, P.R., & Jacobson, G. (2000). Point: Is UNHS worth the cost? *The Hearing Journal, 53*(11), 61, 62, 64–67.

Larson, V.D., Williams, D.W., Henderson, W.G., Luethke, L.E., Beck, L.B., Noffsinger, D., Wilson, R.H., Dobie, R.A., Haskell, G.B., Bratt, G.W., Shanks, J.E., Stelmachowicz, P., Studebaker, G.A., Boysen, A.E., Donahue, A., Canalis, R., Fausti, S.A., & Rappaport, B.Z. (2000). Efficacy of 3 commonly used hearing aid circuits: A crossover trial. *Journal of the American Medical Association, 284,* 1806–1813.

O'Toole, T., Logemann, J.A., & Baum, H.M. (1998). Conducting clinical trials in the public schools. *Language, Speech, and Hearing Services in the Schools, 29,* 257–262.

Palmer, C.V., Adams, S. W., Bourgeois, M., Durrant, J.D., & Rossi, M. (1999). Reduction in caregiver-identified problem behaviors in patients with Alzheimer's disease after hearing aid fitting. *Journal of Speech, Language, and Hearing Research, 42,* 312–328.

Ryals, B.M., Hunter, L., & Roush, J. (2001). Task Force on Research in Audiology: Survey results and discussion. Roundtable presented at the 13th Annual Convention and Exposition of the American Academy of Audiology, San Diego, CA.

Thompson, D.L., McPhillips, H., Davis, R.L., Lieu, T.A., Homer, C.J., & Helfand, M. (2001). Universal newborn hearing screening programs: Summary of evidence. *Journal of the American Medical Association, 286,* 2000–2010.

Walden, B.E. (1997). Toward a model clinical-trials protocol for substantiating hearing aid user-benefit claims. *American Journal of Audiology: A Journal of Clinical Practice, 6,* 13–24.

Walden, B.E. (1999). Hearing aid clinical trials: Good for the manufacturer? The dispenser? The consumer? *The Hearing Journal, 52*(10), 10,12, 14, 16.

Index

F

G

H

U

V

W

System Requirements

75 MHz Pentium Processor or better • Microsoft® Windows® 95/98/2000 or Windows® NT/XP • Microsoft® Word® 97 or higher • CD-ROM drive • SVGA monitor

Set Up Instructions for
Handbook of Outcomes Measurement in Audiology

1. Insert disk into CD-ROM player. The CD should start automatically. If it does not, go to step 2.
2. From my computer, double click the icon for the CD drive
3. Double click the appendices.exe file to start the program

This CD-ROM includes useful outcomes measurement tools for both the student and the practicing audiologist. It is suggested that the reader print all of the forms to compile an accompanying notebook to be used when reading the textbook. Futhermore, practicing audiologists will find that all of the forms are editable and can be personalized with company logos or modified for their individual needs.

Follow these steps to customize the forms included on the CD to accompany
Handbook of Outcomes Measurement in Audiology

a. Open file.
b. Locate the "blinking" cursor and enter the name of your practice or institution.
c. Make changes anywhere on the form by highlighting the text you wish to replace and typing in your own text.
d. Save your custom form to your desktop or hard drive using the "Save As" command from the "File" menu on your toolbar. Be sure to rename the file.